Radionuclide Studies of the Spleen

CRC

Radionuclide Studies of the Spleen

Authors:

Richard P. Spencer, M.D., Ph.D.
Professor and Chairman
Department of Nuclear Medicine
University of Connecticut
School of Medicine
Farmington, Connecticut

Howard A. Pearson, M.D.
Professor and Chairman
Department of Pediatrics
Yale University School of Medicine
New Haven, Connecticut

Published by

CRC PRESS

CRC PRESS, Inc.
18901 Cranwood Parkway · Cleveland, Ohio 44128

Library of Congress Cataloging in Publication Data

Spencer, Richard Paul.
Radionuclide studies of the spleen.

Bibliography
Includes index.
1. Spleen – Diseases – Diagnosis. 2. Radioisotopes in medical diagnosis. I. Title. [DNLM: 1. Spleen – Radiography. WH700 S745r]
RC645.S68 616.4'1 75-4725
ISBN 0-87819-071-6

International Standard Book Number 0-87819-071-6

Library of Congress Card Number 75-4725

Direct all inquiries and correspondence to
CRC PRESS, INC., 18901 Cranwood Parkway, Cleveland, Ohio 44128

PREFACE

Although the spleen has been shrouded in mystery since antiquity, the importance of this large aggregate of lymphoid and reticuloendothelial tissue has been more apparent in recent years. Over 20 years have passed since King and Shumacker first reported the susceptibility of some splenectomized infants to overwhelming infection. Ten years ago, Blaustein published a brief compendium of information on the spleen, and in the ensuing decade, the disciplines and methodologies of hematology and nuclear medicine have resulted in a considerable expansion and revision of concepts of splenic function. We have been fortunate in having had access to a number of illustrative cases which have helped shape our thinking about the spleen and its multiple activities. Indeed, these cases have formed the impetus for this book. We do not claim to have produced an all-inclusive review of the spleen and its functions and malfunctions. We have, however, emphasized how the techniques of hematology and nuclear medicine have been brought to bear on this organ.

Since our focal point has been the spleen, accounts of various diseases are not encyclopedic but rather reflect the role of the spleen in the disorder, as well as our experiences. Not all conceivable topics have been covered. This short volume reflects our own outlook and biases. We have included those subjects which had interest and pertinence from our viewpoint. We are grateful to those who have critically reviewed parts of the manuscript and kept us from further error.

Our thanks are extended to our colleagues, residents, and fellows, whose inquiries have helped refine our thinking about the spleen. Special recognition must be given to the granting agencies which funded the original studies that led to the formulation of our present views.

Richard P. Spencer
Howard A. Pearson

THE AUTHORS

Howard A. Pearson, M. D., is Professor and Chairman of the Department of Pediatrics at the Yale University School of Medicine and Attending Physician at Yale-New Haven Hospital. Dr. Pearson is a graduate of Dartmouth College (1951) and the Harvard Medical School (1954). He had pediatric internship and residency training at the National Naval Medical Center in Bethesda (1954–1957), was a Research Fellow in Hematology at Harvard (1958), and returned to Bethesda as Assistant Head of Pediatrics and Director of Pediatric Hematology until 1961. At the University of Florida School of Medicine (1961–1967), he rose from Assistant to full Professor. He has been Professor of Pediatrics at Yale since 1968 and became Chairman of the Department in 1974. His principal interest is in pediatric hematology.

Richard P. Spencer, M. D., Ph.D., is Professor and Chairman of the Department of Nuclear Medicine at the University of Connecticut School of Medicine. Dr. Spencer is a graduate of Dartmouth College (1951) and the University of Southern California School of Medicine (1954). After a medical internship, he served in the U.S. Navy and was then Associate Professor at the University of Buffalo School of Medicine and Director of Nuclear Medicine at the Veterans Administration Hospital. At the Yale University School of Medicine (1963–1974), he was Director of Nuclear Medicine and became full Professor in 1968. Since 1974, he has been at the University of Connecticut Health Center.

TABLE OF CONTENTS

Chapter 1

HISTORICAL

Because of its size and accessibility, the spleen has been the subject of extensive descriptions since antiquity. The sketchy Egyptian anatomic records make no mention of the spleen, although it must have been noted during mummification. There are elaborate descriptions and discussions by ancient Greek philosophers and physicians.[1] The derivation of the word itself is controversial, some etymologists believing it is derived from a Greek word meaning viscus, others stating that it comes from the verb meaning to draw out.

Hippocrates in 431 B.C. described the splenic configuration and anatomic relationships. Aristotle in 350 B.C. recognized its connections with the portal vein and guessed that it was not essential for the maintenance of life. He also described the comparative anatomy of the spleen and noted its minute size in birds and reptiles. Of interest was the widespread, but mistaken, belief of the ancients that the speedy giraffe was the only animal which lacked a spleen.

The great Galen, in about 150 A.D., more conservatively considered the spleen an "organ full of mystery." He believed that the spleen extracted the "melancholy" from the blood and liver, purified this, and ultimately excreted it into the stomach, apparently through splenogastric veins. Galen's stature was so great that his view was unchallenged for many centuries. The Galenic dogma that the spleen was an excretory organ was finally overthrown, primarily by the careful anatomic dissections and logic of Versalius, who in the 1500s could demonstrate no ductal structures.

There is no mention of the spleen in the Bible, but the Babylonian Talmud unequivocally makes the spleen the seat of merriment and laughter. "The 10 organs that minister to the soul are: the gullet for the passage of food; the windpipe for voice; the liver for anger; the gall for jealousy; the lung to absorb liquids; the stomach to grind food; the spleen for laughter; the kidneys to advise; the heart to give understanding; and the tongue to decide."

Early experimenters recognized that the spleen could be removed without killing an animal. Pliny the Elder, in his "Natural History" of about 50 A.D. as translated by Holland,[2] wrote:

> This member hath a propertie by itself sometime to hinder a man's running: whereupon professed runners in the race that be troubled with the spleen have a devise to burn and waste it with a hot iron. And no marveile: for why. They say that the spleen may be taken out of the body by way of incision and yet the creature live nevertheless. But if it be man or woman that is thus cut for the spleen, he or she looseth their laughter by the means for sure it is that intemperate laughters have always great spleens.

This quotation thus reflects the ancient association of the spleen with physical speed because of the presumed asplenia of the swift giraffe. It might also have been recognized that the physical burden of a massively enlarged spleen would hinder the ability to run swiftly. Also, the Galenic view of the importance of the spleen in extracting melancholy humors from blood is reemphasized. Old ideas, however quaint and unfounded, die hard. For example, in 1925 a German physiologist named Macht reported that rats ran faster after splenectomy, possibly because rats quickly learned what happened when they were caught by a physiologist!

Shakespeare speaks for both of these functions of the spleen:

> Such fantastic tricks as makes the angels weep;
> Who with our spleens, would all themselves laugh mortal.
> (Measure for Measure, II, 2, 72)

> I am scalded with my violent motion,
> And spleen of speed, to see your Majesty.
> (King John, V, 7, 49).

The association of the spleen with laughter and the seat of mirth somehow became reversed, for later "spleen" was equated with ill temper and woe; thus, in the Spectator No. 68, Joseph Addison is described

> In all thy humors,
> Whether grave or mellow
> Thou'rt such a touchy, testy
> pleasant fellow
> Hast so much wit and mirth
> and spleen about thee
> There is no living with thee
> nor without thee.

During the 17th century, authorities such as Harvey, Glisson, Bartholia, and Wharton were interested in the spleen and described the detailed structure of the organ. Malpighi, the great Italian anatomist, first described the Malpighian bodies, to which, however, he erroneously assigned the function of secreting glands. This belief persisted for more than a century. In 1706, Leeuwenhoek, inventor of the microscope, described the fine structure of the spleen. William Hewson, in 1777, wrote that the spleen was concerned with converting the lymph into blood elements and assigned the organ to the lymphatic system. Virchow[3] demonstrated, in 1846, that the Malpighian follicles were concerned with the formation of white blood cells. Ponfick,[4] in 1885, recognized that the spleen could remove various particles, including erythrocytes, from the blood and thus was involved in blood destruction.

The association of the spleen with disease has been recognized for thousands of years. Malaria and other diseases were endemic in ancient Greece and Rome, and splenomegaly was described by Hippocrates. It is said that Roman legionnaires would attempt to dispatch adversaries by striking the left side of the abdomen with the butt of a spear, in order to fracture the nearly universally enlarged spleens of the time.

The prevalence of enlarged spleens in the Mediterranean Basin also probably accounts for the fact that the first description of thalassemia major was made by Cooley in the United States in 1925.[5] Although there is good anthropologic evidence that thalassemia major has been present in the Mediterranean area since ancient times,[6] a sick child with splenomegaly and anemia was presumed to have malaria. Only when transplanted to Detroit did the nonmalarious nature of Cooley's anemia become evident. Splenic disease and splenomegaly were so frequent that physicians in ancient times devised a considerable armamentarium to treat an enlarged organ. The great Jewish physician Maimonides wrote: "A cattle hoof if burned and drunk with orymel will shrink an enlarged spleen and stimulate the desire for coitus." It is unlikely that such potions had much effect, and so it is not surprising that a more activist approach was taken by men of surgical persuasion.

The first splenectomy in a human may have been performed in Naples in 1549. A description is given in a book by an Italian physician, Leonardo Fiorvante. A 24-year-old Greek woman had a spleen so large that " . . . the body could not have held a larger one."[7] At the time of incision "immediately the spleen protruded." The removed organ was said to weigh 32 oz. It should be said that subsequent authors have doubted the veracity of this operation. The discrepancy between the size of the tumor *in situ* and after its removal has caused some to believe it more likely that the so-called spleen was, in fact, an ovarian cyst. However, a splenic cyst seems equally possible.

Better documented splenectomies were reported somewhat later by Cruger in Germany in 1684 and Clarke in England in 1676. These surgeons excised spleens which had protruded through abdominal stab wounds. The first American splenectomy was performed for a similar indication by O'Brien in 1816.[8]

In 1866, Sir T. Spencer Wells,[9] the preeminent English surgeon of the Victorian era, performed a splenectomy on a 34-year-old woman who was "evidently dying from an enlarged spleen." Despite Wells' meticulous technique, the patient died of septicemia 6 days after the operation. The dubious success apparently did not deter others, for in 1882, Collier[10] reviewed the literature and collected 25 cases of splenectomy performed between 1866 and 1881. In 16 cases the indication was "leukocythemia" (leukemia); all of the patients died. During the same interval, nine splenectomies were performed for nonmalignant enlargements, and six patients survived.

The rational use of splenectomy for nontraumatic indications awaited more precise hematologic diagnosis. In 1888, Sir T. Spencer Wells reported performing another splenectomy, this time for "abdominal tumor" in a 22-year-old woman who had a lifelong history of dark urine and frequent attacks of jaundice.[11] An enlarged spleen was removed, and the patient was restored to complete health. Twenty-six years later, this same woman was restudied by Lord Dawson,[12] and her red cells still showed the typically increased osmotic fragility of congenital hemolytic jaundice. By 1920, the curative value of splenectomy in this disease, now better known as hereditary spherocytosis, was firmly established. In 1921 Lord Berkley Moynihan,[13] in an address before the Royal College of Surgeons, was able to define a number of hematologic diseases for which splenectomy might be of value. These included "leukemia, pernicious anemia, Hodgkin's disease, splenic anemia (Banti's disease), haemolytic jaundice, Gaucher's disease, von Jaksch's disease, and polycythemia." Splenectomy was first performed as therapy for purpura hemorrhagica by Kaznelson in 1916.[14]

The term "hypersplenism" was coined by Chauffard.[15] Eppinger in 1913 used the word "hyposplenism,"[16] and in 1955, Dameshek[17] postulated the existence of a state of splenism, presumably eusplenism. An excellent summary of the effects of the spleen on the blood was written by Crosby in 1959.[18]

The association of congenital absence of the spleen with situs inversus and congenital heart disease was reported by Martin in 1826.[19]

The unique role of the spleen in forming antibody in response to particulate, intravenous antigen was demonstrated by Rowley in 1950.[20] A peculiar syndrome of severe and overwhelming infection in the splenectomized child was recognized by King and Schumacher in 1952.[21] The use of thorotrast to outline the spleen on roentgenograms was described by Oka in 1929.[22] Very recently, isotopic techniques have been used to define the concept of "functional asplenia," that is, deficient physiologic function of an anatomically enlarged spleen.[23]

Through more than 2,500 years, the spleen, its function and malfunction, has fascinated physicians. Galen's "organ of mystery" has surrendered many of its secrets. But even today, it holds diagnostic and therapeutic challenges. All is still not known.

REFERENCES

1. **Gray, H.,** *The Structure and Use of the Spleen,* J. W. Parker and Son, London, 1854.
2. *Historie of the World,* commonly called *Naturall Historie,* Holland, P., transl., A. Islip, London, 1601, 343.
3. **Virchow, R.,** Weisses Blut und Milztumoren, *Med. Zeitung.,* 15, 157, 1846.
4. **Ponfick, E.,** Ueber Haemoglobinamie und ihre Folge, *Berl. Klin. Wochenschr.,* 20, 389, 1885.
5. **Cooley, T. B. and Lee, P.,** A series of cases of splenomegaly in children with anemia and peculiar bone changes, *Trans. Am. Pediatr. Soc.,* 37, 29, 1925.
6. **Zaino, E. C.,** Paleontologic thalassemia, *Ann. N. Y. Acad. Sci.,* 119, 402, 1964.
7. **Fioravante, L.,** The history of extirpation of the spleen, Krumbhaar, E. B., transl., *N. Y. Med. J.,* 101, 232, 1915.
8. **O'Brien,** *Med. Chiur. J. Recorder,* 1, 8, 1816 (cited by Krumbhaar, Ref. 7).
9. **Wells, T. S.,** On excision of an enlarged spleen, *Med. Times Gazette,* 1, 2, 1866.
10. **Collier, H.,** Splenectomy: a justifiable operation in leukocythaemia? *Lancet,* 1, 219, 1882.
11. **Wells, T. S.,** Remarks on splenectomy with a report of a successful case, *Med. Chiur. Trans.,* 71, 255, 1888.
12. **Dawson, B.,** In discussion of paper by Thursfield, H. Splenectomy for congenital acholuric jaundice, *Proc. R. Soc. Med.,* 7(1), 84, 1913–14.
13. **Moynihan, B.,** *The Spleen and Some of Its Diseases,* W. B. Saunders, Philadelphia, 1920.
14. **Kaznelson, P.,** Verschwinden der hamorrhagischen Diatheses bei einem Fall von "essentieller Thrombopenie" (Frank) nach Milzexstripation. Splenogene thrombolytische Purpura, *Wien. Klin. Wochenschr.,* 29, 1451, 1916.
15. **Chauffard, M.,** A propos de la communication de M. Vaquez, *Bull. Soc. Med. Hop. Paris,* 24, 1201, 1907.
16. **Eppinger, H.,** Zur Pathologie der Milzfunktion, *Berl. Klin. Wochenschr.,* 50, 1572, 1913.
17. **Dameshek, W.,** Hypersplenism, *Bull. N. Y. Acad. Med.,* 31, 113, 1955.
18. **Crosby, W. H.,** Normal functions of the spleen relative to red blood cells, *Blood,* 14, 399, 1959.
19. **Martin, G.,** Observation d'une deviation organique de l'estomac d'une anomalie dans la situation, *Bull. Soc. Anat. Paris,* 1826, quoted by Ivermark, B. I., *Acta Paediatr. Suppl.,* 104, 441, 1955.
20. **Rowley, D. A.,** The formation of circulating antibody in the splenectomized human being following injection of heterologous erythrocytes, *J. Immunol.,* 65, 515, 1950.
21. **King, H. and Schumacher, H. B.,** Susceptibility to infection after splenectomy performed in infants, *Ann. Surg.,* 136, 239, 1952.
22. **Oka, M.,** Eine neue Method zur roentgenologischen Darstellung der Milz, *Fortschr. Geb. Roentgenstr.,* 40, 497, 1929.
23. **Pearson, H. A., Spencer, R. P., and Cornelius, E. A.,** Functional asplenia in sickle cell anemia, *N. Engl. J. Med.,* 281, 923, 1969.

Chapter 2

EVALUATION OF THE SPLEEN

There is perhaps a rough analogy between the pancreas and the spleen; both organs carry out two distinct types of functions: The pancreas has endocrine and exocrine activities, and the spleen acts as both a biologic filter and as a site of production of lymphocytes and immunologically important molecules. The analogy fails, however, when we note that pancreatectomy is followed by a rapid deterioration due to loss of both exocrine and endocrine functions, while splenectomy is compatible with prolonged survival in most individuals. Indeed, the "nonlethality" of splenectomy may have been partially responsible for the paucity of studies of the organ. In the last several years, the methodologies of hematology and nuclear medicine have provided powerful tools for the delineation of splenic function and pathology.

Although conventionally most essays on the spleen begin with a discussion of splenic morphology, we believe this is not the optimal approach since (during life) the organ is most often evaluated on the basis of its functions, not its histologic and gross anatomic appearance. Morphologic data on the spleen are frequently not available during life.

Splenic tissue may be obtained in three ways:

1. Biopsy or aspiration of splenic tissue.
2. Surgical excision.
3. Autopsy study.

Despite being a routine procedure in some parts of the world, splenic puncture is not widely practiced in the U.S.A. There are multiple contraindications and many ensuing complications. Moeschlin[1] has listed data from which the following precautions concerning splenic biopsy are obtained.

1. Only the enlarged spleen should be punctured.
2. A hemorrhagic tendency contraindicates biopsy of the spleen.
3. Septic splenomegaly and the painful spleen (infarct or capsular "stretching") are contraindications.
4. The unconscious patient should not have a biopsy of the spleen since deep inspiration is needed, and the patient must be able to tell if there is pain.

Spleen biopsy, however, is an interesting and occasionally clinically valuable tool for following the effects of medications on the spleen. It is also used in the tropics for demonstration of parasitic diseases such as malaria and Kala azar.

Surgical removal of the spleen is used both for diagnostic (for example, in Hodgkin's disease) and therapeutic (in idiopathic thrombocytopenic purpura and other disorders) purposes. Histology and chemical response provide data which can be used for determining future therapy effectiveness and prognosis, but the spleen is then not available subsequently for carrying out its multiple functions. Because of these real limitations, a functional approach to the spleen (rather than a morphologic one) is more pertinent and clinically useful.

The principal diagnostic tools for evaluating the spleen can be listed as follows:

1. History.
2. Physical examination.
3. Radiographs: chest and abdominal.
4. Hematologic evaluation ± bone marrow study.
5. Spleen scan.

In some cases additional diagnostic studies may be employed.

1. Barium swallow.
2. Splenoportogram.
3. Arteriogram.
4. Liver biopsy (± spleen biopsy).
5. Immunologic evaluation.
6. Ultrasound scans.
7. Bone marrow scans and dynamic radionuclide angiograms.

The principal clinical findings which call for evaluation of the spleen are

1. Splenomegaly.
2. Hepatomegaly or hepatic disease.
3. Anemia or blood dyscrasia.

4. Lymphoma, leukemia, infectious mononucleosis.

5. Trauma.

6. Left upper quadrant pain or mass.

BASIC WORK-UP

The initial work-up of possible aberrant splenic function includes a complete history (including family history) and physical examination. This is followed by radiographs of the chest and abdomen, a complete hematological evaluation, and a spleen scan. To restate this: history, physical examination, radiographs of chest and abdomen, hematological evaluation, spleen scan. These steps in the evaluation are atraumatic and readily carried out, but when they do not yield fully diagnostic data, they must be supplemented with additional studies. Radiographs of the chest may reveal the presence of disorders which involve both lungs and spleens (such as sarcoidosis) or both mediastinal structures and spleen (Hodgkin's disease, for example).

Silverstein and Maldonado[2] reported on conditions producing *asymptomatic* splenomegaly in patients seen at the Mayo Clinic. Their discussion did not mention the use of spleen scans to determine whether a left upper quandrant mass contained functioning splenic tissue or whether there was an intrasplenic defect. With the nuclear medicine facilities presently available in most medical centers, there appears little point in neglecting this helpful diagnostic study (the limitations, however, are real and will be pointed out). A spleen scan can clearly identify functional splenic tissue. Additional procedures, such as gastrointestinal series or urograms, are usually required only when data are needed as to whether the gastrointestinal or genitourinary systems are also involved by a disease process or are displaced by the spleen.

The most frequent causes of *asymptomatic* splenomegaly, in the patients reported by Silverstein and Maldonado,[2] were as follows:

1. Portal hypertension.
2. Myeloid metaplasia.
3. Gaucher's disease.
4. Splenic cyst.

These four conditions can be thought of as falling into three categories:

1. Splenomegaly due to obstruction of the outflow tract (portal hypertension).
2. Splenomegaly due to infiltration (myeloid metaplasia, Gaucher's disease).
3. Splenomegaly due to intrasplenic mass (splenic cyst).

Bone marrow examination and radiographs of the bones are indicated when myeloid metaplasia is suspected. Splenomegaly, with difficulty in obtaining a bone marrow biopsy, and accompanying evidence of osteosclerosis are the hallmarks of myeloid metaplasia (and bone marrow scans, using a radioactive colloid, can aid in localizing any functional marrow). Since the spleen and bone marrow are reticuloendothelial and erythropoietic organs, they frequently share pathologic processes. Splenomegaly, fractures of bones, avascular necrosis, and expansion of the lower portions of the femurs are seen in Gaucher's disease. Other lipidoses may also be diagnosed by bone marrow studies.

Determination of the site of portal obstruction may require use of splenoportography,[3] and this is discussed further in a later chapter. A barium swallow is often useful in demonstrating esophageal varices, a frequent sequelae of portal obstruction. Interestingly, a "radionuclide splenoportogram" (via intrasplenic injection) has also been described[4] but awaits definitive evaluation. Angiography, of the aorta or splenic vessels, can be of assistance in defining intrasplenic masses.[5] It must be recognized, however, that such radiographic procedures have limitations. Castellino and co-workers[6] discussed their experience with splenic arteriography in 33 patients having untreated Hodgkin's disease. With the exception of filling defects on tomograms (corresponding to focal disease noted in the excised spleen), there was no correlation between the angiographic findings and the presence or absence of Hodgkin's disease in the spleen. There is an additional procedure which may have a role to play in the diagnosis of intrasplenic disease; this is ultrasonic scanning.[7] The ultimate use of the procedure in detecting splenic abnormalities has to be established. Finally, it should be pointed out that the spleen shares the lymphoid hyperreactivity of childhood, and palpably enlarged spleens are frequently found in otherwise healthy children.

HEMATOLOGIC (AND IMMUNOLOGIC) EVALUATION

A complete hematological examination yields important information with respect to splenic functions. Absence of the spleen's function is indicated by intraerythrocytic inclusions, such as Howell-Jolly and Heinz bodies, and siderocytes. Increased numbers of poikilocytes, target cells, and spherocytes are seen in the blood smear of the asplenic individual. Increased numbers of platelets and leukocytes may also be observed.

Splenomegaly of any etiology may result in increased destruction and sequestration of the formed elements of the blood, causing selective cytopenias or pancytopenia. Careful examination of the bone marrow often gives insight into splenic pathology.

The spleen has an immunological function. The antibody response of the asplenic individual to conventional immunization by the intramuscular or subcutaneous route is indistinguishable from that of the person with an intact spleen. However, as Rowley has demonstrated, when asplenic individuals are immunized with particulate antigen by the *intravenous* route, they cannot form antibody. This immunological defect will be described subsequently.

RADIONUCLIDE STUDIES: TERMINOLOGY

In the following discussion, we will employ a number of illustrative radionuclide scans of the spleen. Some were obtained with a gamma ray camera and are referred to as scintiphotos. Others were produced by a rectilinear scanner and are so indicated. In each case, the scan is named from the vantage point of the detector. The nomenclature is shown in Figure 1. By an anterior view (or anterior to posterior, AP), we mean one taken of the anterior aspect of the abdomen while the patient is supine. A posterior view (or posterior to anterior, PA), is obtained from the patient's back while the individual is prone. This view brings the spleen closer to the detector since the spleen is a posterior organ. When a dual-headed scanner is used, the patient lies supine, and dorsal and ventral aspects of the abdomen are scanned at the same time. The views then show a correspondence between the right side on both films. The scans are called anterior for the top view and posterior reverse for that produced by the bottom detector. In the following chapters, we will show few left lateral views of the spleen. The reason is that the massive liver often obscures clear delineation of the spleen when viewed from the left side. Angulated views have been more useful to us and are described below.

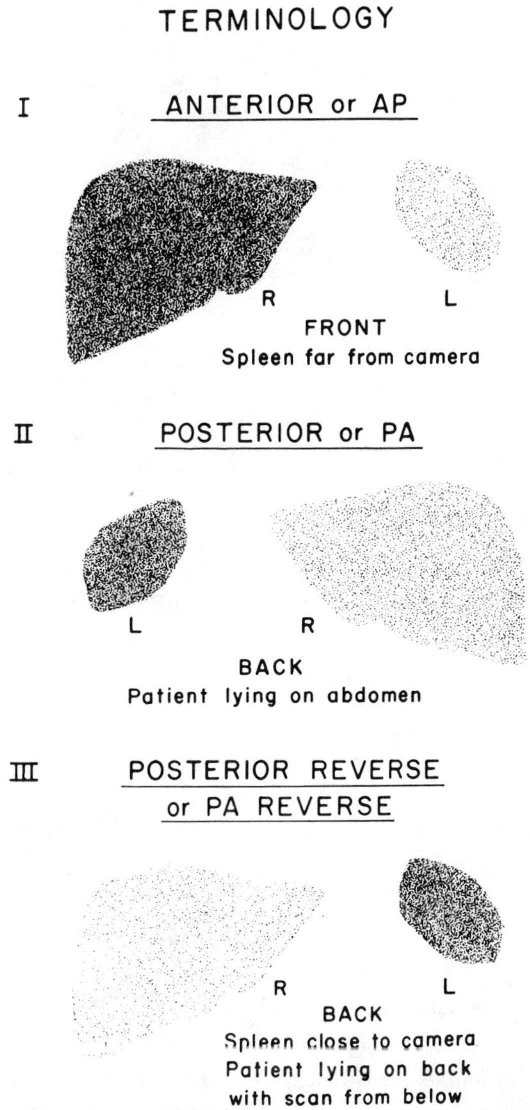

FIGURE 1. The three principal views used in spleen scanning.

Angulated views can be quite helpful in separating the liver from the spleen. Figure 2 depicts a cross section of the human trunk and two schematic detectors to indicate the terminology. At the upper left-hand corner of the diagram, a detector is facing the left side of the body, anterolaterally. Note that it is angulated or

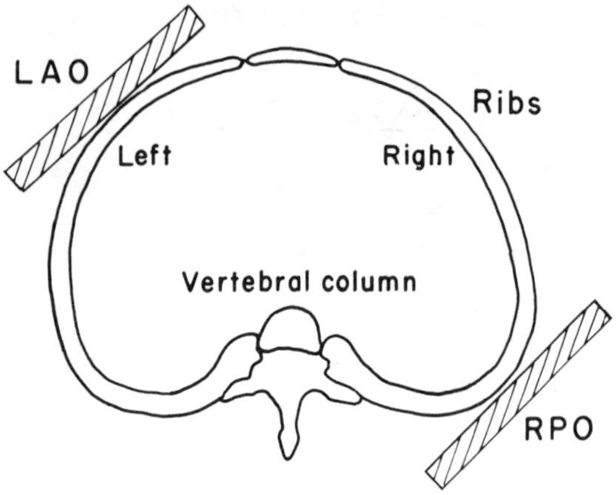

FIGURE 2. Terminology of angulated views (see text), shown on a cross section of the trunk. The viewer is above the sectioned torso, looking towards its feet.

obliqued. The terminology of this view is left anterior oblique or LAO. An example of the usefulness of the LAO projection is shown in Figure 3. Referring back to Figure 2, we can note the second detector pointing toward the right side of the body from a posterior angulated or obliqued position. This is the right posterior oblique or RPO view. Other angulated views are named accordingly. If conventional anterior or posterior views fail to separate hepatic tissue from the spleen (Figure 4), then angulated studies are necessary.

TYPES OF SCANNING AGENTS

Radionuclides used for scanning the spleen can be listed as follows (and see Table 1):

Radioisotopic Visualization of the Spleen

1. Blood pool scan (such as by use of ^{113m}In-transferrin) in the dynamic or static modes.
2. "Negative outlining" by use of ^{75}Se-selenomethionine and ^{131}I-Rose Bengal.
3. Uptake of radioactive colloid.
   a. Small size (0.01 μm, such as ^{198}Au colloid).
   b. Larger size (1 μm, such as ^{99m}Tc-sulfur colloid).
   c. Erythrocytes (7 μm) labeled with ^{51}Cr or other radionuclides and heat denatured.
4. Uptake of ^{67}Ga and other special nuclides.
5. Combined organ scans.

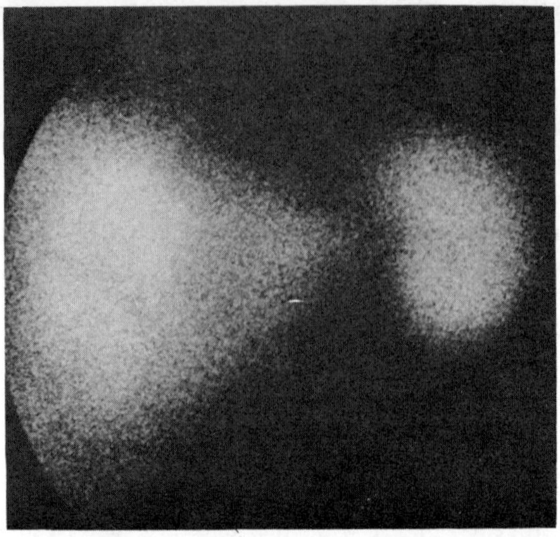

A

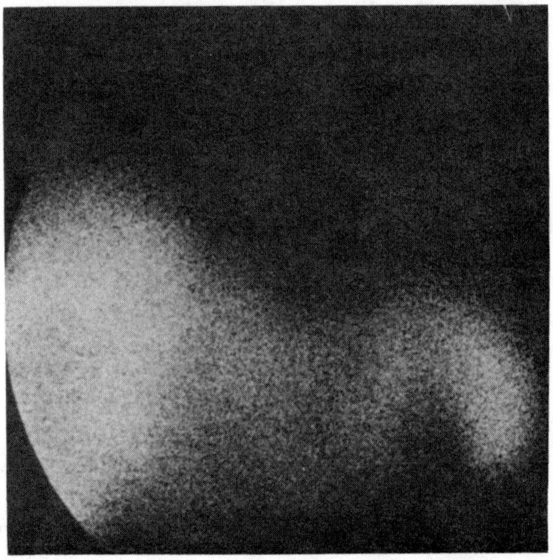

B

FIGURE 3. An anterior spleen scintiphoto (^{99m}Tc-sulfur colloid) in an 81-year-old woman is shown in B. The spleen is not clearly separated from the liver. The other scintiphoto (A) indicates the better separation of the organs achieved on the left anterior oblique view. Case 67-324.

A simple radioisotopic approach to visualization of the spleen is to employ an agent which stays within the vascular compartment for a greater or shorter period. Such a blood pool scan can be done in the dynamic phase or after equilibration. An example of one frame of a dynamic study is shown in Figure 5. A radiolabeled pharmaceutical excreted by the kidneys (^{99m}Tc-diethylenetriamine pentaacetic acid, or DTPA) was injected intravenously and serial scintiphotos obtained. The splenic blood pool can

TABLE 1

A List of Radionuclides Used in Evaluation of the Spleen

Radionuclide	Half-life	Emissions (keV, gamma, unless other shown)	Comment
		Red Cell Labels	
^{51}Cr	27.8 days	320 (9%)	Hexavalent ^{51}Cr, as chromate, binds to hemoglobin and provides a red cell label. The chromate is not reutilized when the cell is lysed. However, some is eluted from red cells. ^{51}Cr-red cells, when heat denatured, accumulate in the spleen. There is a relatively high radiation dose, but it may be a procedure of choice when searching for accessory splenic tissue.
^{197}Hg ^{203}Hg	2.7 days 47.0 days	77 (18%) 279 (77%), beta	The compound 1-mercuri-2-hydroxypropane binds to and denatures erythrocytes. The relatively high radiation dose from ^{203}Hg and the undesirable physical characteristics of the ^{197}Hg emission have limited its use. In addition, there is some accumulation of the Hg in the kidneys, which may obscure accessory splenic tissue.
^{81}Rb	4.7 hr	511 (26%), others	Cells damaged by nonradioactive 1-mercuri-2-hydroxypropane have been reported to take up this label. The radionuclide parent → daughter pair $^{81}Rb \rightarrow {}^{81m}Kr$ ($T\frac{1}{2}$ = 13 sec, 165 keV emission in 65% of the disintegrations) has been used in estimating splenic blood flow.[81]
^{99m}Tc	6.0 hr	140 (90%)	Techniques are being reported for labeling both intact (for blood pool scanning) and denatured erythrocytes (for reticuloendothelial function). This short-lived radionuclide may provide the most useful red cell label for short-term studies.
^{11}C	20.4 min	511 (from positron)	The short half-life and cyclotron production have limited use of this radionuclide. However, ^{11}CO appears to be a ready label for erythrocytes and, hence, a useful blood pool scanning agent (and it has been used in efforts to quantify the number of red cells in the spleen).
^{131}I	8.1 days	364 (82%), others, and beta	The compound *p*-iodophenylhydroxylamine has been reported to bind to hemoglobin. There have not been adequate follow-up studies as to its adequacy as a red cell label.

TABLE 1 (continued)

A List of Radionuclides Used in Evaluation of the Spleen

Radionuclide	Half-life	Emissions (keV, gamma, unless other shown)	Comment
		Radiocolloids	
^{198}Au	2.7 days	412 (95%), others, and beta	This was the first radiocolloid employed clinically. However, the long physical T½ and the beta emission make for a relatively high radiation exposure. The small particle size (under 0.1 μm) resulted in only minimal accumulation by the normal spleen.
^{99m}Tc	6.0 hr	140 (90%)	The short half-life and the nearly ideal gamma ray energy have resulted in the wide use of this radionuclide. There are at least three variants: (1) Technetium-sulfur colloid. The particle size is about 1 μm but is not uniform. About 5% goes to the normal spleen. (2) Technetium-phytate.[82] This is a newer agent, and the full significance for splenic visualization has not been determined. (3) Technetium labeling of albumin microspheres. Here the particle size is relatively uniform; there are as yet insufficient studies to document the advantage of such a preparation.
^{131}I ^{125}I	8.1 days 60.0 days	364 (82%), others, and beta 35	Microaggregates of albumin have been radiolabeled with iodide. The particles are taken up by the reticuloendothelial system, and some of the iodide is then discharged. While of interest in following uptake rates (after a loading dose), the procedure has not gained wide use. The low energy of the ^{125}I emission limits studies to either fixed external counting or to blood sampling.
^{113m}In	1.7 hr	393 (64%)	This radionuclide is readily available from the generator $^{113}Sn \rightarrow {}^{113m}In$. A colloid can be made. In the mouse, about 10% goes to the spleen. The liver radiation dose has been estimated at ~ 0.5 rad/millicurie.
^{51}Cr	27.8 days	320 (9%)	Colloids can be made from ^{51}Cr. Any particular advantages over the short-lived radionuclides have not been demonstrated.

TABLE 1 (continued)

A List of Radionuclides Used in Evaluation of the Spleen

Radionuclide	Half-life	Emissions (keV, gamma, unless other shown)	Comment
		Hematopoiesis	
^{59}Fe	45.0 days	1,095 (56%), 1.292 (44%), others plus beta	The iron radionuclides are of particular interest in the study of hematopoeisis and the search for extramedullary sites. The high energy of the ^{59}Fe emissions make for difficulty in scanning; point-by-point counting can be used. The ^{52}Fe is usable for short-term studies (but not long-term investigations on the rate of entry into erythrocytes). The difficulty of production has restricted its use thus far.
^{52}Fe	8.0 hr	165 (100%), 511 (112%), from positron; daughter radiations	
^{111}In	2.8 days	247 (89%), others	This longer-lived radioisotope of indium shows many properties similar to iron. That is, there is entry into erythropoietic sites (but entry also occurs in the liver and spleen).
		Others	
^{81}Rb-^{81m}Kr	4.5 hr 13 sec	253, others 190	^{81}Rb binds to denatured red cells, which localize in the spleen; ^{81m}Kr is eluted, measuring blood flow.
^{67}Ga	3.2 days	93 (40%), 184 (24%), others	High concentrations occur in many pathologic spleens, following intravenous injection. It may have use in searching for splenic abscesses (as well as in staging Hodgkin's disease).
^{75}Se	120.0 days	136 (57%), 265 (60%), others	In the form of the radiolabeled amino acid, ^{75}Se-selenomethionine, relatively little accumulates in the normal spleen (but the liver is well outlined). Hence, liver tissue can usually be differentiated from the spleen.
^{131}I	8.1 days	364 (82%), others, and beta	The compound ^{131}I-Rose Bengal is accumulated by hepatocytes and not by the spleen (a small amount enters the kidneys, in hepatic obstruction). Hence, it can be used to separate liver and spleen.
^{87m}Sr	2.8 hr	388(80%)	Produced by $^{87}Y \rightarrow {}^{87m}Sr$. There is one report of this bone seeker concentrating in a spleen involved by Hodgkin's disease.
^{133}Xe	5.3 days	81 (37%), beta	Introduced by catheter in the splenic artery the rate of washout can be related to blood flow.
^{113m}In, ^{99m}Tc other			Used as plasma labels in studying blood flow to the spleen. ^{113m}In binds to transferrin.

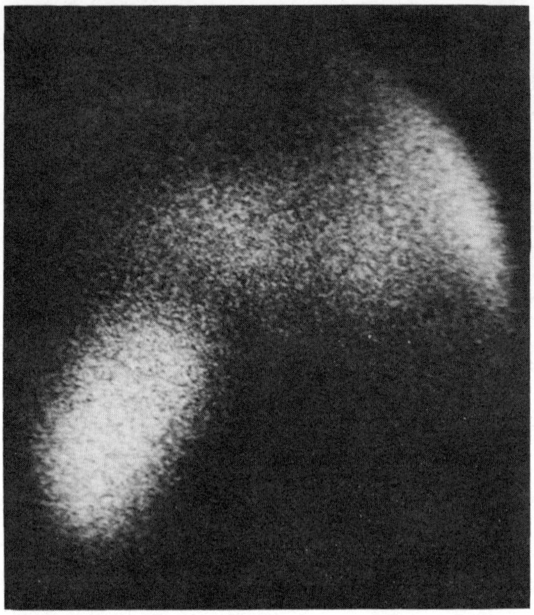

FIGURE 4. Posterior scintiphoto (^{99m}Tc-sulfur colloid) in a 74-year-old man. The first appearance is of an intrasplenic defect. However, on closer scrutiny, it can be seen that hepatic tissue is extending into the left upper quadrant, above the spleen. The "defect" is the space between the liver and spleen. Case 72-670.

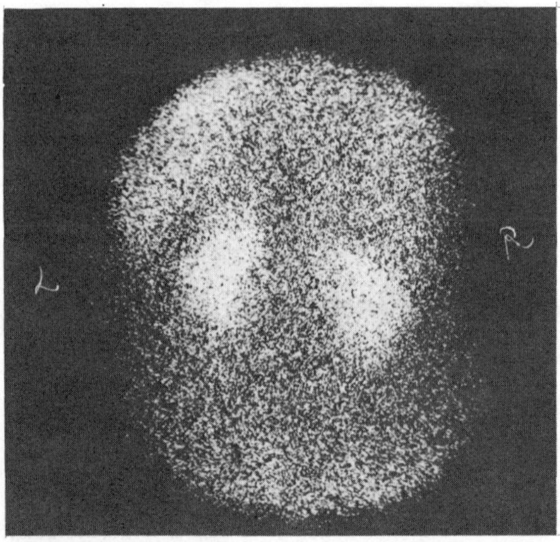

FIGURE 5. Posterior scintiphoto (^{99m}Tc-DTPA) in a 38-year-old woman. This view, at 2 min after injection, is one of a series of photos made during a renal dynamic study. The patient had labile hypertension, hence the interest in renal flow and function. The splenic blood pool can be seen above the left kidney. Case 71-2287.

be seen above the left kidney. Pictures with better resolution can be produced when an agent is used which has a prolonged residence within the vascular tree. Such materials are ^{131}I-albumin (rarely used because of the radiation dose), ^{99m}Tc-albumin, or ^{113m}In-transferrin. Figure 6 shows an anterior radioindium scan. The spleen can be delineated on this anterior view, although the posterior view is preferred since it brings the organ closer to the detector. Figure 7 shows an anterior blood pool scan in a patient who had a splenectomy. There is a relative void in the area formerly occupied by the spleen. Blood pool visualization also has an importance in determining blood flow through the organ; this is further discussed in a following chapter. Fung and co-workers[65] described an "indium scan" of the spleen (whether by use of indium chloride and blood pool visualization or by means of indium colloid was not stated). This showed multiple defects in a case of tuberculosis of the spleen.

Splenic blood pool scanning depends on the anatomic presence of the organ; it does not measure organ function. Two other radionuclides can be employed to outline structures around the spleen, but not the spleen itself. These materials are ^{131}I-Rose Bengal and ^{75}Se-selenomethionine. The Rose Bengal is accumulated in the liver, entering polygonal cells (hepatocytes), and then exiting in the bile. However, little normally enters the spleen, and the splenic area appears as a negative defect on the scan (Figure 8). In obstructive jaundice, some ^{131}I-Rose Bengal is excreted via the urinary tract, and the kidneys can be visualized; these even more markedly contrast with the minimal activity in the left upper quadrant. Figure 9 shows a particularly interesting combination, in that abdominal scans were performed with ^{131}I-Rose Bengal and then with a radioactive colloid (^{99m}Tc-sulfur colloid). Splenic accumulation of the radiocolloid, but not of ^{131}I-Rose Bengal, can be noted. The radiolabeled amino acid, ^{75}Se-selenomethionine, accumulates in the liver and pancreas, as well as in the intestine. Relatively little can be found in the spleen, and it appears as a negative defect on abdominal scans (Figure 10). In one of the early reports on selenomethionine, the following data were given by Blau and Manske:[30]

^{75}Se-Activity (After ^{75}Se-Selenomethionine)

	Percent dose per gram of tissue		
	Spleen	Liver	Pancreas
Dogs, fasted 1 day, material given I.V.	0.008	0.045	0.23

Ben-Porath and Kaplan[31] reported on autopsy data of three patients who died at various times after administration of ^{75}Se-selenomethionine. Converting their data to the same units as above, we can note the following:

^{75}Se-Activity (After ^{75}Se-Selenomethionine)

Percent dose per gram of tissue

	Spleen	Liver	Pancreas
Deceased 3 hr later (carcinoma colon)	0.007	0.0175	0.0135
Deceased 3 days later (bronchogenic carcinoma)	0.009	0.0162	0.0113
Deceased 52 days later (hepatoma)	0.002	0.003	0.0008

Hence, early after administration of ^{75}Se-selenomethionine, in man, the spleen is relatively low in activity as compared with the liver and pancreas. The spleen thus appears as a relative "void" on ^{75}Se-selenomethionine scans (but bowel activity may somewhat interfere).

Radioactive colloids are cleared from the bloodstream by what is referred to as the reticuloendo-

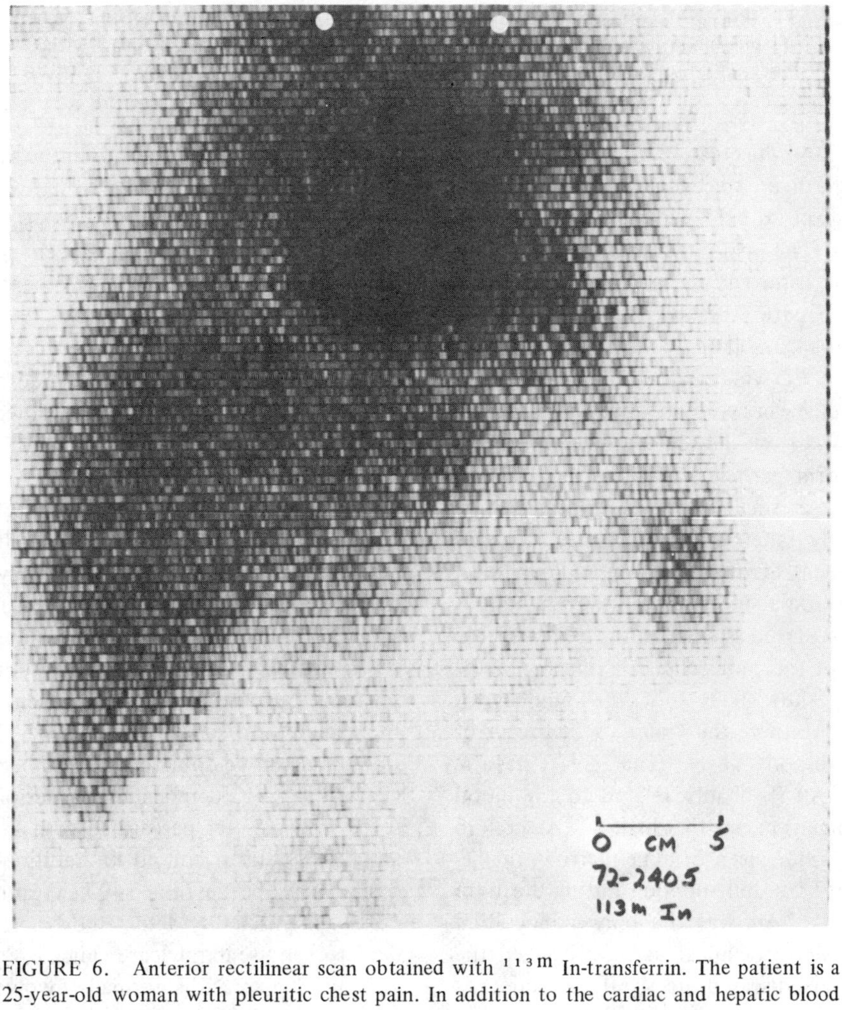

FIGURE 6. Anterior rectilinear scan obtained with ^{113m}In-transferrin. The patient is a 25-year-old woman with pleuritic chest pain. In addition to the cardiac and hepatic blood pools, those of the spleen, kidneys, and aorta can be seen. Case 72-2405.

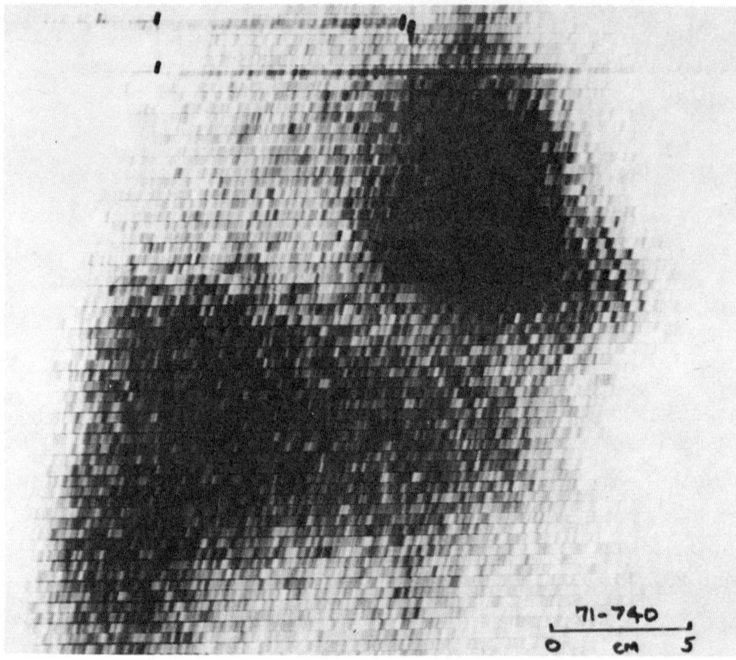

FIGURE 7. Anterior rectilinear scan performed with ^{113m}In-transferrin. No splenic blood pool can be seen. The patient is a 32-year-old woman with Hodgkin's disease who had a prior splenectomy. Case 71-740.

thelial system (and the greatest collections of these cells are in the liver, spleen, and bone marrow). The earliest agent to gain wide use was colloidal gold (^{198}Au). The major part of this material, when injected intravenously, is cleared by the liver. Indeed, hepatic uptake is so rapid that the initial rate of accumulation (when coupled with information on the volume of distribution of the gold radiocolloid) can be used as an approximation of hepatic blood flow. The radiogold, however, is not of a uniform particle size (0.001 to 0.01 μm diameter). These small particles appear to be relatively poorly taken up by the spleen. In this and in subsequent discussions of the radiocolloids, it should be understood that the number of particles administered is small compared with the large number of receptor cells. The limiting factor to uptake is thus likely not the number of receptors but rather the rate of delivery of radiocolloid (blood flow). The great hepatic uptake of ^{198}Au (probably related to the blood flow to that organ) means that little ^{198}Au colloid is taken up by the spleen or bone marrow. Hence, data on spleen size and function during life were limited when ^{198}Au was the only radiocolloid readily available for clinical use. Only when the liver was severely diseased did significant amounts of ^{198}Au colloid accumulate in the spleen or bone marrow (Figure 11). For information purposes, it should be mentioned that studies with loading doses of radiocolloid have been pursued to a limited extent and will be mentioned again shortly.

The addition of ^{99m}Tc-sulfur colloid to the list of agents available for reticuloendothelial system scanning opened a new phase in gathering information about the spleen. First of all, the particle size of this radiocolloid (0.1 to 1 μm) was larger than that of ^{198}Au colloid. A larger fraction is taken up by the spleen. Second, ^{99m}Tc has a shorter half-life (6 hr) than ^{198}Au (2.7 days) and does not have a beta ray emission to contribute to the radiation dose. Hence, considerably more ^{99m}Tc-sulfur colloid can be employed for scanning purposes. Indeed, sufficient amounts of the technetium sulfur colloid can be used so that flow data can be obtained prior to beginning static views. Figure 12 demonstrates anterior liver/spleen scans in a patient, performed with ^{198}Au colloid and ^{99m}Tc-sulfur colloid. In addition to its other desirable properties, the 140 keV gamma ray from ^{99m}Tc is efficiently detected by most scintillation detectors in use in nuclear medicine.

Since the spleen is normally involved in red cell

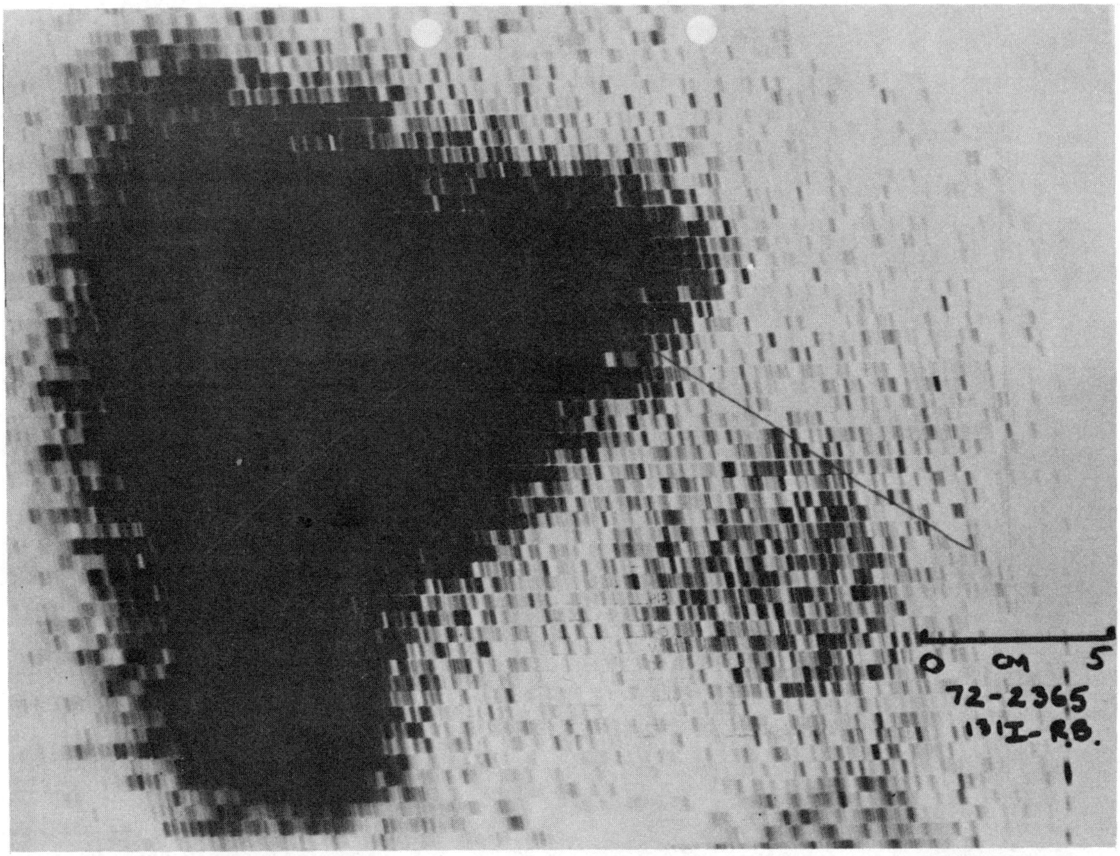

FIGURE 8. Anterior rectilinear scan, performed with Rose Bengal-^{131}I. The patient is a 61-year-old man with carcinoma of the uvula, with spread locally. This scan of the abdomen shows the liver and activity in the intestine (and perhaps kidney as well). There is a relative lack of activity in the left upper quadrant. Case 72-2365.

trapping and destruction, radiolabeled and denatured red cells have been used in spleen scanning. The size of the red cell (7 μm) is, of course, much larger than that of the colloids, and the uptake mechanism may well differ. However, red cell uptake by the spleen can be grossly viewed as in the same class as particulate accumulation. Indeed, ^{51}Cr-labeled and denatured red cells were among the first materials used to delineate the spleen on scan (an example is shown in Figure 13). If erythrocytes are too badly damaged in the denaturation process, or if the spleen is not present, then the radiolabeled cells will accumulate in the liver (Figure 14). Spleen scanning with ^{51}Cr-erythrocytes still finds limited use, especially when searching for accessory splenic tissue following splenectomy (see Chapter 8).

Gallium-67, usually prepared carrier-free as the citrate for intravenous injection, has been widely studied recently as an agent for detecting tumors and staging Hodgkin's disease (and see a discussion in the chapter on leukemias and lymphomas). Splenic concentration of ^{67}Ga can be marked, with values of 1.3 to 11.5% of the administered dose per kilogram of spleen.[29] Despite this uptake, the exact role of ^{67}Ga in evaluating the spleen has still to be defined.

Chaudhuri and co-workers[66] reported an unusual case in which ^{87m}Sr accumulated in the spleen of a patient with Hodgkin's disease. Usually, ^{87m}Sr (like other calcium analogues) seeks bone. The prevalence of splenic entry of ^{87m}Sr and its diagnostic significance are currently unknown.

Scans of the spleen can be combined with those of other organs to obtain information as to the anatomic relations of the structures. Combined lung and liver-spleen scans are often done (Figure 15). There has been less experience with combined kidney-spleen scans.

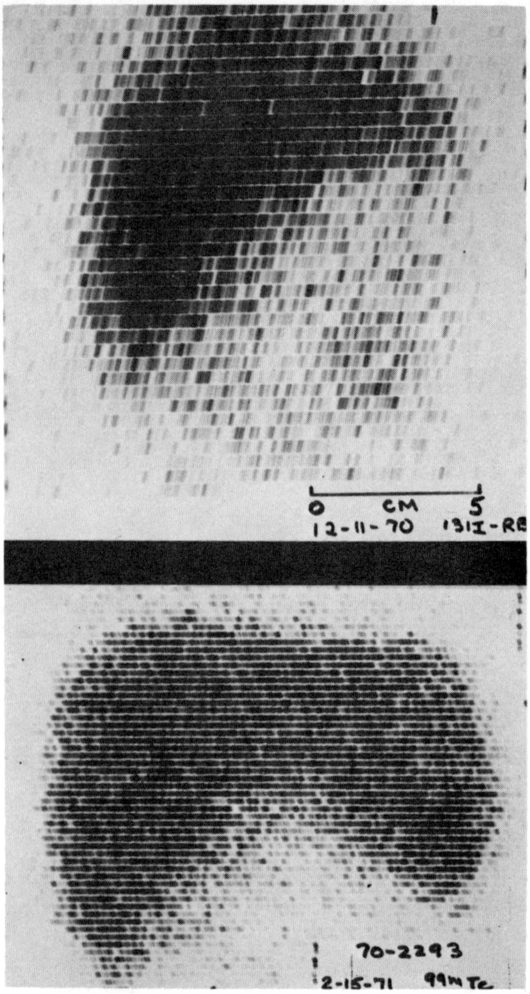

FIGURE 9. Anterior rectilinear scans in a 1-month-old girl. The upper scan was obtained by use of ^{131}I-Rose Bengal. Liver and kidneys (but not spleen) are visible. The lower scan was performed after injection of ^{99m}Tc-sulfur colloid. The spleen can be readily seen. Case 70-2293.

RADIONUCLIDES IN FUNCTIONAL EVALUATION OF THE SPLEEN

The principal functions of the spleen[36] can be listed as follows (and they will be described in greater detail shortly).

1. Hematopoiesis.
2. Erythrocyte destruction.
3. Phagocytosis.
4. Reservoir.
5. Culling and pitting.
6. Possible splenic hormonal control of hematopoiesis.
7. Role in platelet and leukocyte destruction.
8. Immunologic role.

It is in the first three categories and number 7 that the techniques of nuclear medicine have made significant contributions (and in the fourth category, that of reservoir function, radioisotopic studies are just beginning).

Category 1: Hematopoiesis

The spleen is a normal hematopoietic organ during fetal life. At mid-gestation, active blood formation is centered in the liver and spleen. After this time the marrow becomes progressively more important, and, at term, in normal infants, only occasional small nests of hematopoietic cells are found in the spleen. The potential for hematopoiesis remains, for under certain severe hematologic stresses (thalassemia, myeloid metaplasia) hematopoiesis may resume in the spleen.

Following earlier studies by Hahn, a number of investigators (particularly Huff and associates[15]) described iron tracer studies in a variety of diseases which altered iron metabolism. The principal tracer was ^{59}Fe. The point that particularly concerns us is that external monitoring can be utilized to follow the sites of radioiron uptake (and, hence, presumptively in most cases, the sites of erythropoiesis). This is particularly of interest in documenting extramedullary sites of hematopoiesis, such as splenic production of red blood cells. The long physical half-life of ^{59}Fe, and its energetic gamma ray, have limited such studies. A short-lived iron radionuclide (^{52}Fe) is available, but production difficulties have severely restricted its use. More recently, an indium radionuclide (^{111}In, which is handled rather similarly to iron) has been used to delineate areas which accumulate iron.[64] As will be mentioned again later, in many (but not all) instances, the distribution of the erythron (red cell production) parallels the distribution of the fixed phagocytes (reticuloendothelial function) in bone marrow. Hence, the localization of radioactive colloids has been used to follow "erythropoietic areas" in marrow. In animals, following bone marrow irradiation, intravenously injected spleen cells can repopulate the marrow and lead to blood cell production. The spleen cells had thus retained the erythropoietic property they acquired early in fetal development.

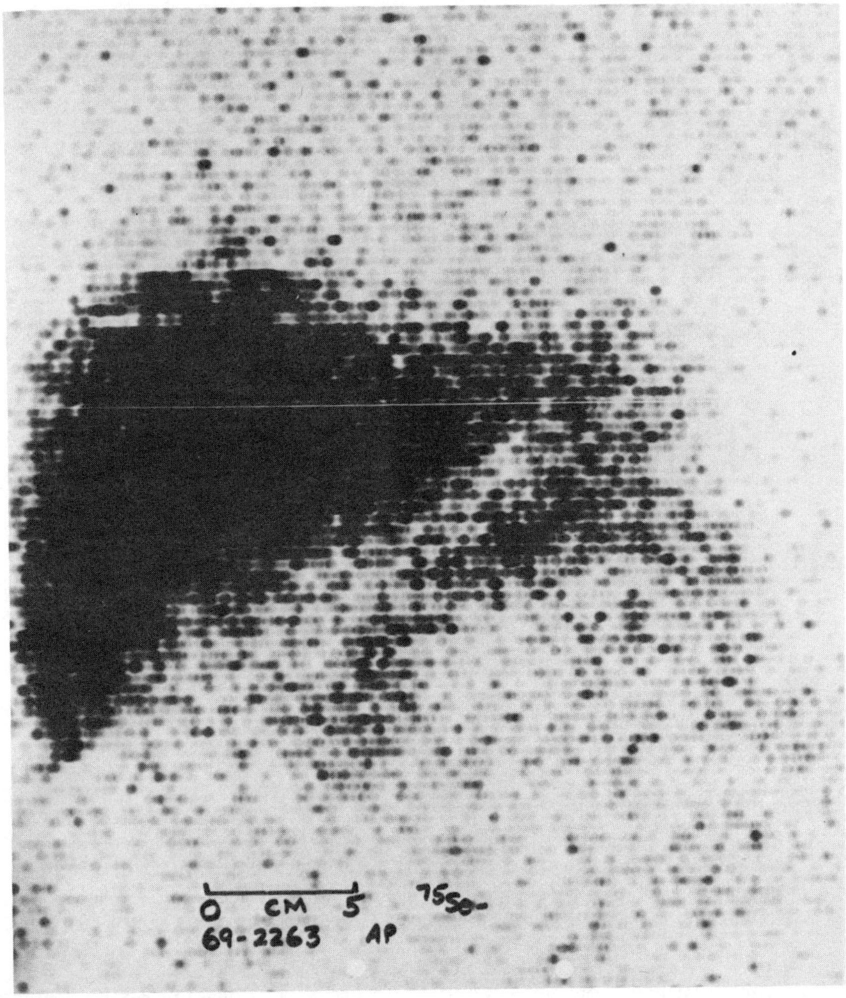

FIGURE 10 Anterior rectilinear scan (^{75}Se-selenomethionine) in a 42-year-old man. The patient, with a known duodenal ulcer, developed severe and atypical abdominal pain. The liver and pancreas can be visualized. There is a "void" in the left upper quadrant, corresponding to the spleen (which normally takes up little of this radionuclide). Case 69-2263.

At present there is no way to ascertain myelopoiesis or thrombopoiesis in the spleen.

Category 2: Erythrocyte Destruction

The finding by Gray and Sterling[8] that hexavalent chromium (^{51}Cr) could radiolabel erythrocytes marked an important step in following sites of red cell destruction. The ^{51}Cr (as sodium chromate) principally binds to the beta chain of hemoglobin[71] and is not reutilized when the erythrocyte is destroyed. This has led to three major uses of ^{51}Cr-erythrocytes: (1) to follow red cell survival (but in addition to ^{51}Cr loss when the red cells are destroyed, some is also lost by elution), (2) to monitor, by means of external probes, sites of red cell sequestration, and (3) to scan the spleen, by means of retained ^{51}Cr, when denatured ^{51}Cr-erythrocytes are injected. D-positive erythrocytes, labeled with ^{51}Cr, can be damaged by incubation with anti-D serum.[9] These damaged cells, following intravenous administration, accumulate in the spleen when the ratio of antibody to RBC is low.[72] A more general approach has been to heat-denature ^{51}Cr-erythrocytes (50°C, 30 min), so that they undergo splenic accumulation after intravenous administration. Higher temperatures gravely damage red cells and result in their removal by the liver. Denaturation of ^{51}Cr-erythrocytes by chemicals (such as *N*-ethylmaleimide) has also been described but is not widely used. The relatively higher radiation exposure from ^{51}Cr has limited such studies, but it may provide information of direct clinical value such as whether splenectomy is likely

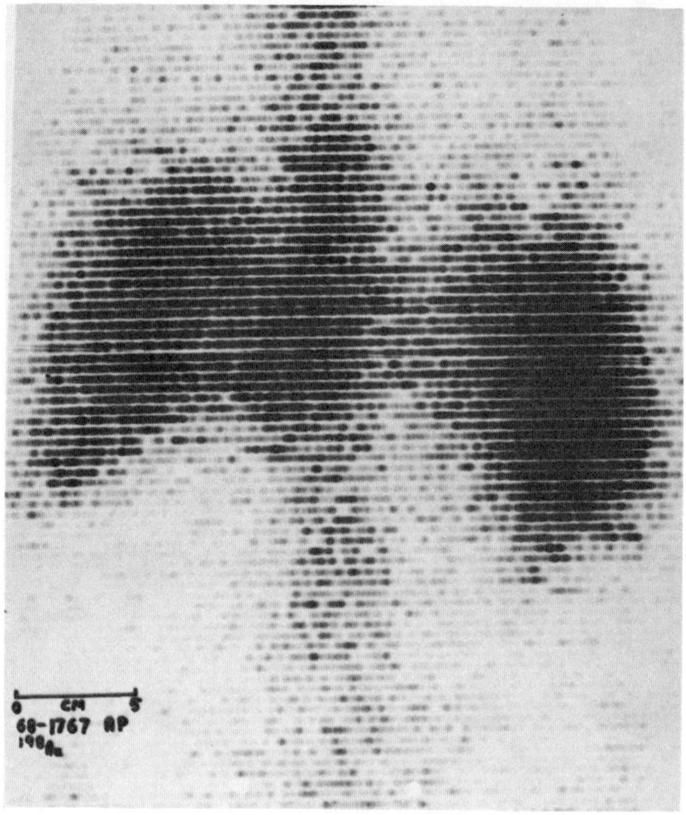

FIGURE 11. Anterior rectilinear scan performed after injection of ^{198}Au-colloid. The patient is a 47-year-old woman with postnecrotic cirrhosis, leukopenia, and thrombocytopenia. In cases of hepatic damage, radiogold accumulates in the bone marrow and spleen. Case 68-1767.

to be beneficial for treatment of hemolytic anemia.[73]

Erythrocytes can be tagged with other radiolabels for splenic scanning. The compound 1-mercuri-2-hydroxypropane, radiolabeled with ^{197}Hg or ^{203}Hg, not only binds to erythrocytes but also denatures them, so that splenic accumulation occurs.[10] It has also been reported that erythrocytes can be denatured with nonradioactive 1-mercuri-2-hydroxypropane and then labeled with a short-lived rubidium isotope (^{81}Rb).[12] In addition, erythrocytes bind carbon monoxide, and CO can be tagged with the short-lived carbon isotope ^{11}C. Some time ago, erythrocyte labeling with an iodine containing compound (*p*-iodophenylhydroxylamine) was reported,[13] but we are not aware of adequate follow-up studies. Erythrocytes can be labeled with the short-lived radionuclide ^{99m}Tc.[11] While this reduces the radiation dose, the radionuclide may be too short lived (T ½ = 6 hr) to allow prolonged studies of erythrocyte survival or sequestration sites.

Category 3: Phagocytosis by Reticuloendothelial Elements

The denatured erythrocytes can be viewed as "large" particles (7 μm) which are trapped by the spleen. Intravenously injected smaller particles are also taken up by splenic tissue. This accumulation of materials, often assayed by uptake of radioactive colloids, is a function of what is referred to as the reticuloendothelial system. The framework for understanding this functionally related collection of cells was laid by Metchnikoff and by Aschoff, and the subject has been reviewed by McIntyre.[16]

Early studies with intravenously administered ^{198}Au-colloid (radiogold) revealed uptake in the human liver.[14] As previously mentioned, the diameter of these particles was about 0.001 to 0.01 μm, and little went to the normal spleen. Increasing the quantity administered (in order to scan the spleen) was not feasible since even the usual liver scanning dose of 250 μCi produced significant radiation exposure, due to the fact that

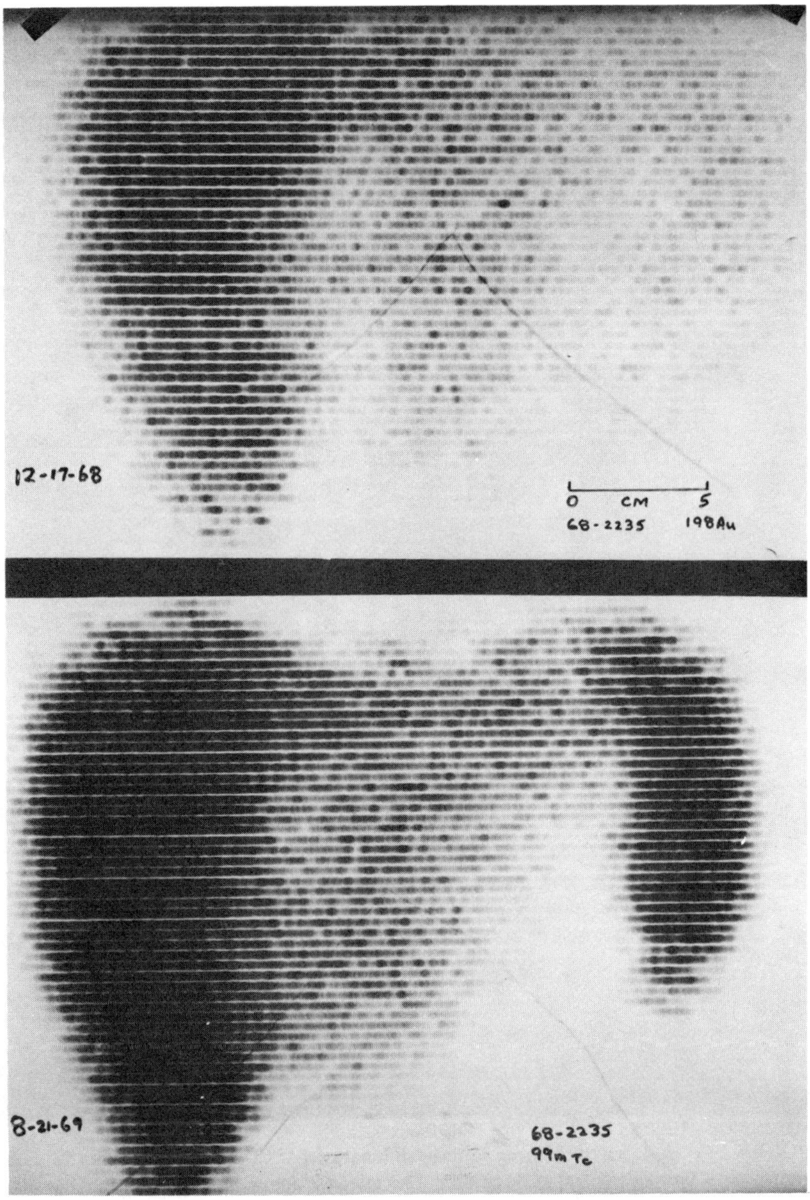

FIGURE 12. Anterior rectilinear scans obtained 8 months apart. The patient is a 20-year-old man with Hodgkin's disease. The upper scan was performed with ^{198}Au. The bottom scan was carried out after injection of ^{99m}Tc-sulfur colloid. The spleen can be clearly visualized with the technetium colloid. Case 68-2235.

^{198}Au had a beta ray emission in addition to the gamma ray and the half-life was relatively long (2.7 days). In various disorders of the liver, splenic uptake of gold radiocolloid was increased,[17] and the organ could be visualized.

The recent availability of radioactive colloids of short-lived materials (such as those labeled with ^{113m}In),[18] and more particularly ^{99m}Tc, has provided a resurgence of interest in scanning the spleen. Since the introduction of ^{99m}Tc sulfur colloid,[19-21] it has become the material of choice in visualizing the distribution of fixed phagocytic (reticuloendothelial) cells. As commonly made, the particles have a size of about 1 μm, and several percent of the administered dose accumulates in the spleen. A recent development has been the preparation of a colloid by reducing pertechnetate ($^{99m}TcO_4^-$) with tin chloride and binding it to small albumin particles. About 4% of this preparation goes to the spleen of rats.[28] There is evidence

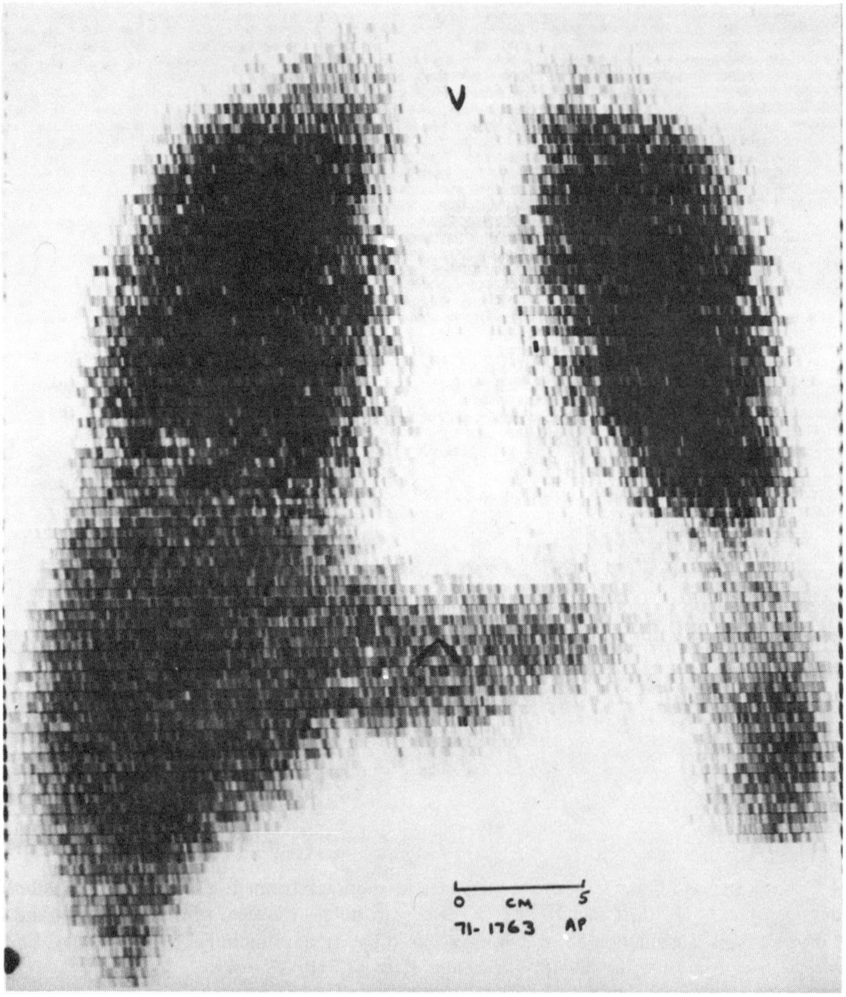

FIGURE 15. Anterior rectilinear scans in a 32-year-old man. The upper portion (lungs) was performed with ^{131}I-macroaggregated albumin. The lower organs (liver and spleen) were visualized by means of ^{99m}Tc-sulfur colloid. Case 71-1763.

is considerably less in man but apparently does occur (at least functionally) as shown by the rise in the platelet count and Factor VIII (antihemophiliac factor) that follows intravenous epinephrene administration (the effect is not observed in splenectomized individuals).[74,80] That the human spleen can contract has also been suggested by observations on the rapid passage of media to the portal vein in splenoportography.[32] Such passage takes about 6 sec, while transit from spleen to liver after splenic artery catheterization takes about 9 sec. There is an additional piece of suggestive evidence. In two children with splenomegaly in sickle cell disease, we noted splenic contraction by means of following movement of the tip of the spleen (the organ was previously labeled with radiocolloid).[33] Long-term changes in splenic size can also occur and are discussed elsewhere.[33,34]

Category 5: Culling and Pitting

These are terms extensively discussed by Crosby.[36,38] By culling is meant that abnormal erythrocytes are selectively removed from the circulation and destroyed by the spleen. Following splenectomy, spherocytes and bizzare poikilocytes appear, the surface area of erythrocytes increases, and "target cells" can be seen. Thus, the spleen may be playing a continual role in processing the red cell membrane (and a splenic effect on the "ripening" of erythrocytes was proposed many years ago).[43] For example, the spleen plays a central part in "conditioning" the surface of red cells in certain cases of liver disease.[84]

By pitting is meant that a variety of intra-erythrocytic inclusions, such as Howell-Jolly bodies, Heinz bodies, and siderocytic inclusions, are taken out (plucked or pitted) of the erythrocytes, without destroying the red cells. An elegant demonstration of this has been described by Crosby.[36] Blood containing large numbers of siderocytes (erythrocytes with iron-staining inclusions) were labeled with ^{51}Cr and were transfused into a patient who had a functioning spleen. The ^{51}Cr in the bloodstream did not change appreciably over the first several hours, indicating that the intact cells were still in the circulation. However, the number of visible siderocytes decreased. Hence, the spleen must have been pitting the cells of the inclusions and then permitting the "cleansed" cells to recirculate. When the ^{51}Cr-siderocytes were introduced into a splenectomized patient, the ^{51}Cr in the circulation, as well as the number of siderocytes, decreased approximately in parallel (no selective pitting of inclusions from the erythrocytes).

A principal indicator of splenectomy is the appearance of Howell-Jolly bodies in a portion of circulating erythrocytes (perhaps 1 to 5 per 1,000). These bodies are remnants of the nucleus, and Crosby[38] has reviewed the history of their discovery. Howell-Jolly bodies apparently are present in all patients who have had splenectomy. However, the presence of these inclusions does not necessarily indicate an anatomically absent spleen. We have shown that the spleen can be physically present but functionless (and see the discussion of "functional asplenia"). It is possible that in still other cases the spleen may be unable to keep up with the pitting of Howell-Jolly bodies when they are produced in overwhelming numbers. Gilbert[43] suggested that such particles are removed from the red blood cells by extrusion. The anatomical basis for this extrusion is found in the squeezing of erythrocytes between endothelial cells of the spleen.[44] The fate of other erythrocytic particles, such as Heinz bodies, has been studied in the spleens of various animals.[69]

Surface vacuoles ("pits") are detected by interference contrast microscopy in over half of the circulating erythrocytes in splenectomized individuals (versus only about 2% of the red blood cells in patients having an intact spleen).[45] Perhaps this relates to splenic "conditioning", repair, or alteration of the red cell membrane. When ^{51}Cr-labeled vacuolated cells are transfused into a normal individual (spleen intact), the vacuoles disappear (nearly all are cleared by 70 hr), while the ^{51}Cr tag remains in the bloodstream. Hence, the vacuoles were removed without destroying the cells. Schnitzer and co-workers,[46] using electron microscopy, concluded that such vacuoles were fused to the surface of red cells, exposing their contents to the outside.

Category 6: Possible Splenic Hormone Control of Hematopoiesis

In occasional cases of aplastic anemia, splenectomy is followed by an increase in the circulating blood count. This could be due to less destruction; there is little hard evidence that the spleen produces a hormone which affects hematopoiesis. Montz and Schneider[68] have reported that after splenectomy, the bone marrow size of man changes. The effect of feeding spleen extracts has been summarized,[75] but it is uncertain whether this has a direct action on hematopoiesis.

Category 7: Role in Platelet and Leukocyte Destruction

Following splenectomy, a thrombocytosis and leukocytosis can occur in man. This has been attributed to a removal of the splenic reservoir rather than a specific increase in survival of platelets. Platelet survival is equal in normal and asplenic individuals. Additional aspects are discussed in a later chapter.

Category 8: Immunologic Role

The spleen has been identified as having roles in determining host resistance. First the spleen is important in antibody synthesis. This activity is not a general phenomenon. Rather, it is restricted to limited and specific circumstances. When an antigen used for immunization is administered by subcutaneous or intramuscular routes, no significant differences can be detected between the asplenic and normal animal or human.[76,77] However, when the antigen is particulate and is given in small amounts by the intravenous route, a clear immunological function of the spleen can be demonstrated. Rowley in 1950 administered heterologous red cells to rats and humans and measured the changes of hemolysins in the serum subsequently. Animals with normal spleens responded rapidly with rises in serum hemolysin titer, whereas those who had been splenectomized showed insignificant changes. The response of splenic antibody production may be very rapid. "Early antibodies" may be detected soon after antigenic challenge,[78] and immunization with killed organisms (as early as 8 hr after challenge with virulent pneumococci) decreases mortality.[79]

A second aspect of splenic function in determining host resistance relates to the spleen as a biological filter – a filter with a precise degree of discrimination. When particulate material such as bacteria or red cells enter the circulation, they are cleared by reticuloendothelial elements in liver, spleen, and bone marrow. By using red cells or bacteria which have been tagged with radioactive isotopes, it is possible to determine the rate and anatomic site of clearance.

In animals immune to bacteria such as pneumococci, the liver by virtue of its large mass of reticuloendothelial tissue is the primary site for clearance of ^{125}I- labeled pneumococci. In the nonimmune animal, the spleen assumes greater importance and may on a weight basis be 10 to 60 times more efficient than the liver.

The same phenomenon can be demonstrated with red cells. Jandl and Kaplan[72] have demonstrated selective splenic activity using ^{51}Cr-tagged RBC which are reacted with antibody. When the ratio of antibody to RBC was low (weak Coombs' test), the spleen removed most of the red cells and was 20 times more active than the liver. When the ratio of antibody to RBC was high (strongly positive Coombs' test), the primary site of red cell clearance was the liver.

The spleen appears to be the crucial first line of defense in cleaning small numbers of bacteria from the circulation in infants who lack specific immunity. This is probably the basis for the syndrome of post-splenectomy overwhelming sepsis. The spleen is also the site of lymphocyte production and may be involved in the genesis of opsonins; both of these activities are of importance in immunology.

ANOTHER VIEWPOINT

Organ imaging by the techniques of nuclear medicine depends on the use of one of the following:

1. Emission scanning.
2. Transmission scanning.
3. Fluorescent scanning.

By emission scanning is meant that a radioactive substance has been administered and that its emissions are detected externally. This is the classical radioisotope scan. Transmission scanning depends on the placing of a source of radioactivity beneath the body and detecting emissions passing through. Less dense areas, such as the lungs, will allow photons to readily pass, while dense areas, such as fluid, soft tissue, or bone, will intercept more photons. Yeh and co-workers[35] combine lung transmission images and liver-spleen emission scans to study ascites and possible subdiaphragmatic abscesses. They suggested that when separation of the lung and liver was seen, lung-spleen visualization should be carried out. If the lung-liver and lung-spleen views showed separation, then ascites was the likely cause. They also noted that lung-spleen separation could not always be correlated with disease states since it occurred in 15% of the control population. Fluorescent scanning depends on the excitation of one or more components present in an organ and detection of the emitted rays (for example, it has been used in quantifying iodine in the thyroid). There has been little application to the study of the spleen.

THE ^{99m}Tc-SULFUR COLLOID SPLEEN SCAN

Intravenous injection of ^{99m}Tc-sulfur colloid is the most common manner of visualizing the spleen by radioisotopic technique. The usual dose is about 2 to 5 millicuries. Disappearance of the radiocolloid from the bloodstream is normally rapid (T½ is about 2 min). There have been no definitive studies to support the contention that the rate of accumulation of the radiocolloid is a quantitative indicator of splenic function.

Indications for a splenic scan are numerous.

1. To visualize the spleen when there is suspected splenic rupture, or left upper quadrant pain.
2. To examine the nature of left upper quadrant masses.
3. To look for accessory splenic tissue (especially post-splenectomy).
4. To look at the distribution of radiocolloid accumulation, especially in evaluating portal hypertension.
5. To aid in the staging of Hodgkin's disease and other lymphomas.

6. To evaluate possible abdominal situs inversus.

7. To serially follow the organ, as during growth or its response to medication.

8. To indicate the location of the spleen prior to radiation therapy (and to follow changes brought about by radiation).

9. To act as a baseline in the evaluation of pancytopenia or depression of individual blood elements. When coupled with data on ^{59}Fe distribution, spleen scans can be utilized in evaluating extramedullary hematopoiesis.

10. To determine whether the spleen is functionally present.

REPORTING THE SPLEEN SCAN

The report of the results of a spleen scan should contain information on several key points. These will be listed and then discussed.

1. Scanning agent used and amount.
2. Functional presence or absence of spleen (and any accessory sites of uptake).
3. Location.
4. Size.
5. Homogeneity of uptake.
6. Any major defects.
7. Count rates over spleen as compared with liver and bone marrow.

Mention of the scanning agent utilized is crucial in properly interpreting the results of spleen scans. While only a small fraction of ^{198}Au-colloid is normally taken up by the spleen, much more of the dose of ^{99m}Tc-S-colloid usually undergoes uptake by splenic tissue. When ^{51}Cr-heat-denatured erythrocytes are employed, nearly quantitative entry into the liver occurs when the spleen is absent (and erythrocyte tagging is still probably the best procedure in searching for splenic absence).

While spleen scans are usually interpreted in terms of gross morphology, we are in reality viewing a representation of the functional activities of the organ. Absence of splenic uptake on a radiocolloid scan can represent either anatomic absence of the organ or functional absence. Hence, reliable evidence for the physical presence of the spleen (by palpation or by radiographic means), without radiocolloid uptake, indicates "functional asplenia." This condition is often associated with hematological disorders.

Congenital absence of the spleen can occur and is frequently part of multiple congenital abnormalities. Polysplenia also occurs, again as part of a syndrome of multiple congenital errors. Hypoplasia of the spleen is also known.

A report of the location of the spleen is of necessity for several reasons. First, the presence of the spleen on the right indicates some degree of situs inversus (in one variant this can be found with sinusitis and bronchiectasis: Kartagener's syndrome). Second, abnormal downward displacement of the spleen can occur in pulmonary diseases or other conditions, causing depression of the diaphragm, as well as when retroperitoneal masses are present (Figure 16). The spleen can be displaced by the stomach, and the converse is also true.

The size of the spleen is certainly a major part of the report of the scan. We usually measure the greatest length and the greatest width (as well as reporting the general shape). Criteria are available for describing the length of the spleen in terms of the normal distribution of sizes in the population (and this is described later). The size of the spleen can be decreased in some vascular disorders and in instances of splenic infarcts. Splenomegaly can be due to a number of conditions, varying from vascular congestion through tumor involvement.

A comment on the homogeneity of splenic uptake of radiocolloid is required since it may provide a clue as to the underlying pathology. Perhaps the most marked inhomogeneities are seen in the thalassemia syndromes, in which splenomegaly, infarcts, and calcium deposition can result in nearly a "patchwork quilt" appearance.

Major defects of the spleen can be singular or multiple and represent regions not accumulating the radiocolloid. Infarcts are common, but cysts, tumors, abscesses, and other space-occupying processes such as hematomas also have to be considered.

Finally, a report must be given as to how much radiocolloid is accumulated in the spleen as compared with the liver and bone marrow. The spleen/liver ratio will vary depending on the radiocolloid used and the view taken (the ratio is higher from the posterior since the spleen is closer to the probe and the liver is farther away). Most radiocolloids presently used (such as ^{198}Au, ^{99m}Tc-S-colloid, ^{113m}In-colloid)[50] accumulate

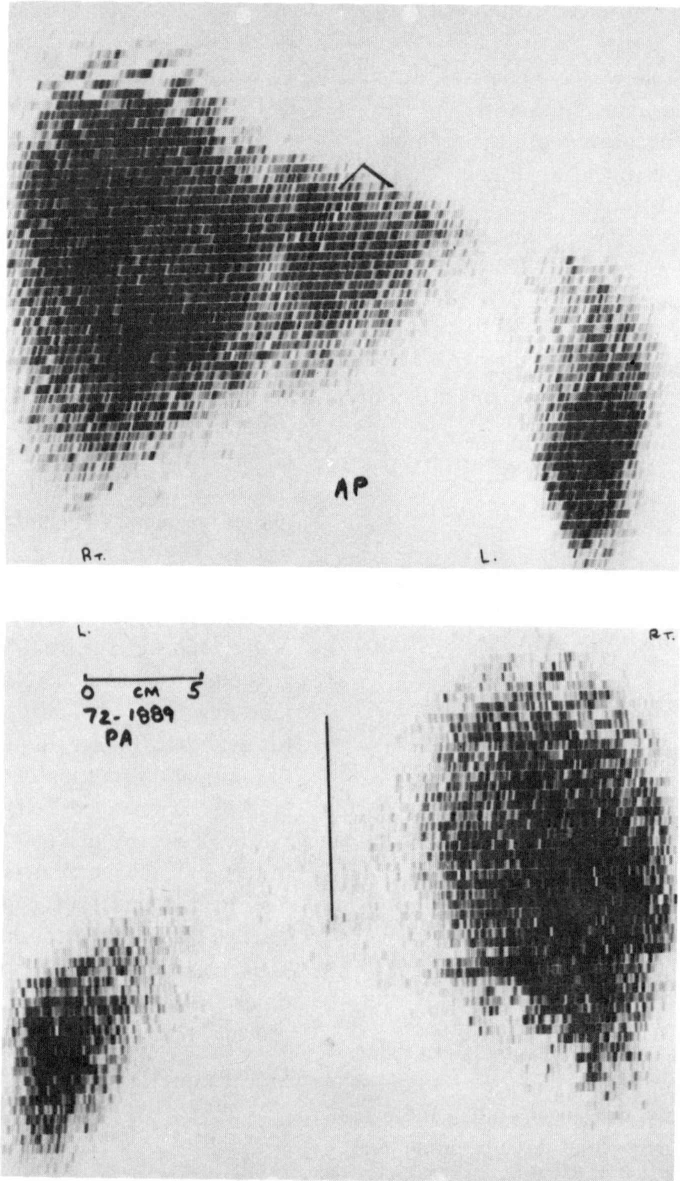

FIGURE 16. Anterior and posterior rectilinear scans (^{99m}Tc-sulfur colloid). The patient is a 24-year-old man with a large left lung lesion. Splenic displacement is pronounced. Case 72-1889.

principally in the liver, and increased uptake in the spleen occurs in hepatic disorders or when the spleen is a major site of extramedullary hematopoiesis.

In each case, the conventional (static) spleen scan must be supplemented by other information to make as definitive a report as possible. Some of the accessory diagnostic aids are the spleen scan-abdominal radiograph overlay (especially when looking for the localization of calcium deposits), splenic blood pool scans, and combined spleen-lung or spleen-kidney scans. The mobility of the spleen must be recalled, along with the ability of the organ to move (and hence to change apparent size and shape) between various views.[83]

The following points may be helpful:

1. Since the spleen is both posterior and lateral, an anterior rectilinear scan may not visualize the organ in any detail on rectilinear scans ("defocused," or not in the focal plane; Figure 17). Left lateral views may sometimes not

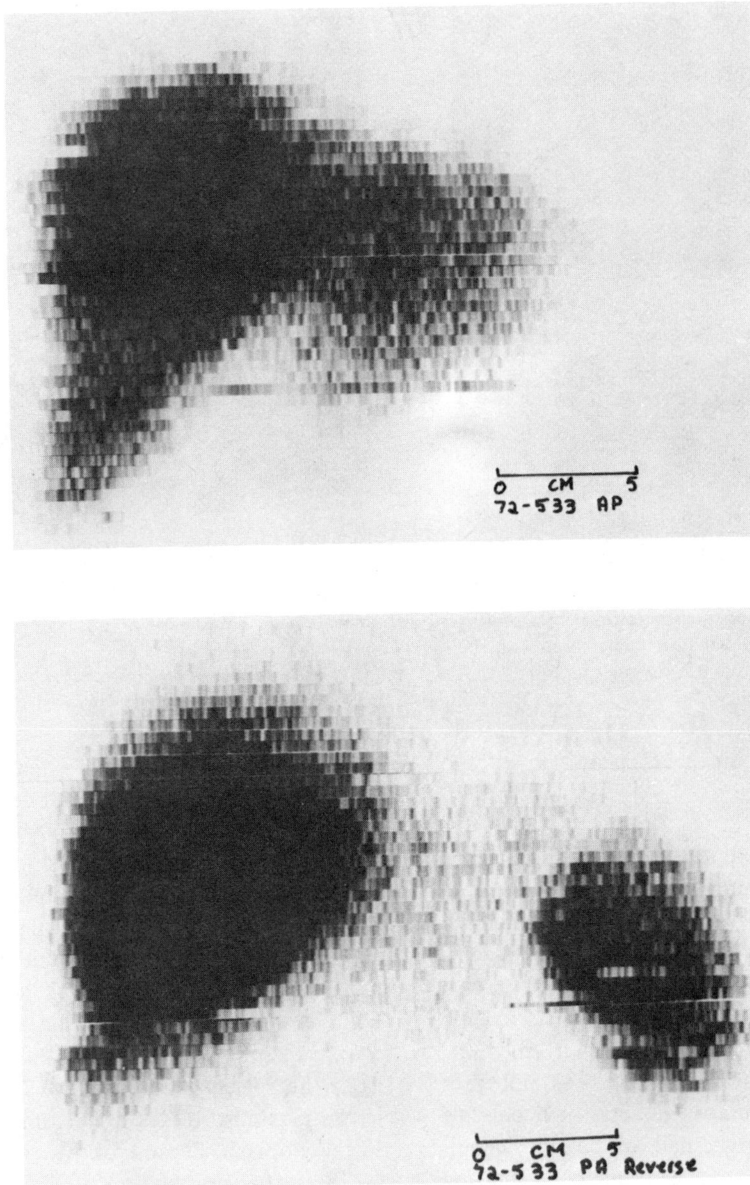

FIGURE 17. Rectilinear scans obtained by use of ^{99m}Tc-sulfur colloid in a 67-year-old woman. The top (anterior view) does not clearly show the spleen. The bottom picture (posterior view reversed) reveals the organ. Case 72-533.

be helpful since an enlarged liver can obscure visualization of the spleen. As splenic enlargement occurs, the organ usually extends anteriorly and inferiorly[49] and may be seen on anterior views.

2. Hepatic tissue may cross midline (Figure 18) and appear to be accessory splenic tissue (especially post splenectomy).[47] In the right lateral decubitus, the spleen may be displaced anteriorly and medially and be obscured by the liver.[48] The left lateral decubitus position may thus be preferable. As mentioned, we have found the left anterior oblique view to often be helpful in seperating the spleen from the liver.

3. Any free technetium accompanying ^{99m}Tc-sulfur colloid will partially appear in the stomach and obscure splenic visualization.[51] When ^{197}Hg mercurihydroxypropane is used to tag erythrocytes for spleen scanning, accumulation occurs in the liver when the spleen is non-functional. In addition, free ^{197}Hg accumulates in the kidneys. In efforts to find accessory splenic tissue, ^{51}Cr-erythrocytes (or perhaps ^{99m}Tc-

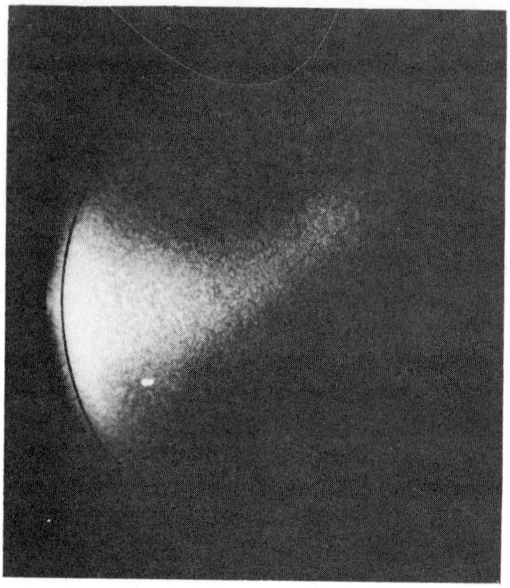

FIGURE 18. Anterior scintiphoto (^{99m}Tc-sulfur colloid) in a 28-year-old man. Hepatic tissue can be seen extending into the left upper quadrant. Case 72-1894.

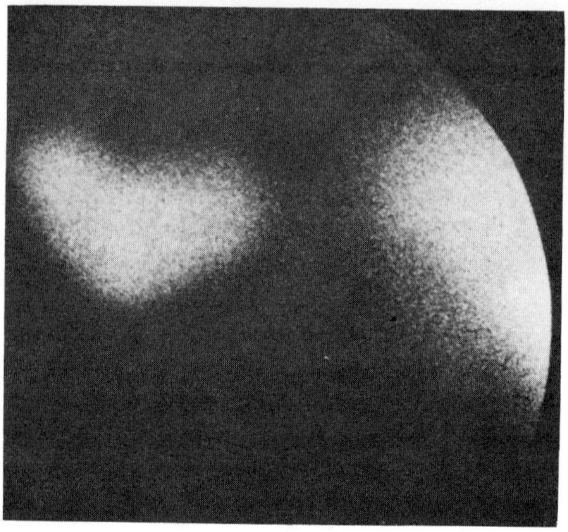

FIGURE 19. Posterior scintiphoto obtained by use of ^{99m}Tc-sulfur colloid. The patient is a 51-year-old woman with diabetes mellitus and weight loss. The spleen is in an angulated or "upside-down" position. Case 73-255.

erythrocytes) which are heat denatured may be the materials of choice.

We have pointed out that radiocolloid scans should have the counting rates (per unit area) recorded over the liver and spleen.[52] Bekerman and Gottschalk[53] have commented on the significance of the liver/spleen uptake of ^{99m}Tc-sulfur colloid. They pointed out that when splenic uptake was diminished as compared with the liver, and when bone marrow uptake was not pronounced, then proliferative diseases or neoplasms of hematopoietic origin had to be considered. Elevated uptake in the spleen and bone marrow occurred in cirrhosis or anemia. Such a comparison of the liver to spleen ratio of activities, from the posterior view, appears to be a simple but useful technique.

Variations in the spleen (such as the degree of rotation, indentations, and lobulations) and the impressions made on it by other organs are considerable. When marked rotation of the spleen is present, the term "upside-down spleen" has been applied.[70] An example is shown in Figure 19. The renal impression on the spleen (and vice versa) can sometimes be appreciated during dynamic kidney studies. A related point is that spleen-visualizing agents that also undergo renal excretion may obscure the scans. Combined spleen scans and kidney scans (posterior) can show the organs in proximity.

The left lobe of the liver extends near, or over, the spleen, making clear anterior delineation of the spleen outline difficult. In many instances this "hepatic walk" or "gratuitous override" can be severe enough to completely hide the spleen on the anterior view. Indeed, these observations should help us recall that the spleen is a *posterior* organ and is best visualized on the posterior and oblique views. Even in the posterior view, however, utilizing ^{99m}Tc-S-colloid, in about 5% of the cases the spleen is obscured by parts of the liver.

We must also recall the proximity of the spleen to the stomach. Because of this, materials secreted by the gastric mucosa ($^{131}I^-$, $^{99m}TcO_4^-$) obscure clear visualization of the spleen. Although the pancreas is usually considerably below the spleen, the splenic vessels run close to the pancreas and can potentially be damaged in the course of pancreatic trauma or disease.

Because of the posterior position of the spleen, it rests close to the posteroinferior portions of the diaphragm and left lung. Hence, pulmonary disorders can depress the spleen (recall Figure 16). Overlays of spleen scans on nonmagnified chest radiographs can also be utilized to define anatomic relations. Anterior, posterior, or lateral combined lung-liver scans can often point out aspects of these relationships. In practice, however, combined lung-liver scans are usually performed in the anterior and right lateral views to search for subphrenic abscesses. The anterior views are obtained by injecting ^{99m}Tc- or ^{131}I-macroagglomerated human serum albumin (for lung visualization) and ^{99m}Tc-S-colloid (for liver and spleen scanning). When ^{99m}Tc-labeled materials and a gamma ray camera are used, views are taken at the technetium channel. However, if two different radionuclides are used, two successive exposures can be superimposed on the same film. For rectilinear scans, anatomic markings are first placed on the dot scan (so that they can be checked at the end to insure lack of motion). The lung scan and liver scan can be obtained in one sequence if the same radionuclide is used for both organs. As mentioned, transmission scans can also be utilized to define the general anatomic relationships. There is little constancy to the splenopulmonic space. More often, the spleen is poorly seen on the anterior lung-liver scan. When faint visualization is coupled with cardiomegaly, little information can be gathered from the anterior view.

Even though the spleen is posterior and retroperitoneal, the organ hangs by a pedicle and is subject to some degree of motion. This must be recalled when the location of the spleen is to be marked on the skin for purposes of defining radiation therapy portals. For example, if the therapy is to be performed with the patient's arms above the head, the scans should also be taken in that position.

ADDITIONAL NOTE ON SPLENOMEGALY

One of the most frequent reasons for examining this organ is the finding of a palpable spleen. Hence, a few remarks will be made on such a physical finding. The first point is that a number of cases of splenomegaly may escape physical examination. The spleen has to be 1½ to 2 times increased in size to be palpable. Splenic enlargement will, however, be detected on radioisotopic scans (*if* the tissue is functional and if the laboratory is aware of the expected range of splenic sizes for the population under study). Secondly, the spleen can be displaced by other structures; hence, simply palpating a spleen does not necessarily mean that it is enlarged. For example, gastric dilation[54] can cause scan-documented displacement of the spleen. Parker and Bennett[55] reported that after the ingestion of one liter of water, variable changes in spleen size and position occurred (perhaps related to fluid in the stomach). Third, the size of the spleen can change (and additional aspects of this will be discussed later). Gould and co-workers[56] have noted liver enlargement (on scintiphotos) during congestive heart failure and an increased uptake of radiocolloid in the spleen. After the restoration of cardiac compensation, the liver decreased in size and the spleen/liver ratio of radioactivity returned toward normal. If we assume that the magnification of the two photos in the article by Gould and co-workers[56] is the same, then the length of the spleen decreased 13% in one patient after the treatment of congestive failure. Dumont and co-workers[57] studied the spleen in four patients who, at death, had congestive heart failure. Two of the spleens were of normal weight (120 g in a patient of age 64 and 145 g in one aged 94). In two younger patients (41, 42 years of age) with congestive failure, the spleens were enlarged (390, 420 g). Dumont and co-workers[57] stated that an examination of splenic hilar lymphatics in patients with congestion of the spleen revealed an increased number of dilated lymphatic vessels (often with contained erythrocytes).

In apparently healthy college freshmen, McIntyre and Ebaugh[58] noted the spleen to be palpable in 2.9%. Over a period of 3 years, 70% of these became nonpalpable, and as many as 10% of children may have a palpable spleen. We must wonder if such cases represented anatomic variants or did indeed harbor disease. The classification of splenomegaly can be made simple or complex. Dameshek[59] provided one classification based on "physiopathologic" criteria and one based on "etiopathologic" data. We can modify this latter grouping to produce the following table.

Major Causes of Splenomegaly

1. Bulk lesions (such as cysts, hematomas).
2. Infections.
3. Granulomas.
4. Neoplasms.
5. Cellular disturbances (such as lipidoses, sarcoid).
6. Hemoglobinopathies, thalassemia, and hemolytic disorders.

7. Circulatory alteration (generalized, or localized such as portal hypertension).

8. Immunologic response.

The relationship of splenomegaly to such findings as fever, pallor and icterus, lymphadenopathy, petechiae and ecchymoses, plethora, bone changes, pancytopenia, and an elevated white cell count has been described by Dameshek.[59] In terms of frequency of being seen in this country, portal hypertension may be the commonest cause of splenomegaly. Globally, malaria may be the most prevalent etiologic factor in splenomegaly. Other frequently encountered causes of splenomegaly are leukemia, lymphoma, Hodgkin's disease, polycythemia vera, idiopathic thrombocytopenic purpura, sickle cell anemia (infants), thalassemia major, hereditary spherocytosis, myeloid metaplasia, schistosomiasis, infectious mononucleosis, subacute bacterial endocarditis, and various infections. As previously mentioned, Silverstein and Maldonado[2] stated that the commonest causes of *asymptomatic* splenomegaly seen at the Mayo Clinic were portal hypertension, myeloid metaplasia, Gaucher's disease, and splenic cyst.

Marsden and Hamilton[61] have listed the commonest causes of splenomegaly in the tropics as parasitic infections (particularly malaria, leishmaniasis, and schistosomiasis), other infections, blood disorders, infiltration of the spleen, congestive splenomegaly, and tropical splenomegaly syndrome. Akinyanju and Lawoyin[62] noted that the commonest causes of splenomegaly in Nigeria were (most frequent to least frequent): hemoglobinopathies, portal hypertension, hepatitis, leukemia, lymphoma, "idiopathic" malaria, septicemia, rheumatoid arthritis, acquired hemolytic anemia, lupus erythematosus, hookworm anemia, and multiple myeloma. In North Africans observed in France,[63] only 12 of 95 cases of splenomegaly had cirrhosis or portal vein thrombosis; many of the others likely had a hemoglobinopathy. Gregory and Klatskin[60] have reported that 15% of 134 patients with biliary tract or pancreatic disease (without evidence of portal obstruction), had a palpable spleen. This might be related to increased resistance to flow within the portal system.

REFERENCES

1. **Moeschlin, S.,** *Spleen Puncture,* Piney, A., transl., Heinemann, London, 1951, 229.
2. **Silverstein, M. N. and Maldonado, J. E.,** Asymptomatic splenomegaly, *Postgrad. Med.,* 48, 80, 1970.
3. **Baron, M. G. and Wolf, B. S.,** Splenoportography, *JAMA,* 206, 629, 1968.
4. **Kuba, J. and Seidlova, V.,** Evaluation of portal circulation by the scintillation camera, *J. Nucl. Med.,* 13, 689, 1972.
5. **King, M. C., Glick, B. W., and Freed, A.,** The diagnosis of splenic cysts, *Surg. Gynecol. Obstet.,* 127, 509, 1968.
6. **Castellino, R. A., Silverman, J. F., Glatstein, E., Blank, N., and Wexler, L.,** Splenic arteriography in Hodgkin's disease. A roentgenologic-pathologic study of 33 consecutive untreated patients, *Am. J. Roentgenol.,* 114, 574, 1972.
7. **Holm, H. H. and Mortensen, T.,** Ultrasonic scanning in diagnosis of abdominal disease, *Acta Chir. Scand.,* 134, 333, 1968.
8. **Gray, S. J. and Sterling, K.,** The tagging of red blood cells and plasma proteins with radioactive chromium, *J. Clin. Invest.,* 29, 818, 1950.
9. **Johnson, P. M., Herion, J., and Mooring, S. L.,** Scintillation scanning of the normal human spleen utilizing sensitized radioactive erythrocytes, *Radiology,* 74, 99, 1960.
10. **Wagner, H. N., Jr., Weiner, I. M., McAfee, J. G., and Martinez, J.,** 1-mercuri-2-hydroxypropane (MHP): a new pharmaceutical for visualization of the spleen by radioisotope scanning, *Arch. Int. Med.,* 113, 696, 1964.
11. **Eckelman, W., Richards, P., Atkins, H. L., Hauser, W., and Klopper, J. F.,** Visualization of the human spleen with ^{99m}Tc-labeled red blood cells, *J. Nucl. Med.,* 12, 310, 1971.
12. **Glass, H. I., de Garreta, A. C., Lewis, S. M., Grammaticos, P., and Szur, L.,** Measurement of splenic red-blood-cell mass with radioactive carbon monoxide, *Lancet,* 1, 669, 1968.
13. **Jackson, H.,** Studies with erythrocytes labeled with radioactive-iodophenylhydroxylamine, *Nature,* 172, 80, 1953.

14. **Stirrett, L. A., Yuhl, E. T., and Cassen, B.,** Clinical applications of hepatic radioactivity surveys, *Am. J. Gastroenterol.*, 21, 310, 1954.
15. **Huff, R. L., Hennessy, T. G., Austin, R. E., Garcia, J. F., Roberts, B. M., and Lawrence, J. H.,** Plasma and red cell turnover in normal subjects and in patients having various hematopoietic disorders, *J. Clin. Invest.*, 29, 1041, 1950.
16. **McIntyre, P. A.,** The reticuloendothelial system: organization and physiology, *Johns Hopkins Med. J.*, 130, 61, 1972.
17. **Magalotti, M. F., Byun, H. H., Des Rosiers, J., Villa, F., Steigmann, F., and Alavi, I. A.,** Significance of splenic concentration of radioactive gold in liver scans, *J. Nucl. Med.*, 8, 390, 1967.
18. **Goodwin, D. A., Stern, H. S., and Wagner, H. N., Jr.,** Colloidal indium-113m for liver, spleen and bone marrow scanning, *J. Nucl. Med.*, 8, 304, 1967.
19. **Harper, P. V., Lathrop, K. A., and Richards, P.,** ^{99m}Tc as a radiocolloid, *J. Nucl. Med.*, 5, 382, 1964.
20. **Petasnick, J. P. and Gottschalk, A.,** Spleen scanning with ^{99m}Technetium sulfur colloid and the scintillation camera, *J. Nucl. Med.*, 6, 362, 1965.
21. **Stern, H. S., McAfee, J. G., and Subramanian, G.,** Preparation, distribution and utilization of technetium-99m sulfur colloid, *J. Nucl. Med.*, 7, 665, 1966.
22. **Scheffel, U., Rhodes, B. A., Natarajan, T. K., and Wagner, H. N., Jr.,** Albumin microspheres for study of the reticuloendothelial system, *J. Nucl. Med.*, 13, 498, 1972.
23. **Benacerraf, B., Biozzi, G., Halpern, B. N., Stiffel, C., and Mouton, D.,** Phagocytosis of heat denatured human serum albumin labeled with I-131 and its use as a means of investigating liver blood flow, *Br. J. Exp. Pathol.*, 38, 35, 1957.
24. **Taplin, G. V., Griswald, M. L., and Dore, E. K.,** Preparation of colloidal suspensions of human serum albumin I-131 for estimating liver blood flow and recticuloendothelial system functions in man, *USAEC Report UCLA-481 (Biology and Medicine)*, June 1961.
25. **Iio, M. and Wagner, H. N., Jr.,** Studies of the reticuloendothelial system (RES). I. Measurement of the phagocytic capacity of the RES in man and dog, *J. Clin. Invest.*, 42, 417, 1963.
26. **Wagner, H. N., Jr., Iio, M., and Hornick, R. B.,** Studies of the reticuloendothelial system (RES). II. Changes in the phagocytic capacity of the RES in patients with certain infections, *J. Clin. Invest.*, 42, 427, 1963.
27. **Briner, W. H.,** Preparation of ^{125}I-labeled microaggregated human serum albumin for use in studies of reticuloendothelial function in man, *J. Nucl. Med.*, 9, 482, 1968.
28. **Lin, M. S. and Winchell, H. S.,** A "kit" method for the preparation of a technetium-tin (II) colloid and a study of its properties, *J. Nucl. Med.*, 13, 58, 1972.
29. **Nelson, B., Hayes, R. L., Edwards, C. L., Kniseley, R. M., and Andrews, G. A.,** Distribution of gallium in human tissues after intravenous administration, *J. Nucl. Med.*, 13, 92, 1972.
30. **Blau, M. and Manske, R. F.,** The pancreas specificity of Se^{75}-selenomethionine, *J. Nucl. Med.*, 2, 102, 1961.
31. **Ben-Porath, M. and Kaplan, E.,** The distribution and concentration of ^{75}Se selenomethionine in man, *J. Nucl. Med.*, 10, 709, 1969.
32. **Dumont, A. E., Martelli, A., and Biris, L.,** Contraction of the spleen following needle puncture: significance in studies of portal hypertension, *Gastroenterology*, 61, 738, 1971.
33. **Spencer, R. P., Lange, R. C., Schwartz, A. D., and Pearson, H. A.,** Radioisotopic studies of changes in splenic size in response to epinephrine and other stimuli, *J. Nucl. Med.*, 13, 211, 1972.
34. **O'Brien, R. T., Pearson, H. A., and Spencer, R. P.,** Transfusion-induced decrease in spleen size in thalassemia major: documentation by radioisotopic scan, *J. Pediatr.*, 81, 105, 1972.
35. **Yeh, E. L., Ruetz, P. P., and Meade, R. C.,** Separation of lung-liver scintiphotos due to ascites – a false positive test for subdiapharagmatic abscess, *J. Nucl. Med.*, 13, 249, 1972.
36. **Crosby, W. H.,** Normal functions of the spleen relative to red blood cells: a review, *Blood*, 14, 399, 1959.
37. **Elenes, N. A., Ewald, R. A., and Crosby, W. H.,** The reservoir function of the spleen and its relation to postsplenectomy anemia in the dog, *Blood*, 24, 299, 1964.
38. **Crosby, W. H.,** Hyposplenism: an inquiry into normal functions of the spleen, *Annu. Rev. Med.*, 14, 349, 1963.
39. **Palmer, D. L., Rifkind, D., and Brown, D. W.,** ^{131}I-labeled colloidal human serum albumin in the study of reticuloendothelial system function. II. Phagocytosis and catabolism of a test colloid in normal subjects, *J. Infect. Dis.*, 123, 457, 1971.
40. **Palmer, D. L., Rifkind, D., and Brown, D. W.,** ^{131}I-labeled colloidal human serum albumin in the study of reticuloendothelial system function. III. Phagocytosis and catabolism compared in normal, leukemic, and immunosuppressed human subjects, *J. Infect. Dis.*, 123, 465, 1971.
41. **Kitani, K. and Taplin, G. V.,** Billiary excretion of ^{99m}Tc-albumin microaggregate degradation products (a method for measuring Kupffer cell digestive function?), *J. Nucl. Med.*, 13, 260, 1972.
42. **Saba, T. M., Kaplan, E., Graham, L., and Cornell, R. P.,** Hepatic phagocytic, metabolic, and blood-flow evaluation by dynamic scintigraphy, *J. Nucl. Med.*, 13, 300, 1972.
43. **Gilbert, Q. O.,** The occurrence of nuclear changes in the red blood cells following splenectomy, *Arch. Int. Med.*, 19, 140, 1917.
44. **Weiss, L. and Tavassoli, M.,** Anatomical hazards to the passage of erythrocytes through the spleen, *Semin. Hematol.*, 7, 372, 1970.

45. **Holroyde, C. P. and Gardner, F. H.,** Acquisition of autophagic vacuoles by human erythrocytes, physiological role of the spleen, *Blood,* 36, 566, 1970.
46. **Schnitzer, B., Rucknagel, D. L., Spencer, H. H., and Aikawa, M.,** Erythrocytes: pits and vacuoles as seen with transmission and scanning electron microscope, *Science,* 173, 251, 1971.
47. **Ball, J. J., Kanzaki, T., Lum, C. H., Jim, R. T. S., and Wong, W. L. H.,** Aberrant liver tissue presenting as accessory spleen on spleen scans following splenectomy, *Hawaii Med. J.,* 30, 393, 1971.
48. **Crandell, D. C., Boyd, M., Wennemark, J. R., and Friedman, B. I.,** Liver-spleen scanning: the left lateral decubitus position is best for lateral views, *J. Nucl. Med.,* 13, 720, 1972.
49. **Petasnick, J. P., and Gottschalk, A.,** Spleen scintiphotography with technetium-99m-sulfur-colloid and the gamma-ray scintillation camera, *J. Nucl. Med.,* 7, 733, 1966.
50. **Szymendera, J., Zoltowski, T., Radwan, M., and Kamiska, J.,** Chemical and electron microscope observations of a safe PVP-stabilized colloid for liver and spleen scanning, *J. Nucl. Med.,* 12, 212, 1971.
51. **Samuels, L. D.,** Visualization of gastric mucosa on ^{99m}Tc-sulfur colloid liver-spleen scans: a puzzling artifact, *J. Nucl. Med.,* 12, 271, 1971.
52. **Spencer, R. P.,** Estimation of functional size of the spleen, *J. Nucl. Med.,* 11, 616, 1970.
53. **Bekerman, C. and Gottschalk, A.,** Diagnostic significance of the relative uptake of liver compared with spleen in ^{99m}Tc-sulfur colloid scintigraphy, *J. Nucl. Med.,* 12, 237, 1971.
54. **Landgarten, S., and Spencer, R. P.,** Splenic displacement due to gastric dilatation, *J. Nucl. Med.,* 13, 223, 1972.
55. **Parker, J. D. and Bennett, L. R.,** Effect of water ingestion on spleen size as determined by radioisotope scans, *Acta Radiol. Diagn.,* 11, 385, 1971.
56. **Gould, L., Collica, C., Comprecht, R. F., Indelicato, R., and Gelsomino, J.,** Scintiphotography in congestive heart failure: the disappearing flying bat pattern, *JAMA,* 219, 1734, 1972.
57. **Dumont, A. E., Pugkhem, T., Grosfeld, J., and Gorstein, F.,** Alterations in splenic hilar lymphatics in patients with congestion of the spleen, *Proc. Soc. Exp. Biol. Med.,* 135, 642, 1970.
58. **McIntyre, O. R. and Ebaugh, F. G., Jr.,** Palpable spleens in college freshmen, *Ann. Intern. Med.,* 66, 301, 1967.
59. **Dameshek, W.,** Splenomegaly: a problem in differential diagnosis, *Med. Clin. North Am.,* 41, 1357, 1957.
60. **Gregory, P. B., and Klatskin, G.,** Splenomegaly in uncomplicated biliary tract and pancreatic disease, *Gastroenterology,* 62, 436, 1972.
61. **Marsden, P. D. and Hamilton, P. J. S.,** Splenomegaly in the tropics, *Br. Med. J.,* 1, 99, 1969.
62. **Akinyanju, O. and Lawoyin, V.,** Aetiology of splenomegaly among Africans in Lagos, Nigeria, *Trop. Geogr. Med.,* 24, 49, 1972.
63. **Paraf, A., Rautaureau, J., and Gouffier, E.,** Splenomegaly in North Africans. Report of 95 cases observed in France, *Sem. Hop. Paris,* 48, 335, 1972.
64. **Lilien, D. L., Berger, H. G., Anderson, D. P., and Bennett, L. R.,** ^{111} In chloride: a new agent for bone marrow imaging, *J. Nucl. Med.,* 14, 184, 1973.
65. **Fung, W. P., Ong, S. C., and Lee, Y. S.,** Splenic tuberculosis presenting as pyrexia of unknown origin, *Med. J. Aust.,* 1, 446, 1973.
66. **Chaudhuri, Ta. K., Chaudhuri, Tu. K., Suzuki, Yl., Go, R. T., and Christie, J. H.,** Splenic accumulation of ^{87m} Sr in a patient with Hodgkin's disease, *Radiology,* 105, 617, 1972.
67. **Hillberg, R. W., Ringle, R. D., and Balcerzak, S. P.,** Howell-Jolly bodies, intracellular or extracellular, *Arch. Intern. Med.,* 131, 236, 1973.
68. **Montz, R., and Schneider, C.,** Eine Methode zur Bestimmung der Grosse des erythropoetischen Knochenmarks beim Menschen aus der Radioeisenkinetik, *Blut,* 21, 283, 1970.
69. **Simpson, C. F.,** Fate of erythrocytes containing Heinz bodies in the spleen and liver of dogs and turkeys, *Vet. Pathol.,* 8, 118, 1971.
70. **Westcott, J. L. and Krufky, E. L.,** The upside-down spleen, *Radiology,* 105, 517, 1972.
71. **Pearson, H. A. and Vertrees, K. M.,** Site of binding of chromium-51 to haemoglobin, *Nature,* 189, 1019, 1961.
72. **Jandl, J. H. and Kaplan, M. E.,** The destruction of red cells by antibodies in man. III quantitative factors influencing the patterns of hemolysis *in vivo, J. Clin. Invest.,* 39, 1145, 1960.
73. **Goldberg, A., Hutchison, H. E., and MacDonald, E.,** Radiochromium in the selection of patients with haemolytic anaemia for splenectomy, *Lancet,* 1, 109, 1966.
74. **Libre, E. P., Cowan, D. A., Watkins, S. P., and Shulman, N. R.,** Relationships between spleen, platelets and factor VIII levels, *Blood,* 31, 358, 1968.
75. **Cooper, M., Briggs, R. S., and Finch, S. C.,** Therapy of refractory idiopathic thrombocytopenic purpura, *Conn. Med.,* 32, 509, 1968.
76. **Saslaw, S., Bournocle, B. A., Wall, R. L., and Doan, C. A.,** Studies on the antibody response in splenectomized persons, *N. Engl. J. Med.,* 261, 120, 1959.
77. **Thurman, W. G.,** Splenectomy and immunity, *Am. J. Dis. Child.,* 105, 138, 1963.
78. **Taliaferro, W. H., and Taliaferro, L. G.,** The dynamics of hemolysin formation in intact and splenectomized rabbits, *J. Infect Dis.,* 87, 37, 1950.
79. **Schulkind, M. L., Ellis, E. F., and Smith, R. T.,** Effect of antibody upon clearance of I^{125} labelled pneumococci by the spleen and liver, *Pediatr. Res.,* 1, 178, 1967.

80. **Schwartz, A. D.,** The splenic platelet reservoir in sickle cell anemia, *Blood,* 40, 678, 1972.
81. **Jones, T., Pettit, J. E., Rhodes, C. G., and Waters, S. L.,** Use of ^{81} Rb-^{81m}Kr ratio for the measurement of spleen blood flow, *J. Nucl. Med.,* 14, 414, 1973.
82. **Subramanian, G., McAfee, J. G., Mehter, A., Blair, R. J., and Thomas, F. D.,** ^{99m}Tc-stannous phytate: a new in vivo colloid for imaging the reticuloendothelial system, *J. Nucl. Med.,* 14, 459, 1973.
83. **Chiles, J. T., Mintzer, R. A., Hoffer, P. B., and Gottschalk, A.,** Documentation of splenic displacement and changes in splenic size, *J. Nucl. Med.,* 14, 386, 1973.
84. **Cooper, R. A., Kimball, D. B., Durocher, J. R.,** Role of the spleen in membrane conditioning and hemolysis of spur cells in liver disease, *N. Engl. J. Med.,* 290, 1279, 1974.

Chapter 3

PRENATAL AND POSTNATAL DEVELOPMENT OF THE SPLEEN

After the first month of gestation, when the human fetus is 8 to 10 mm in length, the primordium of the spleen can be found in the dorsal mesogastrium. This region develops an extensive capillary plexus, and erythrocyte-forming cells appear by about the 4th month of gestation. These events mark the beginning of the hematopoietic function of the spleen. How, or if, the spleen is involved in the prenatal shift in synthesis of hemoglobin from one type to another[105] is unknown. The splenic role in hematopoiesis has been extensively studied in the mouse,[58,59] but human data are much less complete. Hematopoietic activities within the spleen are usually not given up until just following birth. The hematopoietic potential of the spleen stays present, however, and in myeloid metaplasia or other conditions (when bone marrow is involved) the spleen may begin erythrocyte production. The precise stimulus to this extramedullary hematopoiesis has still to be defined.

The spleen, of course, also develops reticuloendothelial activity (and, at birth, the human spleen can concentrate ^{99m}Tc-sulfur colloid). A summary of various aspects of this development (based primarily on uptake of foreign particles) in several species is provided by Solomon.[101] Based on studies by Halpern and associates,[102] a phagocytic index (K) is expressed as

$$K = \frac{\log\left[C_A - C_B\right]}{T_B - T_A} \qquad (1)$$

where C_A and C_B are the concentrations of injected particles at two points in time (T_B and T_A). Assuming that accessory factors, such as opsonins, are not rate limiting, the phagocytic index depends on the quantity (Q) of injected particles.

$$K \cdot Q = \text{constant} \qquad (2)$$

It has been stated that the quantity of particles to be used should be dependent on some increasing physiological parameter, such as the blood volume, in growing animals.[103] It would be of interest to relate the phagocytic index to the total number of reticuloendothelial cells. There is no exact way to do this at present, but a corrected phagocytic index (α) has been proposed.[104]

$$\alpha = \left[\frac{\text{Weight body}}{\text{Weight of liver and spleen}}\right] K^{1/3} \qquad (3)$$

The spleen is dependent on the thymus for development of at least some of its immunocompetent cells. In normal (unsensitized) mice, most of the rosette-forming cells are thymus dependent.[60] A hormone has been isolated from the thymus of mice and termed thymosin.[61] Further studies are needed on its possible interaction with the spleen. In congenitally "nude" mice, the thymus gland is absent, and there are immunological deficiencies. Spleen cells from such "nude" mice do not respond to added sheep erythrocytes. However, incubating the spleen cells with thymus lymphocytes from normal mice restores the response of the spleen cells.[70]

As mentioned previously, development of the human spleen is a continuous process. The germinal centers are formed by the first month after birth.[62] The exact role of various factors in influencing splenic development has still to be determined. Studies on the size distribution of the normal spleen during the postnatal period are of interest[63] since they may permit both a comparison of the spleen with other organs and a search for interrelationships. The role of diet and of bacteria must be sought out. For example, the spleen of conventional pigs (as well as the liver) is larger than that in germfree or contaminated pigs.[64]

Solomon[101] presented a figure of the logarithm of (weight body/weight of liver and spleen) as a function of age in the chicken (prehatching to day 42). The curve could be approximated by a rectangular hyperbola, but the physiological significance is unclear (a further discussion of the development of splenic weight is given later).

Between days 140 and 280 of gestation, there is little evidence for any significant difference in the development of the spleen between male and female human fetuses.[1,2] There is a sex difference later; this will be discussed later. In the human fetus, the weight of the spleen, during the latter half of gestation, is approximately a constant fraction of body weight (see Figure 1, in which data for the human fetus[1] are compared with the rat[3]). Various formulae for prenatal splenic weight have been proposed.[32]

At birth the human spleen is about 4.6 cm in length, 2.7 cm wide, and 1.3 cm thick;[4] the mean weight is some 11 g.[1] The framework for the organ is a collagenous network. There is a capsule covering the organ; the trabeculae enter the spleen. Contained within the spleen is a fine reticular network. This is entwined with lymphatic-like tissue referred to as the white pulp and an unusual lymphatic tissue (the red pulp). At birth, the red pulp constitutes about 86% of splenic weight, connective tissue about 3%, and the white pulp some 4 to 11%.[5-7] The amount of red pulp appears to decrease slightly in the first year and then averages 75 to 83% of the spleen. The relative value of the white pulp may peak between ages 1 to 10 (up to 20%); it then falls to 6 to 9%. Secondary lymphatic nodules form over 29% of the splenic white pulp (age 1 year), and this value decreases dramatically to about 17% at ages 6 to 10, down to 1.5% at ages 21 to 30, and under 1% later in life.[5] Connective tissue, forming only 3.3%

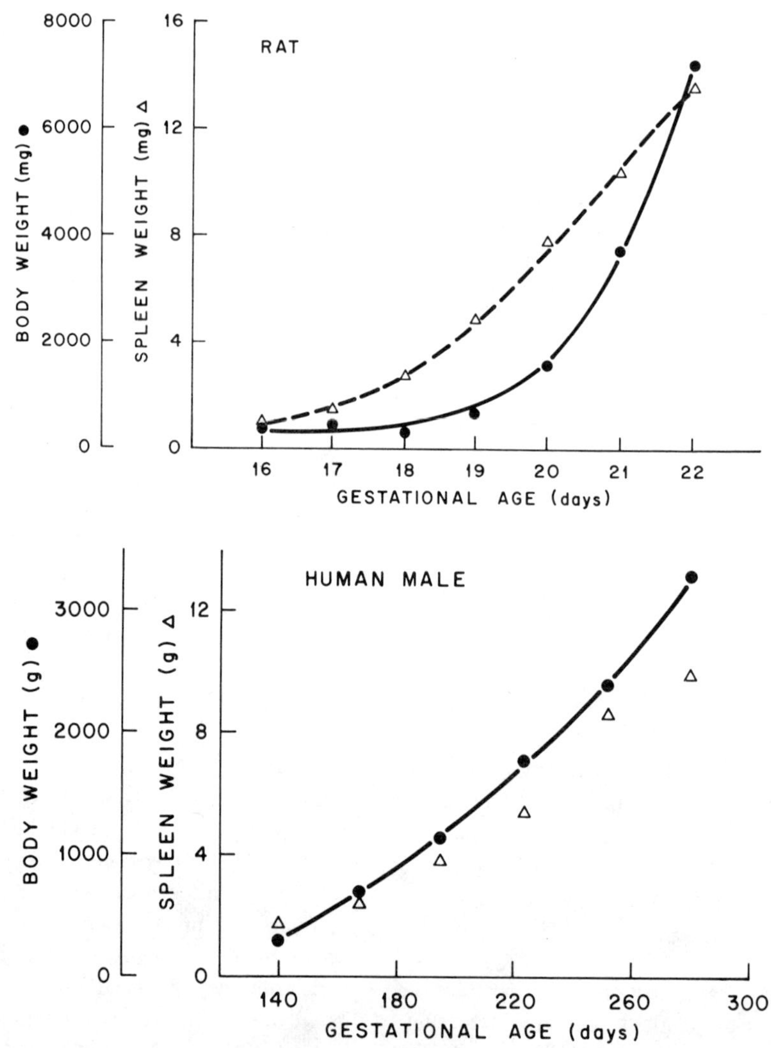

FIGURE 1. Comparison of the prenatal growth of body weight and spleen weight in the rat and the human male. Data were abstracted from References 1 and 3.

of splenic weight at birth, increases with age, up to 11% at age 50. Most of the studies of quantitative splenic histology thus far have been based on a small number of cases and have only infrequently been extended to specific diseases (principally by means of splenic biopsy). There are, however, data available on quanitative changes in the spleens of animals under various conditions.[8-10] Development of the spleen is a continuous process and even progresses following birth, when formation of the Malphigian bodies in the organ has been said to occur.

The specific chemical events occurring during prenatal development of the spleen are little understood. We can perhaps gain a few insights by examining postnatal and adult situations. The spleen can respond to multiple stimuli (and, at least in the frog, it is dependent on the season).[69] Cold and NaCl supplement can affect the spleen of mice.[65] How dehydration or overhydration affects the splenic water content[66] is uncertain. DNA synthesis in the spleen of immature rats is stimulated by giving growth hormone.[11] The spleen also responds to tumors in the host[67] and to foreign antigens.[68] Following administration of sheep erythrocytes to mice, increased metabolic turnover of DNA occurs in the splenic red pulp at times which coincide with maximal development of antibody-producing cells.[12] Splenic DNA of animals can be affected by medications such as 5-fluorouracil,[13] while the number of nucleated cells in the spleen of mice is reduced by hydrocortisone.[14] Using incorporation of 1-^{14}C-leucine into splenic homogenates as a measurement of protein synthesis, the spleens from 2½-month-old rats were noted to be more active (per gram of tissue) than those from rats aged 9 months.[15] Injecting killed *Bordetella pertussis* cells into mice produces splenomegaly, which is associated with increased uptake of radiolabeled phenylalanine[16] and, hence, presumably with increased protein synthesis within the organ. There are multiple enzymes within the spleen, and likely several with similar functions.[17] As yet, no scheme has been evolved for describing the development of enzyme pathways in the spleen. Indeed, splenic enzymes may react differently from those in the liver to various medications.[18]

Growth of the fetal spleen depends on the interaction of genetic factors and the immediate environment, including the availability of nutrients. Passage of materials from the maternal animal to the fetus and the fetal spleen has been documented for a number of substances. Colloidal thorium dioxide (Thorotrast®) is known to accumulate in reticuloendothelial tissue and to produce chronic radiation. When Thorotrast was injected into pregnant rabbits, its degradation products could be detected in the fetus.[19] Maternally administered radioiron (^{59}Fe) crosses the placenta, and the ratio of radioactivity (fetal spleen/entire fetus), increases nearly fivefold between weeks 13 and 22 of gestation in the human.[20] The potassium analogue radiocesium (^{137}Cs) passes from the mother to the fetal dog (and can be noted in the spleen)[21] and so do radiozinc (^{65}Zn)[22] and, of course, tritiated water.[23] Prenatal administration of the alkylating agent 1,4-butanediol dimethanesulfonate (busulfan®) can influence postnatal growth,[25] and detailed studies of the effects of medications on the fetal spleen are needed.

The genetic contribution can be seen in inborn errors of mucopolysaccharide metabolism.[24] Here the liver and spleen, approximately of normal size at birth, can become massively enlarged months to years later. There are few animal models of developmental errors or diseases of the spleen (although splenic tumors can occur).[31] An exception is congenital asplenia in mice.[26,27] In a compendium of animal models of disease, Cornelius does not specifically list the spleen.[28] In newborn lambs, congential splenic defects are unusual and most often consist of displacement, duplication, or rarely hypoplasia.[29] In swine, splenic anomalies are also apparently rare.[30] The spleen has been studied in intrauterine growth retardation in both the pig[33] and the rhesus monkey,[34] but separation of genetic, nutritional, and other factors still has to be accomplished.

SOME CONGENITAL DEFECTS OF THE SPLEEN

A number of splenic defects, apparently congenital, can be studied by means of spleen scans following birth. Among these disorders are the following:

1. Asplenia (Figures 2 and 3).
2. Some instances of functional hyposplenia.
3. Hypoplasia of spleen.
4. Ectopic spleen.

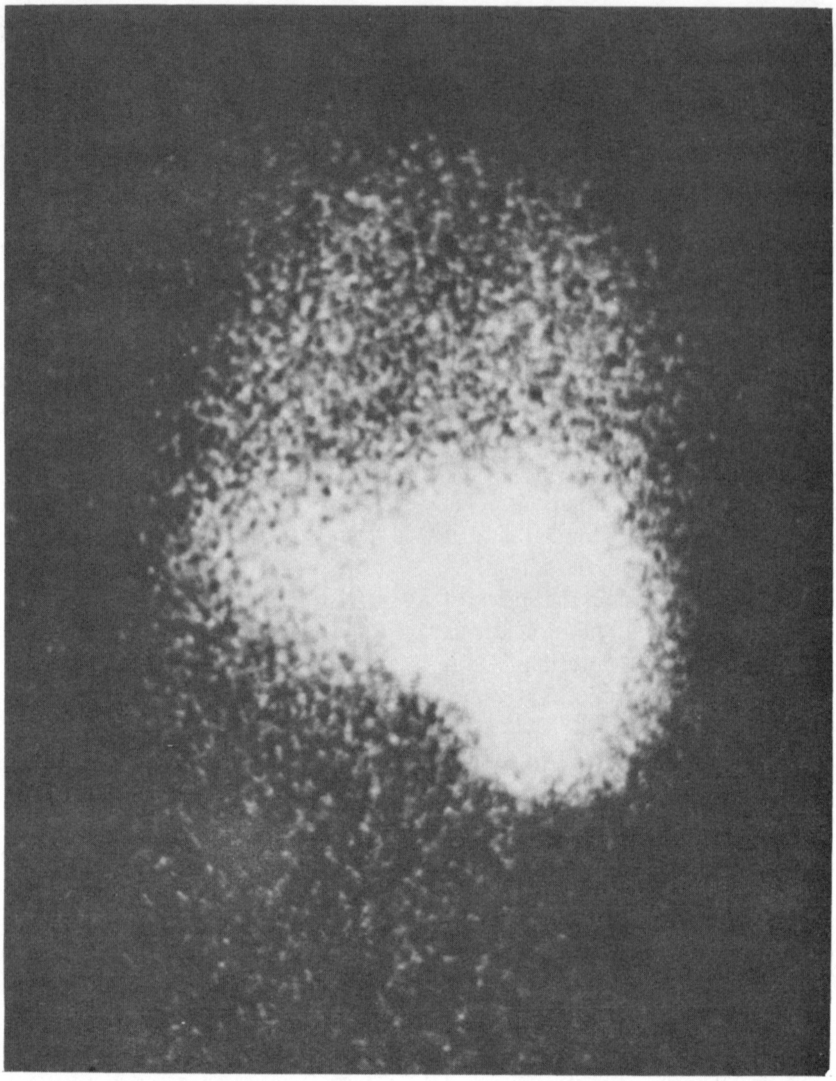

FIGURE 2. Posterior scintiphoto(^{99m}Tc-sulfur colloid) in a 19-month-old boy. No spleen can be seen. Multiple angulated views, as well as repeat studies months later, also failed to define a spleen. Case 70-644.

5. Accessory splenic tissue (discussed in Chapter 8).
6. Polysplenia.
7. Situs inversus (Figure 4).

In the congenital "asplenia syndrome" (Ivemark syndrome), visceral defects occur in association with agenesis of the spleen in many autopsied cases.[35-41, 106-108] Isomerism of the liver and lungs can occur (so-called "bilateral right-sidedness"), and often there is a gastric dextroposition and intestinal malrotation. Complex cardiovascular anomalies may be found (such as pulmonary venous connections, endocardial defects, transposition of vessels, and single ventricle).[42,43] The "bilateral right-sidedness" of the asplenia syndrome can be compared with "bilateral left-sidedness" in the polysplenia-syndrome.[44,56,57] The specific use of spleen scans and radionuclide venography in helping to establish the diagnosis has been reported.[107]

Normally, the spleen is functional at birth, at least in terms of its ability to accumulate a radioactive colloid such as ^{99m}Tc-sulfur colloid. Some infants with cardiac disorders and evidence of hypo- or asplenia (Howell-Jolly bodies) have a functional hyposplenic state.[48] This might be related to the cyanosis or to other functional problems. It resolves after a period of months. That is, all infants with cardiac disorders and

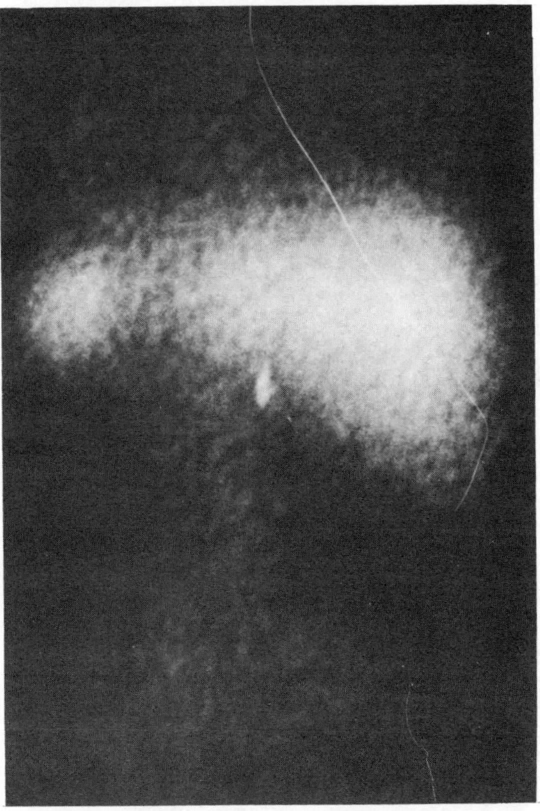

FIGURE 3. Posterior scintiphoto, obtained by use of ^{99m}Tc-sulfur colloid and a diverging collimator, in a 1½-year-old girl. The child had a hypoplastic left heart. The spleen, however, is well seen, and the cardiac disease is not part of the asplenia syndrome. Case 69-2255.

Howell-Jolly bodies do *not* have the "asplenia syndrome." In a later section, functional asplenia, due to sickle cell disease, will be discussed in detail. We have demonstrated that functional asplenia is not present at birth but starts to develop months later, coincident with the postnatal decrease in Hgb F and concomitant increase in Hgb S. A number of other diseases can also produce functional asplenia,[51] but these are believed not to be manifest at birth.

There appears to be a syndrome of congenital hypoplasia of the spleen. Three of five siblings in one family have been described in whom there was absent splenic function (^{198}Au colloid and ^{51}Cr-heat-denatured erythrocytes) and in whom bacteremia occurred.[47] Howell-Jolly bodies appeared in the peripheral blood, and there was failure to synthesize antibody to sheep erythrocytes given intravenously. One spleen weighed 1 g at age 10 months, (versus 11 g at birth expected, with progressive growth in the normal). The children were from a consanguinous marriage; an autosomal recessive inheritance was postulated. Other causes of small spleen are discussed in a later chapter.

Ectopic and accessory splenic tissue can occur. Indeed, about 15% of individuals have more than one spleen (and sometimes more than five spleens can occur). This topic is pursued in Chapter 8. Polysplenia was referred to above.

Abdominal situs inversus, with or without other changes, can occur. Kartagener's[53] recognition of situs inversus, bronchiectasis, and sinusitis has produced many studies on the nature of this triad. Thus far, no specific immunologic defects have been noted,[54] and some patients with the triad may have a normal life expectancy.[55] Techniques for the classification of visceral situs have been described[45,46,52] (Figure 4).

We will briefly comment on some additional congenital defects.

Accessory splenic tissue. The frequency of finding accessory spleens (5 to 10% of autopsy cases) has also been mentioned above. Clark and co-workers[71] have pointed out the angiographic findings of accessory spleens and mentioned that ^{99m}Tc-sulfur colloid scans may be helpful when the accessory tissue is over 2 cm in size. A presumed accessory spleen is shown in Figure 5.

Splenic cysts are discussed in a later chapter.

Gaucher's disease. The spleen can become massive in the course of Gaucher's disease. The removal of a spleen weighing 8,910 g from a 22-year-old woman with the disease has been reported.[72] A spleen scan, revealing an organ of enormous size in Gaucher's disease, is shown in Figure 6. The quantity and composition of the glycosphingolipids in the spleen in Gaucher's disease have been determined.[73] The use of splenic transplantation in an effort to cure the enzymatic defect in Gaucher's disease is dealt with in the section on transplantation. As bone changes can occur in Gaucher's disease,[74] these may be a role for either bone marrow or bone matrix scans.

Cystic fibrosis. Since abnormal liver function tests can occur in the course of cystic fibrosis, Feigelson and associates[75] performed ^{198}Au-colloid liver scans in 14 patients and used ^{99m}Tc-sulfur colloid in 12 others. Thirteen individuals showed hepatomegaly, and six had extrahepatic uptake of the radiogold. In two patients who died, autopsy findings revealed focal biliary cirrhosis. In most of the children we have

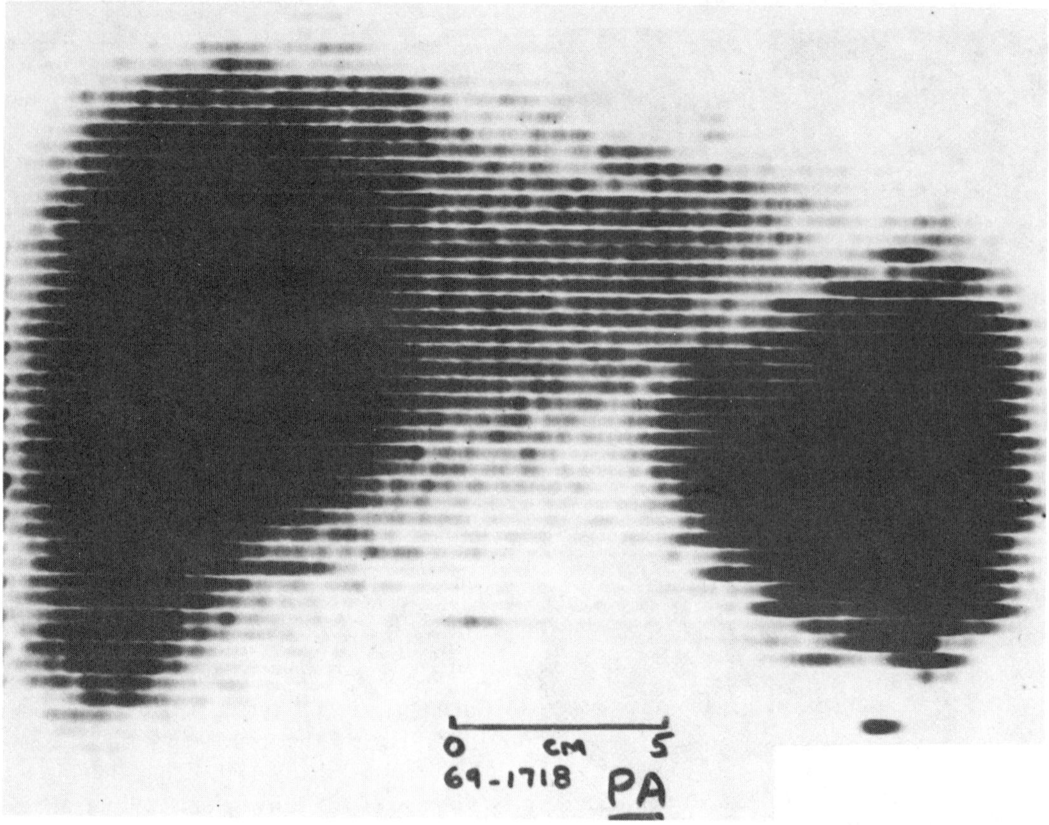

FIGURE 4. This is an oversaturated rectilinear posterior scan (^{99m}Tc-sulfur colloid) obtained in a 12-year-old girl. The spleen and liver are reversed from that normally seen in this view. This situs inversus, plus bronchiectasis and sinusitis, fit the description of Kartagener's syndrome. Case 69-1718.

seen because of cystic fibrosis, the liver-spleen scan has not been remarkable. Occasionally the spleen is enlarged (Figure 7), probably because of portal hypertension secondary to cirrhosis.

Alpha-1-antitrypsin deficiency. This genetically determined disorder is of particular interest to workers in nuclear medicine because of the accompanying pulmonary disease in most cases; the pulmonary problem is usually manifest as an involvement of the lung bases, which is readily seen on a perfusion lung scan. Sharp and associates[110] noted that alpha-1-antitrypsin deficiency was also associated with hepatic cirrhosis. Ryo and co-workers[111] reported abnormal liver scans in two patients with this disease. In one of the two cases, the liver rectilinear scan revealed massive splenomegaly; this was most likely due almost entirely to the hepatic cirrhosis.

Polycystic disease of the liver. There are apparently variants of this entity. However, in the forms associated with cysts of the liver, or of the liver and kidneys,[112–114] we have observed splenomegaly and a shift of radiocolloid to the spleen. Again, this may be secondary to the underlying hepatic disturbance and obstruction of the splenic outflow.

Hereditary splenomegaly with hypersplenism. Rao and associates[115] have described this apparently genetically determined condition. Radionuclide studies have yet to be reported.

Glycogen storage disease. In type I glycogen storage disease, the progressive accumulation of glycogen in the liver produces marked hepatomegaly. Folkman and co-workers[76] have reported that during hyperalimentation therapy, ^{99m}Tc-sulfur colloid liver scans revealed the liver to decrease in size by 30% at 2 weeks and 50% at 4 weeks. The children appeared to benefit from portacaval shunting. Part of the splenomegaly in glycogen storage disease may be secondary to the portal hypertension (Figure 8).

The spleen can also be enlarged in the course of the mucopolysaccharidoses and other congential disorders. In the lipidoses, the spleen can be a

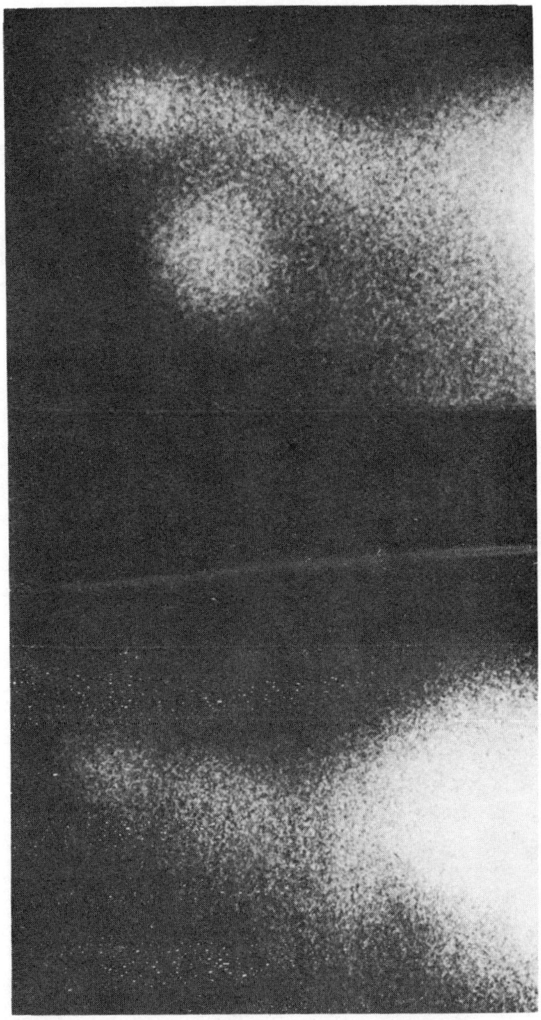

FIGURE 5. Posterior scintiphotos in a 10-year-old boy who had a prior splenectomy during an operation to remove an adrenal tumor. The top scintiphoto (^{99m}Tc-sulfur colloid) clearly shows functional splenic tissue. This was removed during a reexploration procedure, as shown in the bottom view. Case 73-147.

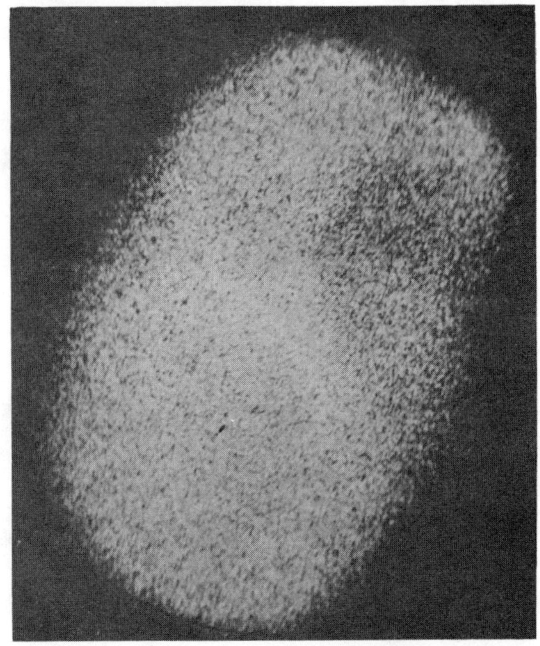

FIGURE 6. Anterior scintiphoto (^{99m}Tc-sulfur colloid) of the spleen, following surgical removal. The patient is a 15-year-old boy with Gaucher's disease. The spleen was 35 cm in length. Prior scans had shown a marked shift of radiocolloid to the spleen, with a spleen to liver ratio (from the anterior) of 1.5 to 1. Observe the large superior defect and the uneven uptake. Case 71-2279.

Adults		Children	
Brain	1.02 N.S.	Brain	0.99 N.S.
Spleen	1.10 N.S.	Spleen	1.27
Kidneys	1.25	Kidneys	1.24
Heart	1.40	Heart	1.33
Pancreas	1.45	Pancreas	1.23
Liver	1.45	Liver	1.29

N.S. = Not significantly different from controls in the original data. Other results were significant at $p < 0.05$.

principal site of lipid deposition. One has to distinguish between primary deposition of an abnormal metabolite in the spleen (the so-called "garbage can" function) and the splenic defect which occurs due to hepatic obstruction and portal hypertension. The spleen may be increasingly employed in determining the presence of various metabolites and enzymes in tissues.[77]

SPLEEN GROWTH

In cases of human obesity, both the number and the size of adipose cells are increased. Naeye and Roode[78] studied the weights of organs in obese adults and obese children and compared them with controls. We have recalculated their data to give the ratio of organ weight in the obese/organ weight in controls. In this series then, obese children had significantly added weight to the spleen, while adults did not. Interestingly, DeLand and Tonkin[109] performed liver-spleen scans in massively obese patients who had jejuno-ileal bypass surgery. In some of the patients there was nearly complete lack of hepatic uptake of the radiocolloid (possibly due to fatty infiltration or metabolic changes), while radiocolloid accumulated in the spleen.

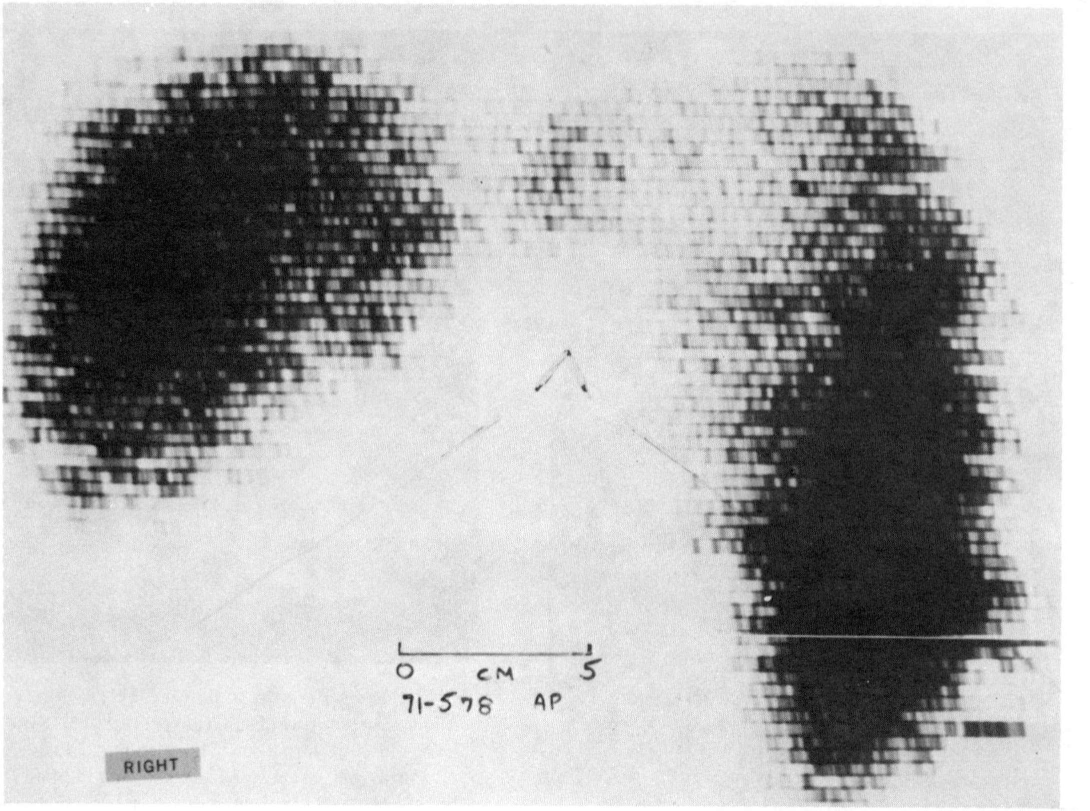

FIGURE 7. Anterior rectilinear scan (^{99m}Tc-sulfur colloid) in an 11-year-old boy with cystic fibrosis. Pancytopenia in this case may have been due to hypersplenism. The splenomegaly may have followed from portal hypertension. Case 71-578.

Some degree of organ enlargement can be noted in certain infants born of diabetic mothers. Frank visceromegaly has been reported in the syndromes associated with fetal hypoglycemia.[79,80] In one of the reports, the spleen was palpable in at least a single case, and the livers were enlarged.[79] We are not aware of studies of splenic function carried out in such infants.

For many animal species, the weight of the spleen can be related to the weight of the body by a power law or allometric relationship[81,82]

$$S = C\,B^{q} \tag{4}$$

or

$$\log S = q \log B + \log C \tag{5}$$

where S is the weight of the spleen, B is the weight of the body, q is the allometeric exponent, and C is the allometric coefficient. The exponent is about 1.02 for mammals. This means that spleen weight is nearly a linear function of body weight in many mammals. Using compiled autopsy data, we showed that the allometric relationship provided a reasonable description of splenic weight in terms of body weight for the human male (age 0 to 30 years).[82] The relationship was

$$S = (3.5 \times 10^{-3})\,B^{0.97} \tag{6}$$

where the weights are in grams.

An interesting concept is to compare the actual weight of the spleen with that predicted on the basis of the allometric equation.[82] We have defined the weight excess (E) as

$$E = A - CB^{q} \tag{7}$$

where A is the actual weight of the organ, and CB^{q} is the allometric expression for splenic weight in terms of body weight. A spleen larger than expected has a positive weight excess, while one smaller than expected has a negative weight excess. Using this expression and literature data on organ changes during estradiol-induced wasting in

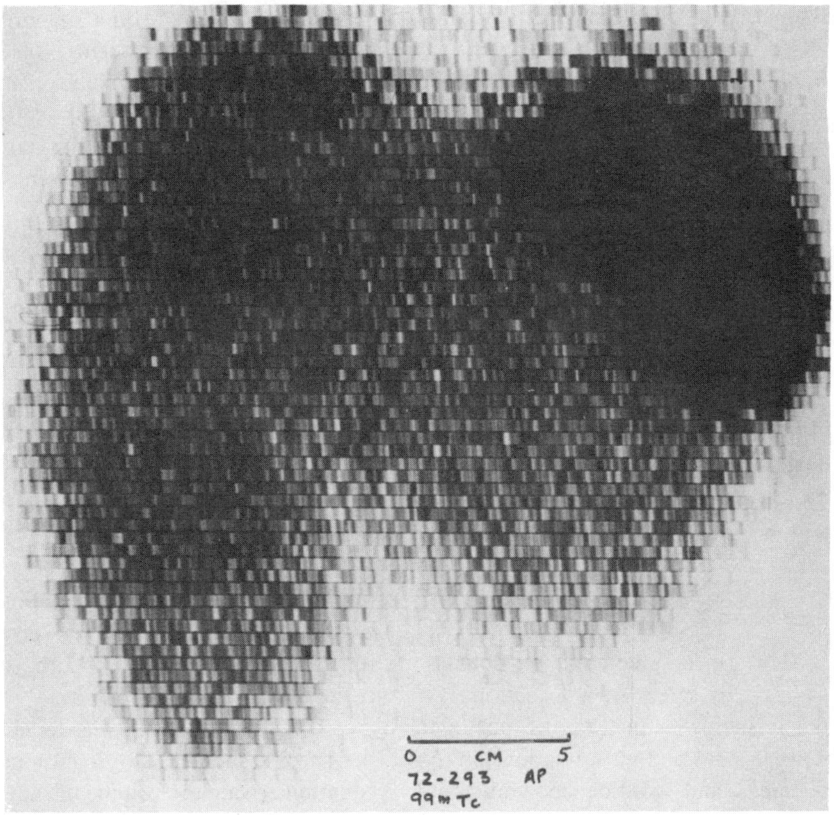

FIGURE 8. Anterior rectilinear scan (^{99m}Tc-sulfur colloid) in a 10-year-old boy with glycogen storage disease. The outline of a slightly enlarged spleen can be noted reinforcing the scan of the left lobe of the liver. Case 72-293.

mice,[83] we showed that there was relatively little change in the size of the spleen. Another approach is to determine the differential growth rate.[82] This is defined by:

$$\text{Differential growth rate} = \frac{1}{W} \cdot \frac{\Delta W}{\Delta t} \qquad (8)$$

where W is the weight of the spleen, and $\Delta W/\Delta t$ is the weight change per unit time. Observe that in Equation 8 the weight units cancel out, and the growth rate is given in terms of 1/time. Between 3 and 5 weeks of age, in mice the spleen grew at a rate of 0.99/week. For estrogen-treated mice, this was slowed to 0.48/week. Expressed in such terms, splenic changes closely mimicked changes in the liver.[82]

SPLEEN SCAN SIZE DURING GROWTH

The growth of the spleen is, of course, accompanied by an enlarging image as far as spleen scans are concerned. Hence, to determine whether a spleen is of normal size, it is imperative to know the age and physical measurements of the child. This topic has still to be fully quantified. In 45 cases[84] (ages 0 to 18.9 years), splenic length in cm (L) in terms of age (A, in years) was described;

$$L = 5.7 + 0.31\ A. \qquad (9)$$

While the correlation coefficient was good (σ = 0.87), the equation tended to overestimate splenic length at birth. From the data of Seltzer and co-workers,[87] we can write for the weight of the spleen (in grams), as a function of age:

$$W = 24 + 7\ A. \qquad (10)$$

If the two populations are comparable, we can combine Equations 9 and 10 to yield:

$$W = 22.6\ L - 104. \qquad (11)$$

This approximately described splenic weight in

children as a function of the scan length of the organ.

In 23 children the relationship between the scan length of the spleen and body height in cm (H) was

$$L = 2.3 + 0.05\ H. \quad (12)$$

At birth (H = 50 cm), the predicted spleen length is 4.8 cm (which is correct). When expressed in terms of body weight (W, in kg), the length of the spleen is described by a straight line, up to about 30 kg body weight, and then by a curvilinear portion that appears to approach an asymptote (and such a behavior follows that of the liver).[88] For birth to 30 kg body weight, in 16 children, the splenic length on scan was given by:

$$L = 4 + 0.22\ W. \quad (13)$$

At birth (W = 3.5 kg), the prediction is a splenic length of 4.8 cm; this agrees with Equation 12. Further work, including estimation of possible differences between boys and girls, relationship to body surface area, and confidence limits, is needed.

"NORMAL" SPLEEN SIZE

There have been many discussions of the size of normal spleen.[85,86] DeLand has pointed out that in adults, the spleen of the male is usually larger than that of the female.[86] Maximum spleen weight is reached at about ages 20 to 29, remains relatively constant between 30 and 59, and then decreases. Palpation and radiography have both been utilized to estimate splenic enlargement.[32] When carefully carried out and when multiple views are employed, spleen scanning can give definitive data as to the size of the functional spleen. Trying to determine the range of normality of the scan size of the spleen is another problem. Sigel and co-workers[90] measured the posterior spleen length during radiocolloid liver imaging. The values for spleen length revealed a normal distribution in 232 of the 294 cases, with a mean value of 10.7 ± 1.7 cm. This agrees with values reported by Larson and associates[91] (26 volunteers, 10. ± 1.5cm). Sigel[90] concluded that spleen sizes above 14 cm (in adults) represented an enlarged organ. From the data of Larson and co-workers,[91] the value of 13 cm can be considered the upper limit of normal. In the adult patients we have been seeing, spleen lengths above 13 cm are viewed as likely enlarged. The introduction of ultrasound for determining spleen size[99] may offer an additional technique for screening large numbers of patients.

ESTIMATION OF SPLENIC WEIGHT FROM SCANS

A voluminous literature has developed around the relationship of roentgenographic and radiographic image sizes to splenic weight. It is not our intent to review all the reports but rather to utilize a few references to emphasize certain key points. In essence, there have been three approaches to the problem.

1. Use of linear equations has inherent simplicity (spleen weight is given as a linear function of scan length, width, surface area, or perimeter).
2. The spleen is considered to conform to the specific model, and dimensions are utilized in equations giving the volume of that model.
3. An exponential relationship is considered to exist between the scan dimensions and the volume or weight of the spleen.

We will discuss each of these approaches in turn. The use of linear equations, employing measurements made on spleen scans (length, width, surface area, or perimeter), is certainly the simplest. There is, however, a severe reservation. The linear equations are usually of the form:

$$W = a \cdot L + b. \quad (14)$$

Here splenic weight (W) is given in terms of scan length (L) and the "constants" a and b. The intercept is not zero. That is, the rigorous prediction would be that at a length equal to zero, the spleen would have weight b. This is certainly unappealing and points out that such equations are really only defined between certain lengths (and certainly do not extend to quite small spleens). Larson and co-workers[91] noted that in 16 spleen scans, with weights confirmed at autopsy or surgery, the posterior length was related to the weight by:

$$W = 71\ L - 537. \quad (15)$$

The intercept is quite a large number. The equation predicts a zero weight for a spleen 7.6 cm in length (and negative weights for still smaller spleens). Whitley and co-workers[92] also noted a good correlation between splenic length (on anteroposterior roentgenograms) and splenic weight. These workers gave as the equation:

$$W = 65\ L - 397. \tag{16}$$

This equation does not work (no weight or negative weight) for spleens with a length of 6.1 cm or smaller. Hence, while linear equations describing splenic weight in terms of dimensions are easy to apply, their limits must be carefully remembered. Equations 15 and 16 give the same answer for splenic weight for a spleen 23 cm in length. At 10 cm length, there is significant disagreement; Equation 15 predicts 173 g, while Equation 16 yields a value of 253 g (which is 46% greater).

The second approach is to assume that the spleen conforms to some sort of model, which can be quantified. For example, Samuels[93] has likened the spleen to a hemiellipsoid. The formula for the weight of such a figure (assuming the density is equal to 1) is

$$W = \frac{2}{3}\ \pi\ a.b.c \tag{17}$$

where a, b, and c are the axes. With rotational symmetry, a = b = width (w), c = height/2 or h/2. Thus,

$$W = \frac{\pi}{3}\ w^2 h \tag{18}$$

or

$$W = 1.047\ w^2 h \tag{19}$$

Samuels had only two cases in which the weight predicted by the formula could be compared with splenic weights at surgery or autopsy. The predictions were inaccurate by 4% in one case and by 13% in the other. Retrospectively applying this formula, to cases we have seen, has not yielded close agreement. It is likely that variations in splenic shape make approximation by an ellipsoid of revolution quite difficult.

Rollo and DeLand[94] considered the spleen to be an ellipsoid segment with thickness h and elliptical semimajor and semiminor axes equal to a and b (posterior and left lateral views are both needed). The weight (if the density was 1) was then given by:

$$W = \frac{\pi}{6}\ (h^3 + 3\ h.a.b). \tag{20}$$

These workers found that using $\pi/7$ gave a closer approximation to the true weight than $\pi/6$. The working equation was thus:

$$W = \frac{\pi}{7}\ (h^3 + 3\ h.a.b). \tag{21}$$

The technique employs both lateral and posterior views of the spleen and hence uses more information than a single view alone. A one view method (posterior) can be used, assuming a = b. Then,

$$W = \frac{\pi}{7}\ (h^3 + 3\ h.a^2). \tag{22}$$

The mean error for the two methods was stated to be ±7.1 and ±6.8% (maximum error 12.8%). The technique has not been widely pursued, and its eventual usefulness is presently unknown.

Whitley and co-workers[92] noted the relationship between the product (P) of splenic length and width and spleen weight.

$$W = 7.73\ P - 122 \tag{23}$$

Mathematically, the equation holds only for products of splenic length and width over 15.8 cm^2.

The third approach is to relate splenic weight to an exponential function of splenic scan measurements. The form at the equation is

$$W = c.\ M^P \tag{24}$$

where M is the measurement and c and P are "constants." There are a few points in favor of such an approach.

1. In some cases, the technique can be dimensionally correct.
2. There is a close similarity between this equation and that of the allometric equation.
3. This equation avoids the major difficulty of the linear equations. That is, when the length or area measurement is zero, the predicted weight is close to zero.

The dimensional relationship between a planar area (A) and a volume (V) is[95]

$$V = c.\ A^{3/2}. \tag{25}$$

This can be used to construct, from the data of Holzbach and co-workers[96] on the lateral scan surface area of the spleen, the formula:

$$W = 0.26\ A^{3/2} \tag{26}$$

or

$$\log W = 1.5 \log A - 0.59 \tag{27}$$

It will be recalled that Whitley and associates[92] had used a linear formula to describe spleen weight from the product (P) of (length $\times$ width) on radiographs. Their data can also be described by:

$$W = 0.7\ P^{3/2}. \tag{28}$$

The maximum difference between this equation and that of Whitley et al.[92] was 7.6% in the range of P from 30 to 100 cm^2. Fischer has also used such an equation (in the form $V = 0.3\ A^{3/2}$) to relate the splenic scan area to organ volume.[100] Blendis, Williams, and Kreel[97] also employed a power function to describe the weight of the spleen in terms of the radiographic area. However, they limited their calculations to grossly enlarged spleens.

CORRECTION OF SPLEEN SCAN IMAGES

In correlating splenic weight with scans, it is important to avoid errors due to:

1. Magnification.
2. Rotation.

Rollo and DeLand[94] have discussed corrections between the posterior and left lateral projections by comparison of the length of the spleen on each view. Blendis and co-workers[97] noted that rotation of the spleen produces little change on the area of the spleen, through an angle of 30°. At 45° from the vertical axis, the apparent surface area can be reduced by about 14%. The great mobility of the spleen, discussed previously, must be recalled.

CORRELATIONS

Blendis and co-workers[97] reported a correlation between the spleen area on radiographs and the body surface area. However, Larson et al.[91] noted no correlation between spleen size and the surface area of the body. Fischer and Wolf[98] put forth an index of spleen size in which the lateral scan surface area/body surface area equaled 3.88×10^{-3} to 4.5×10^{-3}. However, the lateral spleen scan area can vary by at least two fold (Holzbach et al.[96] gave values of 35 cm^2 to 85 cm^2). The data of DeLand[86] suggest a fairly linear relationship between spleen weight and body surface area for the population aged 30 to 59 years.

REFERENCES

1. **Schulz, D. M., Giordano, D. A., and Schulz, D. H.,** Weights of organs of fetuses and infants, *Arch. Pathol.,* 74, 244, 1962.
2. **Gruenwald, P. and Minh, H. H.,** Evaluation of body and organ weights in perinatal pathology. I. Normal standards derived from autopsies, *Am. J. Clin. Pathol.,* 34, 247, 1960.
3. **Sikov, M. R. and Thomas, J. M.,** Prenatal growth of the rat, *Growth,* 34, 1, 1970.
4. **Roessle, R. and Roulet, F.,** Mass und Zahl in der Pathologie, in *Pathologie und Klinik in Einzeldarstellungen,* Vol. 5, Schoff, L. A. et al., Eds., Springer-Verlag, Berlin, 1932, 144.
5. **Hellman, T.,** Die Altersanatomie der Menschlichen Milz, *Z. Menschliche. Verebungs Konstitutionslehre,* 12, 270, 1926.
6. **Hwang, J. M. S., Lippincott, S. W., and Krumbhaar, E. B.,** The amount of splenic lymphatic tissue at different ages, *Am. J. Pathol.,* 14, 809, 1938.
7. **Naeye, R. L.,** New observations in erythroblastosis fetalis, *JAMA,* 200, 281, 1967.
8. **Beran, M. and Tribukait, B.,** The quantitative bone marrow and spleen composition in male NMRI and CBA mice, *Acta Haematol.,* 45, 55, 1971.
9. **Nagy, Z. A. and Feher, G.,** Histometric analysis of the chicken spleen during primary immune response to soluble bovine serum albumin. I. Relationship between quantitative changes of thymus-type and bursa-type splenic lymphocytes and splenomegaly, *Z. Immun. Forsch.,* 143, 223, 1972.
10. **Feher, G. and Nagy, Z. A.,** Histometric analysis of the chicken spleen during primary immune response to soluble bovine serum albumin. II. Mathematical-histometric method for the assessment of quantitative changes of thymus-type and bursa-type lymphocytes, *Z. Immun. Forsch.,* 143, 245, 1972.
11. **Fast, D. K., Garland, M., Thomson, M., and Richards, J. F.,** The effect of growth hormone on DNA synthesis in rat spleen, *Exp. Cell Res.,* 62, 441, 1970.
12. **Pelc, S. R., Harris, G., and Caldwell, I.,** The relationship between antibody formation and deoxyribonucleic acid (DNA) synthesis in mouse spleen during primary and secondary response to sheep erythrocytes (SRC), *Immunology,* 23, 183, 1972.
13. **Suciu, D. and Uray, Z.,** In vivo fragmentation of rat spleen DNA after administration of 5-fluorouracil, *Stud. Biophys.,* 33, 67, 1972.
14. **Vischer, T. L.,** Effect of hydrocortisone on the reactivity of thymus and spleen cells of mice to in vitro stimulation, *Immunology,* 23, 777, 1972.
15. **Kselikova, M.,** Incorporation of 1-^{14}C-leucine into splenic and liver tissue of rats of different age, *Physiol. Bohemoslov.,* 20, 291, 1971.
16. **Finger, H. and Stocker, E.,** Increased protein synthesis of spleen cells after injection of Bordetella pertussis into mice, *Beitr. Pathol.,* 146, 381, 1972.
17. **Verpoorte, J. A.,** Purification of two β-N-acetyl-D-glucosaminidases from beef spleen, *J. Biol. Chem.,* 247, 4787, 1972.
18. **Japundzic, I., Mimic-Oka, J., Japundzic, M., and Szabo, S.,** Influence of spironolactone and dexamethasone on phosphoprotein phosphatase in the rat liver, kidney and spleen, *Eur. J. Biochem.,* 28, 475, 1972.
19. **Einck-Russ Kamp, P., Rajewsky, B., and Stahlhofen, W.,** Cross-placental passage of radium-228 and its daughters after intravenous injection of colloidal thorium dioxide (thorotrast) into rabbits, in *Radiation Biology of the Fetal and Juvenile Mammal,* Sikov, M. R. and Mahlum, D. D., Eds., USAEC CONF-690501, AEC Symp. Ser. #17, 1969, 121.
20. **Dyer, N. C. and Brill, A. B.,** Fetal radiation dose from maternally administered ^{59}Fe and ^{131}I, in *Radiation Biology of the Fetal and Juvenile Mammal,* Sikov, M. R. and Mahlum, D. D., Eds., USAEC CONF-690501, AEC Symp. Ser. #17, 1969, 73.
21. **Tyler, S. A., Kretz, N. D., and Norris, W. P.,** Dependence of ^{137}Cs retention on age in the fetal and juvenile beagle dog, in *Radiation Biology of the Fetal and Juvenile Mammal,* Sikov, M. R. and Mahlum, D. D., Ed., USAEC CONF-690501, AEC Symp. Ser. #17, 1969, 191.
22. **Erdman, H. E., Mahlum, D. D., and Sikov, M. R.,** Age-related differences in zinc metabolism in the rat, in *Radiation Biology of the Fetal and Juvenile Mammal,* Sikov, M. R. and Mahlum, D. D., Eds., USAEC CONF-690501, AEC Symp. Ser. #17, 1969, 207.
23. **Cahill, D. F. and Yuile, C. L.,** Some effects of tritiated water on mammalian fetal development, in *Radiation Biology of the Fetal and Juvenile Mammal,* Sikov, M. R. and Mahlum, D. D., Eds., USAEC CONF-690501, AEC Symp. Ser. #17, 1969, 283.
24. **Neufeld, E. F. and Fratantoni, J. C.,** Inborn errors of polysaccharide metabolism, *Science,* 169, 141, 1970.
25. **Pinto-Machado, J.,** Influence of prenatal administration of busulfan on the postnatal development of mice. Production of a syndrome including hypoplasia of the thymus, *Teratology,* 3, 363, 1970.
26. **Searle, A. G.,** Hereditary absence of spleen in the mouse, *Nature,* 184, 1419, 1959.
27. **Lozzio, B. B.** Hematopoiesis in congenitally asplenic mice, *Am. J. Physiol.,* 222, 290, 1972.
28. **Cornelius, C. E.,** Animal models: a neglected medical resource, *N. Engl. J. Med.,* 281, 934, 1969.
29. **Dennis, S. M.,** Congenital splenic defects in newborn lambs, *Cornell Vet.* 62, 473, 1972.

30. **Selby, L. A., Hopps, H. C., and Edmonds, L. D.**, Comparative aspects of congenital malformations in man and swine, *J. Am. Vet. Med. Assoc.*, 159, 1485, 1971.
31. **Sanders, C. H. and Langham, R. F.**, Myelolipoma of the spleen in a cat, *J. Am. Vet. Med. Assoc.*, 160, 1101, 1972.
32. **Tanimura, T., Nelson, T., Hollingsworth, R. R., and Shepard, T. H.**, Weight standards for organs from early human fetuses, *Anat. Rec.*, 171, 227, 1971.
33. **Widdowson, E. M.**, Intra-uterine growth retardation in the pig. I., *Biol. Neonate*, 19, 329, 1971.
34. **Myers, R. E., Hill, D. E., Holt, A. B., Scott, R. E., Mellits, E. D., and Cheek, D. B.**, Fetal growth retardation produced by experimental placental insufficiency in the rhesus monkey. I., *Biol. Neonate*, 18, 379, 1971.
35. **Ivemark, B. I.**, Implications of agenesis of spleen on pathogenesis of conotruncus anomalies in childhood; analysis of heart malformations in splenic agenesis syndrome, with 14 new cases, *Acta Paediatr.*, 44(Suppl. 104), 1, 1955.
36. **Polhemus, D. W. and Schafer, W. B.**, Congenital absence of the spleen: syndrome with atrioventricularis and situs inversus, *Pediatrics*, 9, 696, 1952.
37. **Freedom, R. M.**, The asplenia syndrome: a review of significant extracardiac structural abnormalities in 29 necropsied patients, *J. Pediatr.*, 81, 1130, 1972.
38. **Holler, J. M., Amplatz, K., and Wolfson, J.**, Malrotation of the bowel in patients with congenital heart disease associated with splenic anomalies, *Radiology*, 99, 393, 1971.
39. **Schumacher, G., Schenck, W., Schlosser, V., Wehinger, H., Gunkel, J., and Schuchmann, L.**, Diagnostic and therapeutic problems in Ivemark's syndrome (asplenia-syndrome), *Mschr. Kinderheilkd.*, 120, 179, 1972.
40. **Esterly, J. R. and Oppenheimer, E. H.**, Lymphangiectasis and other pulmonary lesions in the asplenia syndrome, *Arch. Pathol.*, 90, 553, 1970.
41. **Silver, W., Steier, M., and Chandra, M.**, Asplenia syndrome with congenital heart disease and tetrology of fallout in siblings, *Am. J. Cardiol.*, 30, 91, 1972.
42. **Putschar, W. G. J. and Manion, W. C.**, Congenital absence of the spleen and associated anomalies, *Am. J. Clin. Pathol.*, 26, 429, 1956.
43. **Van Mierop, L. H. S. and Wiglesworth, F. W.**, Isomerism of the cardiac atria in asplenia syndrome, *Lab. Invest.*, 11, 1303, 1962.
44. **Moller, J. H., Nakib, A., Anderson, R. C., and Edwards, J. E.**, Congenital cardiac disease associated with polysplenia: a developmental complex of bilateral "left-sidedness," *Circulation*, 36, 789, 1967.
45. **Van Mierop, L. H. S., Eisen, S., and Schiebler, G. L.**, The radiographic appearance of the tracheobronchial tree as an indicator of visceral situs, *Am. J. Cardiol.*, 26, 432, 1970.
46. **de La Cruz, M. V. and Nadal-Ginard, B.**, Rules for the diagnosis of visceral situs, truncoconal morphologies, and ventricular inversions, *Am. Heart J.*, 84, 19, 1972.
47. **Kevy, S. V., Tefft, M., Vawter, G. F., and Rosen, F. S.**, Hereditary splenic hypoplasia, *Pediatrics*, 42, 752, 1968.
48. **Pearson, H. A., Schiebler, G. L., and Spencer, R. P.**, Functional hyposplenia in cyanotic congenital heart disease, *Pediatrics*, 48, 277, 1971.
49. **Pearson, H. A., Spencer, R. P., and Cornelius, E. A.**, Functional asplenia in sickle cell anemia, *N. Engl. J. Med.*, 281, 923, 1969.
50. **Pearson, H. A., Cornelius, E. A., Schwartz, A., Zelson, J. R., Wolfson, S. L., and Spencer, R. P.**, Transfusion reversible functional asplenia in young children with sickle cell anemia, *N. Engl. J. Med.*, 283, 334, 1970.
51. **Spencer, R. P., Pearson, H. A., and Binder, H. J.**, Identification of cases of "acquired" functional asplenia, *J. Nucl. Med.*, 11, 763, 1970.
52. **Landing, B. H., Lawrence, T. Y. K., Payne, V. C., Jr., and Wells, T. R.**, Bronchial anatomy in syndromes with abnormal visceral situs, abnormal spleen and congenital heart disease, *Am. J. Cardiol.*, 28, 456, 1971.
53. **Kartagener, M.**, Zur Pathogenese der Bronchiektasien bei Situs Viscerum inversus, *Beitr. Z. Klin. Erforsch. Tuberk.*, 83, 489, 1933.
54. **Sharma, O. P.**, Kartagener's syndrome: immunologic studies, *N. Y. State J. Med.*, 72, 1057, 1972.
55. **Miller, R. D. and Divertie, M. B.**, Kartagener's syndrome, *Chest*, 62, 130, 1972.
56. **Rodin, A. E., Sloane, J. A., and Nghiem, Q. X.**, Polysplenia with severe congenital heart disease and Howell-Jolly bodies, *Am. J. Clin. Pathol.*, 58, 127, 1972.
57. **Vaughan, T. J., Hawkins, I. F., Jr., and Elliott, L. P.**, Diagnosis of polysplenia syndrome, *Radiology*, 101, 511, 1971.
58. **Djaldetti, M., Bessler, H., and Rifkind, R. A.**, Hematopoiesis in the embryonic mouse spleen: an electron microscopic study, *Blood*, 39, 826, 1972.
59. **Aggio, M. C., Giusto, N., Bruzzo, M. T., and Montano, M.**, The participation of spleen and bone marrow in mice erythropoiesis as a function of age, *Acta Physiol. Lat. Am.*, 22, 1, 1972.
60. **Bach, J. F. and Dardenne, M.**, Antigen recognition by T lymphocytes. II. Similar effects of azathioprine, antilymphocyte serum, and anti-theta serum on rosette-forming lymphocytes in normal and neonatally thymectomized mice, *Cell. Immunol.*, 3, 11, 1972.
61. **Goldstein, A. L., Guha, A., Latz, M. M., Hardy, M. A., and White, A.**, Purification and biological activity of thymosin, a hormone of the thymus gland, *Proc. Natl. Acad. Sci.*, 69, 1800, 1972.
62. **Kyriazis, A. A. and Esterly, J. R.**, Fetal and neonatal development of lymphoid tissues, *Arch. Pathol.*, 91, 444, 1971.

63. **Schumacher, G. H., Fanghanel, J., and Schultz, E.,** Quantitative Untersuchungen uber das postnatale Wachstum von Rattus norvegicus Berkenhout unter normalen und statisch veranderten Bedingungen.III. Abdominalorgane, *Acta Anat.,* 80, 33, 1971.
64. **Waxler, G. L. and Dress, D. T.,** Comparison of body weights, organ weights and histological features of selected organs of gnotobiotic, conventional and isolator-reared contaminated pigs, *Can. J. Comp. Med.,* 36, 265, 1972.
65. **Mariano, M. and Gomes, M. C. G.,** Influence of exposure to cold and added sodium chloride ingestion on body weight and weights of spleen and kidneys in male mice, *Am. J. Vet. Res.,* 32, 665, 1971.
66. **Jelenko, C., Anderson, A. P. Scott, T. H., Jr., and Wheeler, M. L.,** Organ weights and water composition of the New Zealand albino rabbit (Oryctolagus cuniculus), *Am. J. Vet. Res.,* 32, 1637, 1971.
67. **Edwards, A. J., Sumner, M. R., Rowland, G. F., and Hurd, C. M.,** Changes in lymphoreticular tissues during growth of a murine adenocarcinoma. I. Histology and weight of lymph nodes, spleen and thymus, *J. Natl. Cancer Inst.,* 47, 301, 1971.
68. **Nagy, Z. A. and Feher, G.,** Histometric analysis of the chicken spleen during primary immune response to soluble bovine serum albumin. III. Effect of antigen dose on proliferation of immunologically competent cells using optimal and large quantities of antigen, *Zeit. Immunitaetsforsch.,* 143, 323, 1972.
69. **Meints, R. H. and Carver, F. J.,** Erythropoietic activity in Rana pipiens – the influence of nutrition and season on spleen and peripheral blood activities, *Comp. Biochem. Physiol.,* 42A, 511, 1972.
70. **Bosing-Schneider, R. and Kindred, B.,** Stimulation of "nude" spleen cells in vitro under the influence of thymus lymphocytes, *Cell. Immunol.,* 5, 593, 1972.
71. **Clark, R. E., Korobkin, M., and Palubinskas, A. J.,** Angiography of accessory spleens, *Radiology,* 102, 41, 1972.
72. **Appel, M. F. and Markowitz, A. M.,** Massive splenomegaly in Gaucher's disease, *JAMA,* 217, 343, 1971.
73. **Kuske, T. T. and Rosenberg, A.,** Quantity and fatty acyl composition of glycosphingolipids of Gaucher spleen, *J. Lab. Clin. Med.,* 80, 523, 1972.
74. **Noyes, F. R. and Smith, W. S.,** Bone crises and chronic osteomyelitis in Gaucher's disease, *Clin. Orthoped.,* 79, 132, 1971.
75. **Feigelson, J., Pecau, Y., and Perez, R.,** Liver scanning and liver function in cystic fibrosis, *Acta Pediatr. Scand.,* 61, 337, 1972.
76. **Folkman, J., Philippart, A., Tze, W. J., and Crigler, J., Jr.,** Protacaval shunt for glycogen storage disease: value of prolonged intravenous hyperalimentation before surgery, *Surgery,* 72, 306, 1972.
77. **Bensaude, I., Philippart, M., and Hildebrand, J.,** Alpha-glycosidic configuration in ceramide trihexoside synthesized by rat spleen homogenate, *Biochem. Med.,* 6, 522, 1972.
78. **Naeye, R. L. and Roode, P.,** The sizes and numbers of cells in visceral organs in human obesity, *Am. J. Clin. Pathol.,* 54, 251, 1970.
79. **Combs, J. T. Grunt, J. A., and Brandt, I. K.,** New syndrome of neonatal hypoglycemia; association with visceromegaly macroglossia, microcephally and abnormal umbilicus, *N. Engl. J. Med.,* 215, 236, 1966.
80. **Sotelo-Avila, C. and Singer, D. B.,** Syndrome of hyperplastic fetal visceromegaly and neonatal hypoglycemia (Beckwith's Syndrome): a report of seven cases, *Pediatrics,* 46, 240, 1970.
81. **Stahl, W. R.,** Organ weights in primates and other mammals, *Science,* 150, 1039, 1965.
82. **Spencer, R. P. and Chaudhuri, T. K.,** Quantitative estimates of changes in splenic size during life, *Yale J. Biol. Med.,* 41, 333, 1969.
83. **Reilly, R., Thompson, J., Brelski, R., and Severson, C.,** Estradiol induced wasting syndrome in neonatal mice, *J. Immunol.,* 98, 321, 1967.
84. **Spencer, R. P., Pearson, H. A., and Lange, R. C.,** Human spleen: scan studies on growth and response to medications, *J. Nucl. Med.,* 12, 466, 1971.
85. **Krumbhaar, E. B. and Lippincott, S. W.,** The postmortem weight of the "normal" spleen at different ages, *Am. J. Med. Sci.,* 197, 344, 1939.
86. **DeLand, F. H.,** Normal spleen size, *Radiology,* 97, 589, 1970.
87. **Seltzer, R. A., Kereiakes, J. G., and Saenger, E. L.,** Radiation exposure from radioisotopes in pediatrics, *New Engl. J. Med.,* 271, 84, 1964.
88. **Spencer, R. P. and Banever, C.,** Growth of the human liver: a preliminary scan study, *J. Nucl. Med.,* 11, 660, 1970.
89. **Riemenschneider, P. A. and Whalen, J. R.,** The relative accuracy of estimation of enlargment of the liver and spleen by radiologic and clinical methods, *Am. J. Roentgenol.,* 94, 462, 1965.
90. **Sigel, R. M., Becker, D. V., and Hurley, J. R.,** Evaluation of spleen size during routine liver imaging with ^{99m}Tc and the scintillation camera, *J. Nucl. Med.,* 11, 689, 1970.
91. **Larson, S. M., Tueli, S. H., Moores, K. D., and Nelp, W. B.,** Dimensions of the normal spleen and prediction of spleen weight, *J. Nucl. Med.,* 11, 341, 1970.
92. **Whitley, J. E., Maynard, C. D., and Rhyne, A. L.,** A computer approach to the prediction of spleen weights from routine films, *Radiology,* 86, 73, 1966.
93. **Samuels, L. D.,** Estimation of spleen weight from posterior radioisotope scans, *J. Assoc. Can. Radiol.,* 20, 192, 1969.
94. **Rollo, F. D. and DeLand, F. H.,** The determination of spleen mass from radionuclide images, *Radiology,* 97, 583, 1970.

95. **Spencer, R. P.,** Relationship of surface area on roentgenograms and radioisotopic scans to organ volumes, *J. Nucl. Med.,* 8, 785, 1967.
96. **Holzbach, R. T., Clark, R. E., Shipley, R. A., Kent, W. D., III, and Lidsay, G. E.,** Evaluation of spleen size by radioactive scanning, *J. Lab. Clin. Med.,* 60, 902, 1962.
97. **Blendis, L. M., Williams, R., and Kreel, L.,** Radiological determination of spleen size, *Gut,* 10, 433, 1969.
98. **Fischer, J. and Wolf, R.,** Quantitative estimation of spleen size by scintigraphy, *German Med. Month.,* 9, 63, 1964.
99. **Kardel, T., Holm, H. H., Rasmussen, S. N., and Mortensen, T.,** Ultrasonic determination of liver and spleen volumes, *Scand. J. Clin. Lab. Invest.,* 27, 123, 1971.
100. **Fischer, J.,** Die Milzszintigraphie als Methode zur funktionellen Milzanalyse, in *Die Milz,* Lennert, K. and Harms, D., Eds., Springer-Verlag, Berlin, 1970.
101. **Solomon, J. B.,** *Foetal and Neonatal Immunology,* American Elsevier, New York, 1971, 3.
102. **Halpern, B. N., Benacerraf, B., and Biozzi, G.,** Quantitative study of the granulopoetic activity of the reticuloendothelial system. I. The effect of the ingredients present in india ink and of substances affecting blood clotting in vivo on the fate of carbon particles administered intravenously in rats, mice and rabbits, *Br. J. Exp. Pathol.,* 34, 426, 1953.
103. **Benacerraf, B. Biozzi, G., Halpern, B. N., and Stiffel, C.,** Physiology of phagocytosis of particles by the reticuloendothelial system, in *Physiopathology of the Reticuloendothelial System,* Halpern, B. N., Benacerraf, B., and Delafresnaye, J. F., Eds., Blackwell, Oxford, 1957, 52.
104. **Benacerraf, B., Kivy-Rosenberg, E., Sebestyen, M. M., and Zweifach, B. W.,** The effect of high doses of X-irradiation on the phagocytic, proliferative, and metabolic properties of the reticulo-endothelial system, *J. Exp. Med.,* 110, 49, 1959.
105. **Hollenberg, M. D., Kaback, M. M., and Kazazian, H. H., Jr.,** Adult hemoglobin synthesis by reticulocytes from the human fetus at midtrimester, *Science,* 174, 698, 1971.
106. **Kessler, H. and Smulewicz, J. J.,** Microgastria associated with agenesis of the spleen, *Radiology,* 107, 393, 1973.
107. **Freedom, R. M. and Treves, S.,** Splenic scintigraphy and radionuclide venography in the heterotaxy syndrome, *Radiology,* 107, 381, 1973.
108. **Freedom, R. M. and Fellows, K. E., Jr.,** Radiographic visceral patterns in the asplenia syndrome, *Radiology,* 107, 387, 1973.
109. **DeLand, F. H. and Tonkin, A.,** Serial liver scanning as an index of hepatic function following jejuno-ileal bypass surgery, *J. Nucl. Med.,* 14, 390, 1973.
110. **Sharp. H. L., Bridge, R. A., Krivit, W., and Freiter, E. F.,** Cirrhosis associated with alpha-l-antitrypsin deficiency: a previously unrecognized inherited disorder, *J. Lab. Clin. Med.,* 73, 934, 1969.
111. **Ryo, U. Y., Moses, D. C., and Milam, W. F.,** Abnormal liver scans in patients with alpha-l-antitrypsin deficiency, *J. Nucl. Biol. Med.,* 18, 39, 1974.
112. **Blyth, H., and Ockemden, B. G.,** Polycystic disease of kidneys and liver presenting in childhood, *J. Med. Genet.,* 8, 257, 1971.
113. **Lanson, S. Z., Frieden, J. H., and Bierman, H. R.,** Polycystic disease of the liver, *JAMA,* 215, 793, 1971.
114. **Lieberman, E. Salinos-Madrigal, L., Gwinn, J. L., Brennon, L. P., Fine, R. N., and Landing, B. H.,** Infantile polycystic disease of the kidneys and liver, *Medicine,* 50, 277, 1971.
115. **Rao, L. M., Shahidi, N. T., and Opitz, J. M.,** Hereditary splenomegaly with hypersplenism, *Clin. Genet.,* 5, 379, 1974.

Chapter 4

SPLENECTOMY AND BLOOD VOLUME CHANGES

While removal of the spleen is often necessary, and in some cases can be life saving, the full implications and possible consequences of splenectomy must be considered in every case. The indications for splenectomy are usually classified as hematologic reasons, traumatic reasons, and miscellaneous reasons.[1] We have worked with a slightly different classification, recognizing that the spleen is sometimes removed for diagnostic purposes.

Splenectomy for Diagnosis

1. Staging of Hodgkin's disease.
2. Unexplained lesion in the spleen.

Splenectomy for Therapy ("Medical Disorders")

1. "Hypersplenism."
2. Hemolytic anemias, especially hereditary spherocytosis and hereditary elliptocytosis, autoimmune hemolytic anemia, and nonspherocytic hemolytic anemia.
3. Tumors or cysts in spleen.
4. Idiopathic thrombocytopic purpura.
5. Abscess.
6. ? Chronic lymphatic leukemia.

Splenectomy for Therapy ("Surgical Disorders")

1. Splenic laceration, rupture, or hematoma.
2. Torsion or major vascular impairment.
3. Surgical trauma.
4. Necessity for adequate exposure of structures in left upper quadrant.
5. As part of shunting procedure.
6. Splenic vein thrombosis and bleeding varices.
7. To relieve mechanical problems of massive splenomegaly, as in Gaucher's disease, thalassemia major, myeloid metaplasia.

It should be apparent that in some cases these categories may not be clear cut; they represent a first guide to a clinical approach. In the category "Medical Disorders," spherocytosis and idiopathic thrombocytopenic purpura are the most commonly encountered entities (and in Hodam's[1] discussion of splenectomy for hematologic reasons, these two disorders accounted for 90 of the 121 cases). In the report by Schwartz and co-workers,[2] spherocytosis and idiopathic thrombocytopenic purpura represented the reasons for 103 of their 200 splenectomies. In both spherocytosis and idiopathic thrombocytopenic purpura, splenectomy can provide prolonged beneficial results.[18,19] Lammi and Lovric,[74] in an epidemiologic study of children with idiopathic thrombocytopenic purpura, noted that splenectomy was usually curvative in those with long standing, symptomatic disease. Interestingly, the prognosis was not related to the size of the spleen. Christensen and associates[3] noted that while there is general agreement on the need for splenectomy in hereditary spherocytosis, in other instances of hemolytic anemia the use of splenectomy presumes that the spleen is playing the major role in red cell trapping. It is apparent that more definitive criteria are needed for the diagnosis of hypersplenism and for the determination of which patients will be benefited by splenectomy (and see the discussion of hypersplenism in a separate chapter). Lennert[71] has described the indications for splenectomy in children. While splenectomy is usually considered contraindicated or of no value in sickle cell disease, there may be a use if specific criteria are met. Stevens[10] reported splenectomy (and survival) in a 12-year-old male with sickle cell anemia, who had trapping of 40% of his red blood cell mass in a 970-g spleen. The second case involved a woman who had a ^{51}Cr-erythrocyte survival time of only 4 days (normal = 28 days) and a spleen/liver ratio of 2 to 1. This hemolytic crisis of sickle cell anemia was treated successfully by splenectomy.

Crosby has also provided a summary of some of the hematologic indications for splenectomy.[17] He makes the point that there are occasions when splenectomy has desirable but remote effects (for example, aplastic anemia may be benefited in some cases; a splenic hormone affecting the bone marrow has not been clearly demonstrated).

The role of splenectomy in the treatment of

portal hypertension is open to much debate. The splenic artery can be ligated in man and the spleen still retained during use of the splenic vein for splenorenal anastomosis.[20] The overall 5-year survival following splenectomy for portal hypertension, in 32 patients, was only 20%.[21] Splenectomy, and coronary vein ligation, has been employed in an effort to control esophageal varices[22] (and splenectomy has also been used in the therapy of splenic vein thrombosis and bleeding varices).[72] Gehrmann and Elbers[23] mention that splenectomy is indicated when hepatic cirrhosis is accompanied by increased splenic trapping of ^{51}Cr-platelets. Splenectomy, for portal hypertension, can be followed by gastrointestinal bleeding.[59]

Use of splenectomy in other disease states is briefly tabulated below.

Lymphoma and Leukemia – Of about 1,000 patients with malignant lymphoma reported by O'Brien and associates,[9] 18 had splenectomies for hypersplenism. The operative mortality (death within 30 days of operation) was 39%. Splenectomy appeared to be without therapeutic value in Hodgkin's disease but may relieve hypersplenic symptoms. While splenectomy is apparently without therapeutic benefit on the basic process in Hodgkin's disease,[9] removal of the spleen has been employed as a tool in staging (Figure 1). It is recognized that preoperative classification is frequently changed on the basis of the operative findings.[12] In one series, no patient was observed to have extrasplenic abdominal Hodgkin's disease without the spleen being involved.[13] Crosby[17] states that splenectomy should be performed in Hodgkin's disease when hypersplenism is detected. A further discussion is given in the chapter on the lymphomas.

The occurrence of lymphosarcoma, principally involving the spleen, has been noted[4] (and the diagnosis established by splenectomy). Three patients had splenomegaly, while eight had both splenomegaly and pancytopenia. The blood picture improved following splenic removal. In 6 of the 11 patients subjected to splenectomy, a blood picture of lymphatic leukemia developed. O'Brien and co-workers[9] noted that splenectomy might be useful for treating the hypersplenism of lymphosarcoma. There is some evidence that splenectomy favorably influenced not only the hypersplenism but also the underlying lymphosarcoma.[11] Lymphosarcoma and lymphatic leukemia have been noted in the dog,[5] with splenectomy offering clinical improvement. Christensen and co-workers[3] state that splenectomy in chronic lymphatic leukemia may be useful when there is massive splenomegaly, as well as anemia, thrombocytopenia, and systemic signs.

In chronic granulocytic leukemia, splenectomy has not usually been viewed as a treatment of choice; splenic radiation and cytotoxic drugs have been utilized in therapy. However, in the chronic phase of the disease, with thrombocytopenia, Canellos and co-workers[6] reported a postoperative increase in the platelet count following splenectomy. When the platelet count tends to be seriously depressed by chemotherapy in chronic granulocytic leukemia, splenectomy might be indicated. More recently, Schwarzenberg and co-workers[75] have presented a discussion of possible uses of splenectomy in the disease.

Histiocytic Medullary Reticulosis – Evidence is scanty. However, in one patient, splenectomy was followed by survival for nearly 2 years.[16]

Thrombotic Thrombocytopenia Purpura (TTP) – Affected patients have thrombocytopenia with purpura, hemolytic anemia, fever, and renal and neurological disorders. While steriods have been employed in the treatment of TTP, at least one series reported encouraging results with splenectomy.[34]

Tropical Splenomegaly Syndrome – Splenectomy in this disorder is apparently well tolerated. However, the size of the liver continues to increase (with continued hepatic sinusoidal infiltration with lymphocytes and hyperplasia of Kupffer cells).[14] Perhaps this is related to the basic stimulus that is causing hypertrophy of the reticuloendothelial system.

Hemodialysis – Hartley and co-workers[15] noted four patients on hemodialysis who had anemia with extracorpuscular hemolysis (shortened ^{51}Cr-erythrocyte survival half-time) and evaluated spleen/liver ^{51}Cr ratios. The patients were benefited by splenectomy.

Felty's Syndrome – Splenomegaly and neutropenia occurs in about 1% of patients with rheumatoid arthritis. Splenectomy alleviated the neutropenia in 10 of 15 cases in one series.[25]

Hemophilia – The normal spleen is likely a site of production of antihemophiliac globulin (factor VIII). Splenectomy has been accomplished in some hemophiliacs because of bleeding and rupture.[43] There are too few cases to allow us to

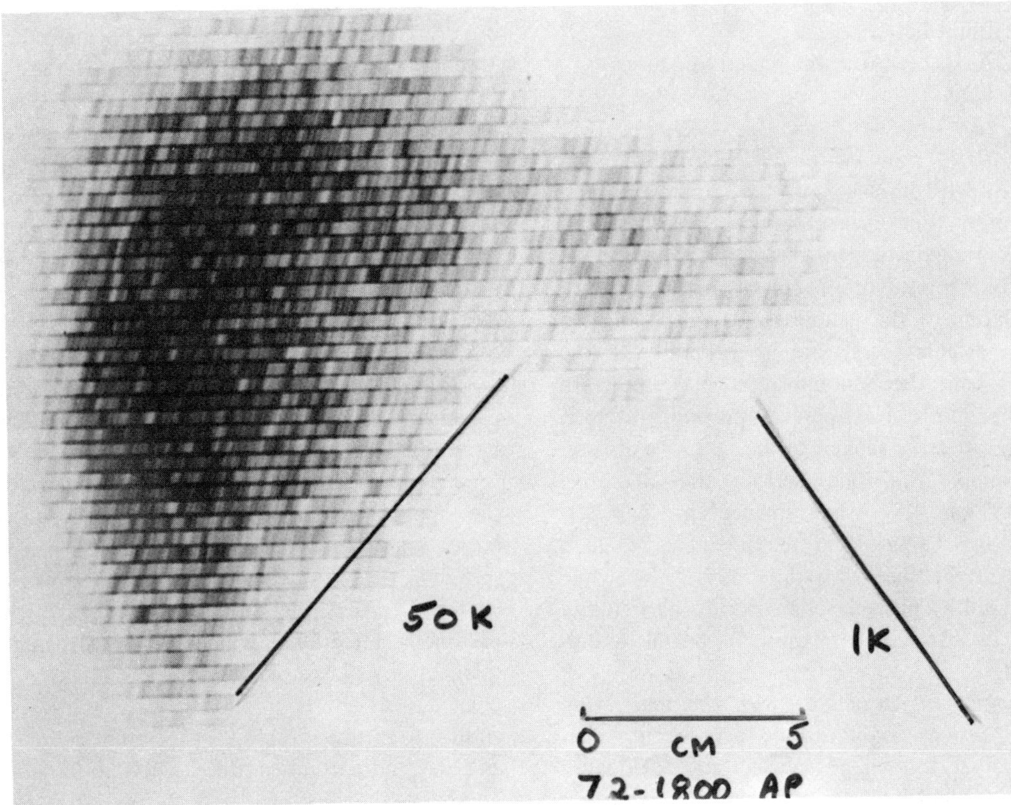

FIGURE 1. Anterior rectilinear scan (^{99m}Tc-sulfur colloid) in a 30-year-old female. The patient had Hodgkin's disease diagnosed 1 year previously and then underwent splenectomy. The count ratio (liver/"spleen") per unit area was 50 to 1. Case 72-1800.

determine whether splenectomized hemophiliacs are more susceptible to infections.

Renal Transplants – Beneficial effects of splenectomy on human kidney transplant recipients could not be confirmed in a more recent study.[78]

Surgical Trauma – Olsen and Beaudoin[7] reviewed 584 instances of splenectomy and noted that 121 (or 21%) were necessitated by surgical injury to the spleen. Complications were severe, perhaps due in part to the underlying disease that necessitated the abdominal operation.

Nearby Tumor – The spleen may have to be removed if adherent to a tumor or an adjacent organ which is being extirpated. The significance of perisplenic lymph node enlargement is less clear. Bengmark and co-workers[8] have discussed the role of splenectomy in operations for gastric cancer.

Relative Contraindications – There are some disorders in which splenectomy has not consistently produced useful clinical results. Crosby[17] lists several of these as hereditary hemolytic disorders of moderate or minimal extent (pyruvate-kinase deficiency, hemoglobin C, hemoglobin-S-C, thalassemia minor, thalassemia-hemoglobin S), acute leukemia, acute myelofibrosis, paroxysomal nocturmal hemoglobinuria, and agranulocytosis.

Absolute Contraindications – Diseases in which splenectomy has been marked by postoperative worsening[17] include:

1. Wiskott-Aldrich syndrome and allied inherited thrombocytopenias.
2. Sex-linked hypochromic anemia.
3. Thrombocythemia.

In the last two disorders, thrombosis can develop postoperatively. Many workers have found that pancytopenia is a contraindication to splenectomy (and to other operations) because of the bleeding tendency. Platelet transfusions and attention to controlling bleeding vessels may be effective.

Complications – The complications which follow, or are associated with, splenectomy can be divided into three classes.

1. Immediate.
2. Associated with the underlying disease.
3. Late.

Immediate complications. Reynolds[24] has recommended drainage of the pancreatic and splenic areas after splenectomy. This was based on his findings of elevated amylase levels in peritoneal fluid after removal of the spleen (perhaps due to manipulation of the pancreas). It will be recalled that the splenic vessels are in proximity to the pancreas, and their mobilization may result in pancreatic insult. The operative mortality of splenectomy is largely related to the causative disease. For example, in one series[1] the operative mortality was 2.5% when splenectomy was performed for hematologic reasons, 17.5% when carried out because of trauma, and 20.5% when necessitated by miscellaneous reasons (particularly disease in contiguous organs or portal hypertension).

Complications associated with the underlying disease. Septic complications can occur postoperatively, following splenectomy. Hodam[1] noted an incidence of postoperative sepsis in nearly 14% of patients who underwent splenectomy. These were attributed to postoperative complications and to the debilitating nature of the underlying disorder. In myeloid metaplasia and in Wiskott-Aldrich and related syndromes,[26] the infections can be severe. An increase in the circulating blood elements, that occurs after splenectomy, is usually well tolerated.[1] However, as mentioned, in sex-linked hypochronic anemia and thrombocythemia, splenectomy can be followed by thromboses.[17]

Late complications. In Chapter 2, functions of the spleen were listed as:

1. Hematopoiesis.
2. Erythrocyte destruction.
3. Phagocytosis.
4. Reservoir.
5. Culling and pitting.
6. Possible splenic hormonal control of hematopoiesis.
7. Role in platelet and leukocyte destruction.
8. Immunologic role.

Loss of functions 1, 2, 4, 6, and 7 does not appear to be life threatening. The bone marrow usually carries out hematopoiesis normally in the absence of the spleen (functions 1 and 6). Following splenectomy, erythrocyte survival is not prolonged (function 2). There is some type of delicate mechanism that continues erythrocyte destruction at the normal rate after splenectomy. Loss of the reservoir function of the spleen (function 4) appears to be of little importance in man. Function 7 (role in platelet and leukocyte destruction) seems to go on readily in the absence of the spleen.

The effects of splenectomy are apparently principally manifested through lack of functions 3, 5, and 8. Loss of the culling and pitting functions provides one of the hallmarks of splenectomy – the appearance of intraerythrocytic inclusions. More important, there is apparently a corresponding loss of the ability to clear various bacterial forms. The ultimate is perhaps seen in bartonella infections, which are exacerbated by splenectomy. Loss of the filtering function and phagocytosis, when coupled with the loss of ability to form antibodies to certain particulate antigens, compromises the ability to combat a number of diseases.

King and Shumacker[27] were the first to note the susceptibility of infants to infection, following splenectomy. An enormous literature has evolved the subject. We will summarize pertinent parts of the data.

1. The original report was of meningitis or meningococcemia, developing 6 weeks to 3 years after splenectomy.[27] In two cases the meningococcus was isolated, while in one, Hemophilus influenzae appeared to be the causative organism (and in two instances, no organism was identified).

2. However, in most series of postsplenectomy infections in infants or children, the pneumococcus is the responsible microorganism.

3. There are statements that splenectomy, when carried out because of trauma in childhood (that is, without other underlying disease), does not lead to increased risk of infection.[28] There are still other case reports that cause us to be concerned.[29,35] However, Donaldson and her co-workers[73] noted that the fatality rate did not differ between patients with lymphoma and others who developed bacteremia after splenectomy.

4. Of particular importance is recognition of the high rate of infection not only in those who had the spleen surgically removed but also in

individuals with cogential absence of the spleen, cogenital hypoplasia of the spleen, or nearly absent spleen function due to infarcts (as in sickle cell disease).

5. Trauma, as an indication for splenectomy, is relatively infrequent when major series are examined. We must therefore consider why infections, particulary those with the pneumococcus or meningococcus, occur in splenectomized children.

There are several relevant observations in the literature.

1. In rabbits, the spleen is more efficient in nonimmune clearance of ^{125}I-labeled pneumococci than the liver (uptake/g).[30] Splenectomy hence eliminates a portion of the mechanism for removing pneumococci. It has been hypothesized that in the rat, the spleen plays a key role in the clearance of pneumococci and the early immunologic response.[66]

2. Opsonins are necessary for the phagocytosis of pneumococci by leukocytes. In sickle cell disease (with nearly absent splenic function due to infarction), the requisite heat labile opsonizing factor is decreased.[31] Interestingly, heat stable opsonin (required for phagocytosis of salmonella) is normal in sickle cell disease. We can extrapolate that the opsonizing factor for pneumococci is also decreased or absent after splenectomy. Johnston and associates[76] found that sera from 28 patients with sickle cell disease permitted normal phagocytosis of pneumococci *if* the bacteria has been sensitized by antibody. However, if the antibody used was decreased, then a defect was apparent. This could not be attributed to a deficiency of antibody or complement. If activation of the complement sequence was prevented, serum did not adequately allow fixation of the opsonin C3 to bacteria. Bogart and co-workers[32] prepared pneumococci labeled with ^{59}Fe. Clearance of pneumococci from the blood of rats was measured by both the disappearance rate of ^{59}Fe and blood culture. When tested 5 days after splenectomy, the splenectomized rats had a delay in clearance as compared with controls. This delay was partially overcome if preopsonized pneumococci were injected. The overall effect did not persist, and 3 months after splenectomy, rats had normal rates of clearance.

The above finding of impaired clearance of pneumococci immediately after splenectomy, but normal clearance 3 months later, correlates with clinical observations. The time of major risk of infections is the early postsplenectomy period.[33] There does not seem to be agreement, however, whether postsplenectomy patients should be maintained on antibiotics for a period of 2 years. In summary, then, postsplenectomy infections (largely pneumococcal) are highest in infants, in individuals with underlying diseases, and in the first 2 postoperative years. Other hyposplenic states also show an increased risk of infections.[35] For example, in sickle cell disease, the risk of bacterial meningitis is some 300 times that of the usual pediatric population.[36] Serious infection can apparently occur after splenectomy performed for staging Hodgkin's disease,[69] but there are views that differ.[73] There has been much debate as to whether such patients should be maintained on prophylactic antibiotics.[70] We will recapitulate that splenectomy alters a number of functions.

1. The spleen's ability to filter out certain bacteria is lost.

2. Splenic production of opsonins is eliminated.

3. Splenectomy reduces or eliminates the ability of human subjects to produce antibodies to intravenous heterologus erythrocytes.[37] This role of the spleen in responding to injected foreign red cells can be found in much of the phylogenetic tree (and it occurs in the lizard).[67] The small, infarcted spleen in sickle cell disease apparently has lost the ability to respond to heterologous red cells.[38]

4. Splenectomy is followed by the appearance of abnormal erythrocytes[39] in the peripheral circulation. This may be related to loss of the ability to "cull" deranged cells from the bloodstream or to the removal of the spleen's ability to process red cell membranes.

5. Intraerythrocytic inclusions, particulary Howell-Jolly bodies (nuclear remnants), appear after splenectomy. All splenectomized individuals show Howell-Jolly bodies. However, the presence of Howell-Jolly bodies does not always guarantee that the spleen is absent (it may be functionally absent, or such a large number of these inclusions might potentially be produced that the spleen may be unable to clear them all). The normal spleen has

the ability to "pit" red cells of these inclusions (that is, to remove the inclusions without destroying the red cells).

6. Leukocytes and thrombocytes become elevated after splenectomy. In rats, the elevated values tend to return toward normal after a number of weeks.[40]

7. In mice, splenectomy is followed by decreased ability to produce interferon following intravenous injection of *E. coli* endotoxin.[42] Three days post splenectomy, there was almost no interferon production. By 6 weeks after the operation, interferon production was approaching control levels.

8. Changes occur in blood proteins after splenectomy.

a. Coagulation changes (at least in the rat) following splenectomy are real but minimal.[41] This function has also been studied in the human after splenectomy.[68]

b. Immunoglobulin levels change after splenectomy. In rabbits, the increase in IgG (after removal of the spleen) has been attributed to increased production by other immunocompetent tissues.[44] Thalassemic subjects (β-thalassemia major) both with and without splenectomy were noted to have increased levels of IgG, IgA, and IgM,[45] as compared with normal controls. IgA and IgG levels were highest in the splenectomized thalassemic patients, while IgM was reported to be the same in both splenectomized and nonsplenectomized thalassemics. Wasi and co-workers[46] also noted higher IgA, IgG, and IgM in nonsplenectomized thalassemics. They reported, however, that in splenectomized thalassemics, IgA was increased, while IgM was depressed. They postulated that the spleen was a site of production of IgM and that a decrease in this immunoglobulin may be partly responsible for infections following splenectomy.

After splenectomy, fever may develop. In some cases this may be related to white cell aggultinins.[79] The following have been seen.

1. In dogs, the spleen plays a role as a reservoir for blood elements. The packed cell volume in dogs increases after feeding, but the effect is abolished by splenectomy.[47] In the dog, the spleen also influences the platelet response to bleeding.[45]

2. A number of reports have dealt with the relationship of the spleen to tumorigenesis. For example, in certain female mice carrying the mammary tumor virus, splenectomy decreased the incidence and age of onset of mammary tumors.[49] However, splenectomy did not affect the incidence of lymphomas or mammary tumors in urethan-treated mice[50] or the incidence of leukemia in male mice of the ICRC strain.[51] Splenectomy increased the rate of regression of sarcoma 180 in some strains of mice.[58]

3. In mice, splenectomy renders the animals more susceptible to hepatic amyloidosis following casein injection.[52]

4. Albright and co-workers[53] noted that when the spleens of aged mice were transferred into middle-aged recipients, there was life shortening. Also, splenectomy of aging mice prolonged their lives. What the age-related factors (? immunological) might be is not presently known.

5. The differences between the hematologic responses of splenectomized and nonsplenectomized patients with Hodgkin's disease, following irradiation, have been documented.[54] The spleen plays a complex role in radiation protection.[55]

6. Splenectomy may be followed by an effect on liver microsomal enzymes.[56] The spleen, however, is not needed for erythropoietin to carry out its effects on bone marrow.[57]

BLOOD VOLUME IN SPLENOMEGALY

In the section on polycythemia vera, it is pointed out that in that disease, the ratio of whole body hematocrit (determined by means of ^{51}Cr-erythrocytes and ^{131}I-human serum albumin) to the peripheral hematocrit is about 0.92.[60] This result was indistinguishable from that obtained in control subjects. Hence, in polycythemia vera, the spleen does not concentrate erythrocytes at the expense of plasma. This, however, is not the case with many other causes of splenomegaly. Donaldson and co-workers[61] noted that in 65 patients with splenomegaly due to a number of disorders, there was red cell trapping in the spleen and hemodilution of the circulating erythrocytes in an expanded plasma volume. The ultimate prognosis depended on the nature of the primary disease process.

Splenomegaly is often associated with what is called a "hemodilution anemia." That is, there is hypervolemia due to an increase in the plasma volume (Blendis and co-workers[62] have reviewed the early history of recognition of this disorder). A summary of 96 cases collected by Blendis and co-workers (as follows) indicates that in blood dyscrasias there is frequently anemia, but a reduction in red cell mass occurs in only a small percentage of cases.

	Blood dyscrasias	Cirrhosis
Cases	46	50
Anemic	37	20
Percent anemic	80%	40%
Number with reduced red cell mass	3	7
Percent with reduced RBC mass	7%	14%

At splenectomy, the enlarged spleens contained an expanded red cell pool but only 30% of the calculated excess plasma volume. We can make this clearer by the following tabulated data (recall that the hematocrit of blood in the normal spleen does not differ markedly from the whole body hematocrit).

Peripheral venous hematocrit (13 cases)	32
Splenic hematocrit (drip blood)	52
Spleen contained (% of red cell mass)	25
Spleen contained (% of plasma volume)	8

Hence, there was excess red cell pooling in the spleen or, to put it another way, excess plasma in the vascular tree. There was, in the blood dyscrasia patients, a close correlation ($\sigma = 0.83$) between the plasma volume (P, in ml/kg) and the weight of the spleen (S, in kg/m^2). The relationship was approximately

$$P = 38 + 33.2\ S. \qquad (1)$$

With a normal spleen weight (0.1 kg/m^2, from the values of 0.17 kg spleen/1.7 m^2 surface area), the plasma volume would be about 41 ml/kg. With a spleen of 2.5 kg/m^2, the plasma volume would be up to 120 ml/kg. In all the patients with blood dyscrasias, standing upright for 30 min produced a fall in the plasma volume, with a rise in the peripheral venous hematocrit. This was likely due to plasma pooling in the legs since the ankle circumference increased. Toghill and Green[63] noted that the splenic red blood cell pool increased with spleen size (8.9% of total red cells in approximately normally sized spleens, up to 17.5% in greatly enlarged spleens). Christensen[77] correlated splenic content of ^{51}Cr-erythrocytes with that in the cardiac blood pool and with the size of the spleen (determinedly ultrasonic scanning or by splenectomy).

Blendis and associates[62] measured splenic blood flow by the ^{133}Xe method and surface counting when studying the hemodilution anemias. They noted an increased blood flow through these spleens and a correlation ($\sigma = 0.73$) between the plasma volume (V, in liters) and the total splenic blood flow (B in ml/min). The relationship was approximately

$$V = 3.0 + 0.0014\ B. \qquad (2)$$

At a splenic blood flow of 200 ml/min, the plasma volume was 3.3 1. However, when the splenic blood flow was 1,200 ml/min, the plasma volume was 4.7 l.

Other studies have also shown a significant increase in the plasma volume in patients with splenomegaly from multiple causes. Bowdler[64] has noted that the venous hematocrit was not a good indicator of red cell mass in such patients. The plasma volume and the total blood volume showed positive correlations with the size of the spleen. Bowdler[64] suggested that the important factors were the intrasplenic blood volume and the elevated splanchnic blood volume from portal hypertension.

Webber and Garnett[65] also noted the expanded blood volume in splenomegaly and stated that the ^{133}Xe rebreathing technique showed elevated splenic blood flow (up to half of the cardiac output in such cases). The enlarged spleen was likened to an arteriovenous shunt. In patients with an elevated blood volume (in terms of volume/body weight), the exchangeable sodium (mEq/kg) was elevated. Diuretics resulted in a decrease in the blood volume and in the exchangeable sodium. Hence, part of the increase in blood volume may be due to sodium retention; this could be secondary to the failing heart resulting from the spleen acting as an arteriovenous shunt.

REFERENCES

1. **Hodam, R. P.,** The risk of splenectomy. A review of 310 cases, *Am. J. Surg.*, 119, 709, 1970.
2. **Schwartz, S. I., Bernard, R. P., Adams, J. T., and Bauman, A. W.,** Splenectomy for hematologic disorders, *Arch. Surg.*, 101, 338, 1970.
3. **Christensen, B. E., Hansen, L. K., Kristensen, J. K., and Bidebdek, A.,** Splenectomy in haematology. Indications, results and complications in 41 cases, *Scand. J. Haematol.*, 7, 247, 1970.
4. **Skarin, A. T., Davey, F. R., and Moloney, W. C.,** Lymphosarcoma of the spleen, *Arch. Intern. Med.*, 127, 259, 1971.
5. **Carrig, C. B. and Penny, R. H. C.,** Treatment of lymphosarcoma in the dog by splenectomy: a case report, *Vet. Rec.*, 86, 26, 1970.
6. **Canellos, G. P., Nordland, J., and Carbone, P. P.,** Splenectomy for thrombocytopenia in chronic granulocytic leukemia, *Cancer,* 29, 660, 1972.
7. **Olsen, W. R. and Beaudoin, D. E.,** Surgical injury to the spleen, *Surg. Gynecol. Obstet.*, 131, 57, 1970.
8. **Bengmark, S., Domellof, L., and Olsson, A. M.,** The role of splenectomy in stomach cancer operations, *Digestion,* 4, 314, 1971.
9. **O'Brien, P. H., Hartz, W. H., Jr., Derlacki, D., and Graulich, K.,** Splenectomy for hypersplenism in malignant lymphoma, *Arch. Surg.*, 101, 348, 1970.
10. **Stevens, A. R., Jr.,** Splenectomy in sickle cell anemia, *Arch. Intern. Med.*, 125, 883, 1970.
11. **Hyatt, D. F., Skarin, A. T., Moloney, W. C., and Wilson, R. E.,** Splenectomy for lymphosarcoma, *Surg. Gynecol. Obstet.*, 131, 928, 1970.
12. **Lowenbraun, S., Ramsey, H., Sutherland, J., and Serpick, A. A.,** Diagnostic laparotomy and splenectomy for staging Hodgkin's disease, *Ann. Intern. Med.*, 72, 655, 1970.
13. **Aisenberg, A. C., Goldman, J. M., Raker, J. W., and Wang, C. C.,** Spleen involvement at the onset of Hodgkin's disease, *Ann. Intern. Med.*, 74, 544, 1971.
14. **Hamilton, P. J. S., Stuiver, P. C., and Ziegler, J. L.,** Splenectomy in tropical splenomegaly syndrome: a five year follow-up, *J. Trop. Med.*, 74, 230, 1971.
15. **Hartley, L. C. J., Innis, M. D., Morgan, T. O., and Clunie, G. J. A.,** Splenectomy for anemia in patients on regular haemodialysis, *Lancet,* II, 1343, 1971.
16. **Goldman, J. M., Jacobson, B. M., and James, G. W., III,** Splenectomy for histiocytic medullary reticulosis, *Postgrad. Med. J.*, 47, 671, 1971.
17. **Crosby, W. H.,** Splenectomy in hematologic disorders, *N. Engl. J. Med.*, 286, 1252, 1972.
18. **Orringer, E., Lewis, M., Silverberg, J., and Rosenbach, L.,** Splenectomy in chronic thrombocytopenic purpura, *J. Chron. Dis.*, 23, 117, 1970.
19. **Baird, R. N., MacPherson, A. I. S., and Richmond, J.,** Red-blood-cell survival after splenectomy in congenital spherocytosis, *Lancet,* II, 1060, 1971.
20. **Haller, J. D., Glick, H., Hallman, G. L., and Cooley, D. A.,** Portal decompression by side-to-side splenorenal venous anastomosis, *Arch. Surg.*, 102, 316, 1971.
21. **Poilleux, J., Bouvresse, M., and Hivet, M.,** Place de la splenectomic dans le traitment de l'hypertension portale, *Ann. Chir.*, 25, 1309, 1971.
22. **Smith, G. W.,** Splenectomy and coronary vein ligation for the control of bleeding esophageal varices, *Am. J. Surg.*, 119, 122, 1970.
23. **Gehrmann, G. and Elbers, C.,** Thrombopenisches hyperspleniesyndrom bei splenomegaler leberzirrhose, *Deutsch. Med. Wochenschr.*, 95, 1429, 1970.
24. **Reynolds, B. M.,** Observations on postsplenectomy drainage and its significance, *Surgery,* 68, 783, 1970.
25. **Moore, R. A., Brunner, C. M., Sandusky, W. R., and Leavell, B. S.,** Felty's syndrome: long-term follow-up after splenectomy, *Ann. Intern. Med.*, 75, 381, 1971.
26. **Weiden, P. L. and Blaese, R. M.,** Hereditary thrombocytopenia: relation to Wiskott-Aldrich syndrome with special reference to splenectomy, *J. Pediatr.*, 80, 226, 1972.
27. **King, H. and Shumacker, H. B., Jr.,** Splenic studies. I. Susceptibility to infections after splenectomy performed in infants, *Ann. Surg.*, 136, 239, 1952.
28. **Orlando, J. C. and Moore, T. C.,** Splenectomy for trauma in childhood, *Surg. Gynecol. Obstet.*, 134, 94, 1972.
29. **Maron, B. J. and Maloney, J. R.,** Septicemia following traumatic or incidental splenectomy, *Johns Hopkins Med. J.*, 130, 266, 1972.
30. **Schulkind, M. L., Ellis, E. P., and Smith, R. T.,** Effect of antibody on clearance of ^{125}I labelled pneumococci by the spleen and liver, *Pediatr. Res.*, 1, 178, 1967.
31. **Winkelstein, J. A. and Drachman, R. H.,** Deficiency of pneumococcal serum opsonizing activity in sickle cell disease, *N. Engl. J. Med.*, 279, 459, 1968.
32. **Bogart, D., Biggar, W. D., and Good, R. A.,** Impaired intravascular clearance of pneumococcus type 3 following splenectomy, *J. Reticuloendethel. Soc.*, 11, 77, 1972.
33. **Eraklis, A. J., Kevy, S. V., Diamond, L. K., and Gross, R. E.,** Hazards of overwhelming infection after splenectomy in childhood, *N. Engl. J. Med.*, 276, 1225, 1967.

34. **Bernard, R. P., Bauman, A. W., and Schwartz, S. I.,** Splenectomy for thrombotic thrombocytopenic purpura, *Ann. Surg.,* 169, 616, 1969.
35. **Bisno, A. L.,** Hyposplenism and overwhelming pneumcoccal infection: a reappraisal, *Am. J. Med. Sci.,* 262, 101, 1971.
36. **Lukens, J. N.,** Hemoglobin S, the pneumococcus, and the spleen, *Am. J. Dis. Child.,* 123, 6, 1972.
37. **Rowley, D. A.,** The formation of circulating antibody in splenectomized human beings after intravenous injection of heterologous erthrocytes, *J. Immunol.,* 64, 515, 1950.
38. **Schwartz, A. D. and Pearson, H. A.,** Imparied antibody response to intravenous immunization in sickle cell anemia, *Pediatr. Res.,* 6, 145, 1972.
39. **Smith, C. H. and Khakoo, Y.,** Burr cells: classification and effects of splenectomy, *J. Pediatr.,* 76, 99, 1970.
40. **Widmann, W. D., Laubscher, F. A., Davidson, S. J., and Grenoble, R. A.,** Effects of splenectomy and splenosis on the blood and platelet count and red cell morphology, *Milit. Med.,* 136, 15, 1971.
41. **Pudlak, P., Farska, I., Brabec, V., and Pospisilova, V.,** Coagulation findings in rats with experimental hypersplenism and their changes after splenectomy and after administration of adrenaline, *Thromb. Diath. Haemorrh.,* 23, 593, 1970.
42. **Ito, Y., Kunii, A., Mori, N., and Nagata, I.,** Effects of splenectomy on production of endotoxin-type interferon in mice, *Virology,* 44, 638, 1971.
43. **Baron, J. M., Kingdon, H. S., Block, G. E., and Gottschalk, A.,** Splenectomy in a hemophiliac, *Surg. Clin. North Am.,* 50, 205, 1971.
44. **Bednarik, T. and Cajthamlova, H.,** Zur Frage des erhohton IgG-Spiegels nach der splenektomie, *Z. Immun. Forsch.,* 141, 378, 1971.
45. **Setianidis, B., Mihas, A., and Angelopoulos, B.,** Serum immunoglobulins in β-thalassemia after splenectomy, *Acta Haematol.,* 46, 267, 1971.
46. **Wasi, C., Wasi, P., and Thongcharoen, P.,** Serum-immunoglobulin levels on thalassemia and the effects of splenectomy, *Lancet,* II, 237, 1971.
47. **Reece, W. O. and Snodgrass, R. R.,** Effect of splenectomy on postfeeding changes in packed cell volume of dogs, *Am. J. Vet. Res.,* 33, 635, 1972.
48. **Ljungqvist, V.,** The platelet response to haemorrhage in splenectomized dogs, *Acta Chir. Scand.,* 137, 97, 1971.
49. **Squartini, F. and Bolis, G. B.,** Mammary tumorigenesis in splenectomized mice, *Tex. Rep. Biol. Med.,* 28, 115, 1970.
50. **Porta, G. D., Colnaghi, M. I., and Parmi, L.,** Influenza della timectemia, della splenectemia e del cortisone sulla cancerogenesis, *Tumori,* 56, 121, 1970.
51. **Pai, S. R. and Ranadive, K. J.,** Influence of splenectomy on the development of leukemia in male mice of the ICRC strain, *Life Sci.,* 10, 475, 1971.
52. **Dreher, R.,** Experimentelle amylosdose bei splenktomiesten mausen, *Z. Immunitaetsforsch. Allerg. Klin. Immunol.,* 140, 1, 1970.
53. **Albright, J. F., Makinodan, T., and Deitchman, J. W.,** Presence of life-shortening factors in spleens of aged mice of long life span and extension of life expectancy by splenectomy, *Exp. Gerontol.,* 4, 267, 1969.
54. **Salzman, J. L. and Kaplan, H. S.,** Effect of prior splenectomy on hematologic tolerance during total lymphoid radiotherapy of patients with Hodgkin's disease, *Cancer,* 27, 471, 1971.
55. **Smith, L. H. and McKinley, T. W., Jr.,** Recovery from radiation injury with and without bone marrow transplantation: effects of splenectomy, *Radiat. Res.,* 44, 248, 1970.
56. **Brodeur, J. and Marchand, C.,** Effect of splenectomy on the activity of drug metabolizing enzymes in the liver of rats, *Can. J. Physiol. Pharmacol.,* 49, 161, 1971.
57. **Gutinsky, A.,** Failure of splenectomy to alter the response to erythropoietin, *Acta Physiol. Latinoam.,* 21, 48, 1971.
58. **Rumi, L., Pasqualini, C. D., and Rabasa, S. L.,** Growth of sarcoma 180 in splenectomized mice bearing diffusion chambers containing spleen or tumor cells, *Eur. J. Cancer,* 7, 551, 1971.
59. **Berchtold, R. and Scharer, K.,** Zur problem der postsplenektomieblutung, *Schweiz. Med. Wochenschr.,* 100, 2105, 1970.
60. **Bowdler, A. J.,** Plasma volume and splenomegaly in polycythaemia vera, *Br. J. Haematol.,* 22, 331, 1972.
61. **Donaldson, G. W. K., MacArthur, M., MacPherson, A. I. S., and Richmond, J.,** Blood volume changes in splenomegaly, *Br. J. Haematol.,* 18, 45, 1970.
62. **Blendis, L. M., Ramboer, C., and Williams, R.,** Studies on the haemodilution anemia of splenomegaly, *Eur. J. Clin. Invest.,* 1, 54, 1970.
63. **Toghill, P. J. and Green, S.,** The influence of spleen size on the distribution of red cells and plasma, *J. Clin. Pathol.,* 25, 270, 1971.
64. **Bowdler, A. J.,** Blood volume studies in patients with splenomegaly, *Transfusion,* 10, 171, 1970.
65. **Webber, C. E. and Garnett, E. S.,** Sodium retention associated with splenomegaly, *J. Nucl. Med.,* 11, 646, 1970.
66. **Leung, L. S. E., Szal, G. J., and Drachman, R. H.,** Increased susceptibility of splenectomized rats to infection with Diplococcus pneumoniae, *J. Infect. Dis.,* 126, 507, 1972.
67. **Kanakambika, P. and Muthukkaruppan, V.,** Effect of splenectomy on the immune response in the lizard, Calotes versicolor, *Experientia,* 28, 1225, 1972.

68. **Prentice, C. R. M., Hassanein, A. A., McNicol, G. P., and Douglas, A. S.,** Studies on blood coagulation, fibrinolysis and platelet function following exercise in normal and splenectomized people, *Br. J. Haematol.,* 23, 541, 1972.
69. **Ravry, M., Maldonado, N., Velez-Garcia, E., Montalvo, J., and Santiago, P. J.,** Serious infection after splenectomy for the staging of Hodgkin's disease, *Ann. Intern. Med.,* 77, 11, 1972.
70. **Levin, M. L.,** Penicillin after splenectomy? *Ann. Intern. Med.,* 77, 1002, 1972.
71. **Lennert, K. A.,** Indikationen zur splenektomie im kindesalter, *Z. Kinderchir.,* 11, 297, 1972.
72. **Yale, C. E. and Crummy, A. B.,** Splenic vein thrombosis and bleeding esophageal varices, *JAMA,* 217, 317, 1971.
73. **Donaldson, S. S., More, M. R., Rosenberg, S. A., and Vosti, K. L.,** Characterization of postsplenectomy bacteremia among patients with and without lymphoma, *N. Engl. J. Med.,* 287, 69, 1972.
74. **Lammi, A. T. and Lovric, A.,** Idiopathic thrombocytopenic purpura: an epidemiologic study, *J. Pediatr.,* 83, 31, 1973.
75. **Schwarzenberg, L., Mathe, G., Pouillart, P., Weiner, R., Locour, J., Genin, J., Schneider, M., deVassal F., Hayat, M., Amiel, J. L., Schlumberger, J. R., Jasmin, C., and Rosenfeld, C.,** Hydroxyurea, leucophoresis, and splenectomy in chronic myeloid leukaemia at the problastic phase, *Br. Med. J.,* 1, 700, 1973.
76. **Johnston, R. B., Jr., Newman, S. L., and Struth, A. G.,** An abnormality of the alternate pathway of complement activiation in sickle-cell disease, *N. Engl. J. Med.,* 288, 803, 1973.
77. **Christensen, B. E.,** Erythrocyte pooling and sequestration in enlarged spleens, *Scand. J. Haematol.,* 10, 106, 1973.
78. **Opelz, G. and Terasaki, P. I.,** Effect of splenectomy on human renal transplants, *Transplantation,* 15, 605, 1973.
79. **Mo-Wah, C., and McFadzean, A. J. S.,** Post splenectomy fever. Trans. Royal Soc. Trop. Med. Hgy., 68, 437, 1975.

Chapter 5

SPLENIC ATROPHY AND FUNCTIONAL ASPLENIA

THE SMALL OR ATROPHIC SPLEEN

If we recognize that the normal spleen is of a general (but age- and sex-related) size, then the small spleen must arouse our interest both as to the mechanisms of production and any resultant functional changes. There are a number of known causes of a "small" or atrophic spleen. In some of these disorders, it is uncertain whether the spleen reaches a normal size and then involutes or whether there has been developmental failure.

1. Familial hypoplasia.[1]
2. In some cases of Fanconi's anemia.[8]
3. In sickle cell disease.[2]
4. Following thorotrast administration.[3]
5. Resulting from antineoplastic agents and radiation.[3]
6. In celiac disease.[4,5]
7. Accompanying dermatitis herpetiformis.[6]
8. In thrombocythemia.[7]
9. Possibly following steroid use.[9]
10. Accompanying pneumococcal infections.
11. Possibly following chronic blood removal.[10]
12. In marasmus.[13]

Familial hypoplasia of the spleen has been described.[1] Three children of a consanguinous marriage were affected (and had severe bacterial infections). The parents and two other siblings were not involved, as judged by apparently normal splenic uptake of ^{198}Au-colloid and ^{51}Cr-denatured red cells. The spleens in the affected children seemed to have red and white pulp but were quite small. Howell-Jolly and Heinz bodies were present in the peripheral blood. Antibodies were not produced against intravenously injected sheep erythrocytes.

In the genetically determined disease, Fanconi's anemia, there is a high incidence of quite small spleens.[8] Garriga and Crosby commented that this might be due to dystrophy of tissues with a mesenchymal origin. In sickle cell disease, the spleen is close to normal at birth and may even become enlarged in the first few years of life. Vascular blockade and infarction lead to a reduction in the size of the organ. In addition, there is often a more considerable loss of splenic ability to extract a radiocolloid from the bloodstream (functional asplenia).[2] The multiple infarcts of sickle cell disease can eventually result in a small and atrophic spleen with loss of nearly all splenic activities. Vascular blockade may also be the reason for the small spleen observed in thrombocythemia.[7]

Thorotrast administration can result in a reduction in spleen size, likely through the effects of chronic radiation (and this is discussed in the section of the effects of medication on the spleen). In the resultant spleen of small size, ability to accumulate a radioactive colloid may be lost.[3] This result can probably be related to reticuloendothelial blockade and to chronic radiation. Effects of radiation and antienoplastic in reducing splenic size and function[3] are described in other sections.

Splenic atrophy occurs in many cases of malabsorption. This is manifested by the peripheral appearance of Howell-Jolly bodies and by a decreased rate of clearance of ^{51}Cr-denatured erythrocytes (and a small or functionless organ on scan).[4,5] The mechanism of production is unknown. In dermatitis herpetiformis, with an enteropathy resembling celiac disease, splenic atrophy can occur.[6] Recently, three cases of ulcerative colitis and hyposplenism have been reported (presence of Howell-Jolly bodies and lack of splenic uptake of ^{51}Cr-heat-damaged red cells).[37]

The finding of a small spleen, after overwhelming infections (particularly pneumococcal invasion), raises multiple questions as to cause and effect. Perhaps the spleen represents an analogue (of organ destruction) to adrenal involvement in the Waterhouse-Friedricksen Syndrome. It might also be that splenic dysfunction occurs, and then overwhelming infection follows, due to the loss of splenic trapping.

Of great interest in the observation by de Langen that after rabbits are bled a small amount each day (for months), the spleen is found to be atrophic.[10] We have seen no further reports on this phenomenon. Perhaps when (as Crosby[11] suggested) the hemolytic function was not needed, the spleen became reduced in size. It is known that there can be a proliferative response of the reticuloendothelial systems of the liver and spleen in hemolysis.[12] Whether there is involution under reduced stress is still uncertain. When expressed in terms of percent of expected spleen weight for a particular crown/heel length, the spleen in children with marasmus was quite small.[13] Functional studies (in terms of radiocolloid uptake) have not been reported.

APPROACHES TO REDUCTION OF SPLENIC SIZE AND FUNCTION

In Chapter 4 we noted some of the alterations produced by removal of the spleen. Recognizing the variety of postsplenectomy complications, our attention must focus on alternatives to splenectomy. In essence, we are looking for techniques which will reduce splenic size and function, short of total removal of the organ. We will mention eight different approaches, which are in various stages of evaluation.

1. **Splenic artery ligation** – In man and dog, the splenic artery can be ligated without gross infarction of the organ. Haller and co-workers[14] have ligated the splenic artery and preserved the spleen, while employing a splenorenal anastomosis. However, they did not report on changes in the size of the spleen postoperatively. We have followed a patient with hypersplenism and Hodgkin's disease whose spleen could not be surgically removed because of the adherence of a tumor mass. Splenic artery ligation was followed by both a decrease in the size of the spleen and an alleviation of the hypersplenism.[15] We have since followed two additional cases. One, with hypersplenism and pancytopenia, is described in the section on myeloid metaplasia. The other patient also underwent splenic artery ligation successfully, with remission of hypersplenism. There are, however, two points that will have to be fully explored.

1. While the hypersplenism remits following splenic artery ligation, the underlying cause of the hypersplenism has not been attacked.

2. It is possible that the remaining circulation to the spleen will, at some later time, permit the hypersplenism to recur.

Splenic artery ligation must be viewed as a promising approach to hypersplenism, when pancytopenia or adherent tumor prevent splenectomy. After the hypersplenism has abated, a second operation might be indicated. Rather than ligate the splenic artery, it might be occluded by embolization via a catheter.[38,39] This approach avoids the use of foreign chemicals and deserves further evaluation. Use of vessel blockade by microspheres or electrocoagulation should also be considered.

2. **Chemical or physical alteration of splenic vessels** – If the splenic artery cannot be surgically interrupted, can it be effectively occluded by other techniques? Two early studies suggest that the answer might be affirmative. Viamonte and co-workers[16] occluded splenic artery flow for 30 hr (without adverse effects) by means of a balloon on the catheter. How long an occlusion would be needed to correct hypersplenism is unknown. Indeed, because of the collateral supply, additional blood vessels might have to be occluded in order to have a therapeutic effect. The feasibility of leaving a balloon in the artery has not been determined. Chemically obstructing the splenic artery is another alternative. Lowman and associates[17] have studied the ability of allylamine to produce intracranial vascular lesions when introduced into vessels. The allylamine molecule ($CH_2 = CH \cdot CH_2 \cdot NH_2$) is a singly unsaturated aliphatic amine. When applied to vessel walls, it causes a necrotizing arteritis. Studies are just beginning as to whether it will be an effective agent for occluding the splenic artery or smaller tributaries. The entire area of physical or chemical occlusion of the splenic artery is in need of intense investigation.

3. **Partial splenectomy** – If only a small quantity of splenic tissue can carry out essential activities, why not leave a small portion of the spleen behind during splenectomy? There has been no adequate study of partial splenectomy, although the procedure was first suggested about 50 years ago (deBoer and Downie[18] have referred to some of the literature). One problem has been local hemostasis. This can be overcome in the dog

by use of appropriate techniques,[18] but it is uncertain how successful the procedure would be with the human spleen.

4. **Induced splenosis** – The implanting of small amounts of splenic tissue in the abdomen (splenosis) can occur after surgery or apparently spontaneously (likely following splenic trauma). The splenic tissue that successfully implants appears capable of carrying out normal spleen activites (such as clearing Howell-Jolly bodies).[19] If the specific details of how much splenic tissue to implant and the most opportune sites are worked out (high yield of takes and low incidence of complications such as rupture or obstruction), then splenectomy and production of splenosis with small fragments of the patient's spleen might have merit (splenosis is discussed in another section).

5. **External radiation** – We have discussed external radiation of the spleen in a separate section. There has been understandable reluctance to use external radiation of the spleen in nonmalignant conditions. However, when the patient's condition makes splenectomy (for hypersplenism) unfeasible, external radiation might be considered. Sommer and Kontras,[20] for example, have reported on the successful treatment of hypersplenism in a 12-year-old girl with sickle cell disease by use of 1,150r. Potential damage to the kidney or other structures must be considered.

6. **Internal radiation** – Ariel and Padula[21] pointed out that surgical splenectomy carries a risk and that external radiation might irradiate the kidneys and lungs. In the treatment of Hodgkin's disease they therefore utilized ^{90}Y (T½ = 64 hr, 2.27 meV beta ray) microspheres, delivered by arterial catheter, to irradiate the spleen. The radiation dose was calculated to be about 50,000 rd when 50 to 100 mCi of ^{90}Y was employed. Ariel and Padula[21] reported that scans revealed a decrease in the size of the spleen after the internal radiation. We assume, since the spleens continued to have the ability to accumulate ^{99m}Tc-sulfur colloid, that they retained some of their functions. There might be variants on the delivery of therapeutic amounts of radioactive materials via the splenic artery. Gianturco and co-workers[22] injected powdered tantalum intravenously and noted uptake in the liver and spleen of animals. Slow direct injection into the splenic artery might be a technique for localizing the material (and its labeled analogue) almost exclusively in the spleen. Doppman and associates[23] utilized silicone rubber preparations for performing transcatheter embolization. It is possible that therapeutic quantities of radionuclides could be incorporated into the preparation and used for therapy of the overactive spleen.

7. **Intrasplenic injection** – Many materials, when injected directly into the spleen, rapidly pass through the circulation of the organ to the venous drainage and on to the liver. This is true for inert radioopaque agents and for most of the ^{133}Xe injected into the spleen. Roser and Ford[24] have reported, however, that ^{32}P colloidal chromic phosphate (^{32}P has a T½ of 14.3 days and a beta ray of 1.7 meV maximum), when injected directly into the spleen, is largely retained by that organ. ^{185}W, in the form of tungsten trioxide, also was retained by the spleen, following intrasplenic injection (^{185}W has a T½ of 75 days and a beta ray of 0.43 meV maximum). Both of these agents produced lymphocytopenia in the rat when introduced into their spleens. Furthermore, removal of the spleen, after production of lymphocytopenia by ^{185}W, resulted in the return of peripheral lymphocytes. This suggests that irradiation of circulating lymphocytes, by the radionuclide in the spleen, was the major cause of the depressed lymphocyte count. The immunological competence of rats with intrasplenic ^{185}W was much less than controls but more than that of splenectomized rats.[25] The procedure of intrasplenic injection of radionuclides deserves further study.

8. **Chemical splenectomy** – A very desirable solution to the problem of retaining part of the spleen, while destroying most of its function, would be a chemical whose effects could be titrated. Emulsions of fatty acid esters are known to be toxic when given systemically. A principal effect is damage to the spleen. Prosnitz and co-workers[26] have summarized the literature on the use of the fatty acid esters, particularly ethyl palmitate. They worked out a dosage schedule and showed that ethyl palmitate produced focal hemorrhagic lesions in the rodent spleen after a single dose. Repeated injections of ethyl palmitate resulted in an atrophic spleen. As the chemically affected spleen changes in size, so does its ability to carry out various functions. For example, when the related compound ethyl stearate is used in mice, there is apparently diminished ability of the spleen to respond to injected heterologous erythrocytes.[27] These studies have to be systema-

tized and then developed to a useful state in dogs, monkeys, and, finally, man. Chemical splenectomy is a desirable, and perhaps reachable, goal.

FUNCTIONAL ASPLENIA

The concept of a spleen being anatomically present, but functionally absent, was first put forth in 1969. The evidence came from several lines, but the final documentation depended on radioisotopic techniques (lack of uptake of radiocolloid). There are many indications of splenic hypofunction in sickle cell anemia. Principal among these is the finding of Howell-Jolly bodies (intraerythrocyte inclusions) in the peripheral blood. The presence of these bodies had been considered as due to the outpouring of immature red cells from the base marrow into the circulation. Another explanation was thought to be possible, namely, that the spleen in most children with sickle cell anemia was not functioning.

The initial study covered 12 children (ages of 0.7 to 14 years) who had a hemoglobin S-F pattern and (in 11 of the 12), Howell-Jolly bodies on blood smears treated with Wright's stain. Following intravenous injection of ^{99m}Tc-sulfur colloid (particle size about 1 μm; about 10 μCi/kg body weight), anterior and posterior spleen and liver scans were attempted. In nine of the children there was a palpable spleen, and in eight, radiographic evidence of splenomegaly was present. Yet despite the physical presence of the organ, in 11 of the 12 children, we could not demonstrate any appreciable uptake of the radiocolloid.[28] As our thinking about functional asplenia evolved, we were able to set up necessary requirements for its diagnosis.

1. The spleen had to be physically present (demonstrated by palpation, by radiographic means, or by blood pool scans).
2. The batch of radioactive colloid used had to be well accumulated by a normal spleen. That is, at least one individual with a normally functioning spleen had to receive the same test batch to demonstrate that the radiocolloid was behaving properly.
3. A third aspect, of course, is that there had to be evidence of hyposplenism, particularly the presence of Howell-Jolly bodies.

A number of points were immediately raised.

1. At what age did functional asplenia arise in sickle cell anemia?
2. Was the disorder reversible?
3. Were all splenic functions lost, or was there a disassociation of activities?
4. Did functional asplenia occur in other diseases?

The answer to the first question has become clear. The spleen in sickle cell disease is functional at birth. Ability to accumulate ^{99m}Tc-sulfur colloid is lost months to years following birth. A close correlation exists between the ability of the spleen to accumulate radioactive colloid and the level of circulating hemoglobin F. When the production of hemoglobin F is lost, circulating Hb S-F is replaced by S-S. With this change, the spleen of many of the affected youngsters begins to lose the ability to take up the radiocolloid.

The actual mechanism of production of functional asplenia cannot be the multiple infarcts produced by the occasionally occluded circulation of the spleen. The reason for this is that functional asplenia occurs in many cases with a massively enlarged spleen, as well as in those which are contracted due to infarction and scarring. In some cases of functional asplenia, due to hemoglobin S-S in young children, a transient reversal of the lack of uptake of ^{99m}Tc-sulfur colloid can be brought about by transfusion of whole (nonsickle) blood.[29,30] Our observations on this can be summarized as follows:

1. The reversal does not occur after transfusion of normal whole plasma, suggesting that a circulating opsonin is not deficient. However, erythrocytes can adsorb many foreign proteins, and this point should not be considered entirely settled.
2. Children with specific protein deficiencies (hemophilia, agamma globulinemia, and others) do not have functional asplenia. Any opsonin required can not yet be related to a major protein (but may be a glycoprotein).[40] This discussion is continued in a later chapter.
3. Transfusion of nonsickle whole blood does transiently reverse the functional asplenia in some cases. This suggests a washing away of obstructed cells from the sinusoids. The effect lasts while the hemoglobin S level is depressed.

The third point, as to whether all splenic activities are lost, cannot be answered with certainty. We know that the spleen affected by functional asplenia can not pit erythrocytes of their inclusions. In addition, these youngsters do not form antibodies to injected foreign red cells. They have not been challenged, however, by radiocolloids of different particle sizes (particularly because of the inability to make uniformly sized sterile and pyrogen-free particles of a variety of sizes and tagged with short-lived radionuclides). The size of the spleen that we see on a ^{99m}Tc-sulfur colloid scan is the functional size of the organ.[31] We do not yet know whether this functional size (for radiocolloid uptake) corresponds to the size for other functions, or whether there is a disassociation of activities. Since all cases of splenic inability to accumulate radioactive colloid are associated with circulating Howell-Jolly bodies, we can ask if the reverse is also true (that is, do circulating Howell–Jolly bodies always denote an inability of the spleen to take up radioactive colloid?). The answer to this is negative. We have described patients who, after hematological stress, showed numerous Howell-Jolly bodies but still had the ability to accumulate radioactive colloid in the spleen.[36] Since this may represent an inability of the spleen to keep up with a tremendous load of Howell-Jolly bodies, the term "overload syndrome" was suggested.

Functional asplenia has been identified in other diseases (for example, in thorotrast intoxication)[32] and likely occurs in some cases of celiac disease (see preceding section). Principles for the production and reversal of functional asplenia still have to be worked out. There are other aspects of the disorder that will deserve intensive study. For example, a transient hyposplenia has been demonstrated in some cases of cyanotic congenital heart disease.[33] Again the stresses triggering the disorder can only be vaguely appreciated at this time. We have also described an interesting case of persistent neutrophilic leukocytosis with functional asplenia.[34] Perhaps the splenic dysfunction permitted elevated neutrophil levels. Finally, functional asplenia as discussed above was an isolated absence of reticuloendothelial function in the spleen, while the liver (and presumably other reticuloendothelial sites) was grossly normal. We have observed a case of familial erythrophagocytic lymphohistiocytosis[35] in which nearly all reticuloendothelial function was lost. This was a generalized disorder, with the spleen but one of the sites of the abnormality. The significance of functional asplenia lies not only in the explanation of circulating Howell-Jolly bodies but also in the association with the apparent loss of ability to filter out bacteria. The resultant occasionally overwhelming infection is dealt with in Chapter 4.

REFERENCES

1. **Kevy, S. V., Tefft, M., Vawter, G. F., and Rosen, F. S.,** Hereditary splenic hypoplasia, *Pediatrics,* 42, 752, 1968.
2. **Pearson, H. A., Spencer, R. P., and Cornelius, E. A.,** Functional asplenia in sickle cell anemia, *N. Engl. J. Med.,* 281, 923, 1969.
3. **Spencer, R. P., Pearson, H. A., and Binder, H. A.,** Identification of cases of "acquired" functional asplenia, *J. Nucl. Med.,* 11, 763, 1970.
4. **Ferguson, A., Hutton, M. M., Maxwell, J. D., and Murray, D.,** Adult coeliac disease in hyposplenic patients, *Lancet,* 1, 163, 1970.
5. **Marsh, G. W. and Stewart, J. S.,** Splenic function in adult coeliac disease, *Br. J. Haematol.,* 19, 445, 1970.
6. **Pettit, J. E., Hoffbrand, A. V., Seah, P. P., and Fry, L.,** Splenic atrophy in dermatitis herpetiformis, *Br. Med. J.,* 2, 438, 1972.
7. **Marsh, G. W., Lewis, S. M., and Szur, L.,** The use of ^{51}Cr-labelled heat-damaged red cells to study splenic function. II. Splenic atrophy in thrombocythaemia, *Br. J. Haematol.,* 12, 167, 1966.
8. **Garriga, S. and Crosby, W. H.,** The incidence of leukemia in families of patients with hypoplasia of the marrow, *Blood,* 14, 1008, 1959.
9. **Arroyo, H. and Aubert, L.,** Hypotrophie splenique au cours de la polyarthrite rhumatoide, *Nouv. Presse Med.,* 1, 876, 1972.
10. **de Langen, C. D.,** Function of the spleen and blood, *Acta Med. Scand.,* 115, 271, 1943.

11. **Crosby, W. H.**, Normal functions of the spleen relative to red blood cells: a review, *Blood,* 14, 399, 1959.
12. **Jandl, J. H., Files, N. M., Barnett, S. B., and McDonald, R. A.**, Proliferative response of the spleen and liver to hemolysis, *J. Exp. Med.,* 122, 299, 1965.
13. **Smythe, P. M., Schonland, M., Brereton-Stiles, G. G., Coovadia, H. M., Grace, H. J., Loening, W. E. K., Mafoyane A., Parent, M. A., and Vos., G. H.**, Thymolymphatic deficiency and depression of cell-mediated immunity in protein-calorie malnutrition, *Lancet,* 2, 939, 1971.
14. **Haller, J. D., Glick, H., Hallman, G. L., and Cooley, D. A.**, Portal decompression by side-to-side splenorenal venous anastomosis, *Arch. Surg.,* 102, 316, 1971.
15. **Nuland, S. B., Cornelius, E. A., and Spencer, R. P.**, Scan evidence of organ involution and improvement of hypersplenism in Hodgkin's disease following splenic artery ligation, *J. Nucl. Med.,* 11, 693, 1970.
16. **Viamonte, M., Jr., Danner, P., Warren, W. D., and Fomon, J.**, A new technique for the assessment of hyperkinetic portal hypertension, *Radiology,* 96, 539, 1970.
17. **Lowman, R. M., Solitaire, G. B., and McAllister, W. B.**, Experimental production of intracranial vascular lesions. Allylamine-induced vascular lesions of the brain and intracranial infarction, *Acta Radiol. (Diagn.),* 9, 383, 1969.
18. **deBoer, J. and Downie, H. G.**, Partial splenectomy in dogs: an experimental tool for studies of the spleen, *Can. J. Physiol. Pharmacol.,* 49, 1110, 1971.
19. **Widmann, W. D., Laubscher, F. A., Davidson, S. J., and Grenoble, R. A.**, Effects of splenectomy and splenosis on the blood and platelet count and red cell morphology, *Milit. Med.,* 136, 15, 1971.
20. **Sommer, A. and Kontras, S. B.**, Splenomegaly with hypersplenism in sickle cell anemia treated by radiation – case report, *Pediatrics,* 48, 457, 1972.
21. **Ariel, I. M. and Padula, G.**, Are laprotomy and splenectomy necessary for patients with Hodgkin's disease? *J. Nucl. Med.,* 12, 412, 1971.
22. **Gianturco, C., Ruskin, B., Steggerda, F. R., and Takeuchi, T.**, A feasibility study of splenohepatography with tantalum metal and tantalum peroxide, *Radiology,* 102, 195, 1972.
23. **Doppman, J. L., Zapol, W., and Pierce, J.**, Transcatheter emoblization with a silicone rubber preparation: experimental observations, *Invest. Radiol.,* 6, 304, 1971.
24. **Roser, B. and Ford, W. L.**, Prolonged lymphocytopenia in the rat. The depletion of blood and thoracic duct lymphocyte populations following injection of β-emitting colloids into the spleen or lymph nodes, *Aust. J. Exp. Biol. Med. Sci.,* 50, 165, 1972.
25. **Roser, B. and Ford, W. L.**, Prolonged lymphocytopenia in the rat. The immunological consequences of lymphocyte depletion following injection of ^{185}W tungsten trioxide into the spleen or lymph nodes, *Aust. J. Exp. Biol. Med. Sci.,* 50, 185, 1972.
26. **Prosnitz, L., Kawasaki, S.**, Cohen, G. S., **Dineen, J. L., Perille, P. E., and Finch, S. C.**, Ethyl palmitate induced splenic destruction, *J. Reticuloendothel. Soc.,* 6, 487, 1969.
27. **Melnick, H. D. and Friedman, H.**, The immunosuppressive effect of RES "blockade" with ethyl stearate emulsion on cellular formation of antibody to sheep erythrocytes, *Proc. Soc. Exp. Biol. Med.,* 133, 423, 1970.
28. **Pearson, H. A., Spencer, R. P., and Cornelius, E. A.**, Functional asplenia in sickle-cell anemia, *N. Engl. J. Med.,* 281, 923, 1969.
29. **Pearson, H. A., Spencer, R. P., Cornelius, E. A., Treves, S. and Lange, R. C.**, Functional asplenia in sickle-cell anemia – a reversible defect, *J. Nucl. Med.,* 11, 349, 1970.
30. **Pearson, H. A., Cornelius, E. A., Schwartz, A. D., Zelson, J. R., Wolfson, S. L., and Spencer, R. P.**, Transfusion reversible functional asplenia in young children with sickle cell disease, *N. Engl. J. Med.,* 283, 334, 1970.
31. **Spencer, R. P.**, Estimation of functional size of the spleen, *J. Nucl. Med.,* 11, 616, 1970.
32. **Spencer, R. P., Pearson, H. A., and Binder, H. A.**, Identification of cases of "acquired" functional asplenia, *J. Nucl. Med.,* 11, 763, 1970.
33. **Pearson, H. A., Schiebler, G. L., and Spencer, R. P.**, Functional hyposplenia in cyanotic congenital heart disease, *Pediatrics,* 48, 277, 1971.
34. **Spencer, R. P., McPhedran, P., Finch, S. C., and Morgan, W. S.**, Persistent neutrophilic leukocytosis associated with idiopathic functional asplenia, *J. Nucl. Med.,* 15, 224, 1971.
35. **O'Brien, R. T., Schwartz, A. D., Pearson, H. A., and Spencer, R. P.**, Reticuloendothelial failure in familial erythrophagocytic lymphohistocytosis, *Pediatrics,* 81, 543, 1972.
36. **Spencer, R. P. and Pearson, H. A.**, Splenic radiocolloid uptake in the presence of circulating Howell-Jolly bodies, *J. Nucl. Med.,*15, 294, 1974.
37. **Ryan, F. P., Smart, R. C., Preston, F. E., and Holdsworth, C. D.**, Hyposplenism in ulcerated colitis. *Lancet,* 2, 318, 1974.
38. **Maddison, F. E.**, Embolic therapy of hypersplenism, *Invest. Radiol.,* 8, 280, 1973.
39. **Tadavarthy, S. M., Knight, L., Ovitt, T. W., Snyder, C., and Amplatz, C.**, Therapeutic transcatheter arterial embolization, *Radiology,* 111, 13, 1974.
40. **van Oss, C. J., Gillman, C. F., Bronson, P. M., and Border, J. R.**, Opsonic properties of human serum alpha-2 HS glycoprotein, *Immunol. Commun.,* 3, 329, 1974.

Chapter 6

MALARIA, BARTONELLOSIS, AND BABESIOSIS

The two infections malaria and bartonellosis are considered together because of the similar properties of intraerythrocytic infestation and splenomegaly. Indeed, once the splenic processing of the infected erythrocytes is understood, we will have a clearer idea of the overall functioning of the organ.

BARTONELLOSIS

Bartonellosis, spread by the sand fly, is due to a motile, pleomorphic bacillus, termed *Bartonella bacilliformis*. The Gram-negative organism causes a disease which is limited to parts of the Andes mountains in South America. Apparently related organisms can produce illness in Southeast Asia.[1] After an incubation period of about 3 weeks, the disease begins with fever and pain. Even in the early phase of the disorder, blood cultures are positive. After this stage, two clinical forms of illness develop (Oroya fever or verruga peruana). Their interrelationship was proven by the self-experimentation of Daniel Carrion.[2] In the Oroya fever type, 90% of the erythrocytes may be invaded by *Bartonella bacilliformis* organisms. Fever, weakness, and pallor result from massive destruction of red cells by the parasites. The erythrocyte count can fall by nearly one million cells per mm^3 for 3 or 4 days. Smears of peripheral blood reveal multiple changes. Howell-Jolly bodies appear in erythrocytes, suggesting a functional inability of the spleen to "pluck" these inclusions from the red blood cells. Nucleated erythrocytes, stippled red cells, Cabot rings, and a leukocytosis also can be noted. Bacilli occur in monocytes and also within fixed cells of the reticuloendothelial system. The spleen may show colonylike masses of the *Bartonella* organism,[3] perhaps garnered from trapped erythrocytes. Electron microscopic studies have been reported to show that in three cases (with over 70% of the erythrocytes parasitized), the bartonellosis organism was indenting (or in) the erythrocyte and was not superfically on its surface.[4]

Whether splenic failure is partially responsible for the secondary infections that occur in the course of bartonellosis is uncertain at present. A superimposed infection with *Salmonella* is frequently associated with a fatal outcome. While splenomegaly is usually described in bartonellosis, the autopsy on Daniel Carrion had been reported as showing a spleen diminished in size.[2] This might represent the final stage of the disease, with the added complications of weight loss, dehydration, and secondary infections. The ability of the spleen to accumulate radiolabeled colloid during the course of bartonellosis has not been evaluated. Animal models may have use in defining some of these relationships. Related organisms (for example, *Haemobartonella muris*, which infects rats) have been investigated. Erythrocytes from splenectomized and infected rats were collected (with red cell infestation in four groups averaging 8%, 26%, 51%, and 70%). The cells were tagged with ^{51}Cr and injected into recipient rats. Loss of ^{51}Cr from the circulation was proportional to the degree of parasitemia only during the first 24 hr.[5] It is likely that not all parasitized erythrocytes are recognized as being irreversibly damaged. Finch and Jonas[34] have demonstrated activation of latent *Hemobartonella muris* infection in rats after an injection of ethyl palmitate (which tends to ablate the spleen). In some splenectomized animals, anemia may develop due to the unmasking of a *Bartonella* infection.[37]

MALARIA

Although accurate statistics are difficult to obtain, it is likely that malaria is the commonest cause of splenomegaly in the world. In a village in Vietnam, 70 to 90% of children and adolescents had splenomegaly; many had demonstrable malarial infections.[29] Blaustein[22] has stated that malaria is the commonest cause of spontaneous rupture of the spleen. Croft and Dawson[23] have reported spontaneous subcapsular hematoma in malaria. The causative organisms are four species of the protozoan genus *Plasmodium* (*P. vivax, P. malariae, P. falciparum, P. ovale*). After spreading to man by the mosquito, the first stage of infection is development of the parasite in the liver ("exoerythrocytic"). Erythrocyte infestation follows, and the parasites asexually reproduce within circulating red cells (Figure 1). So-called

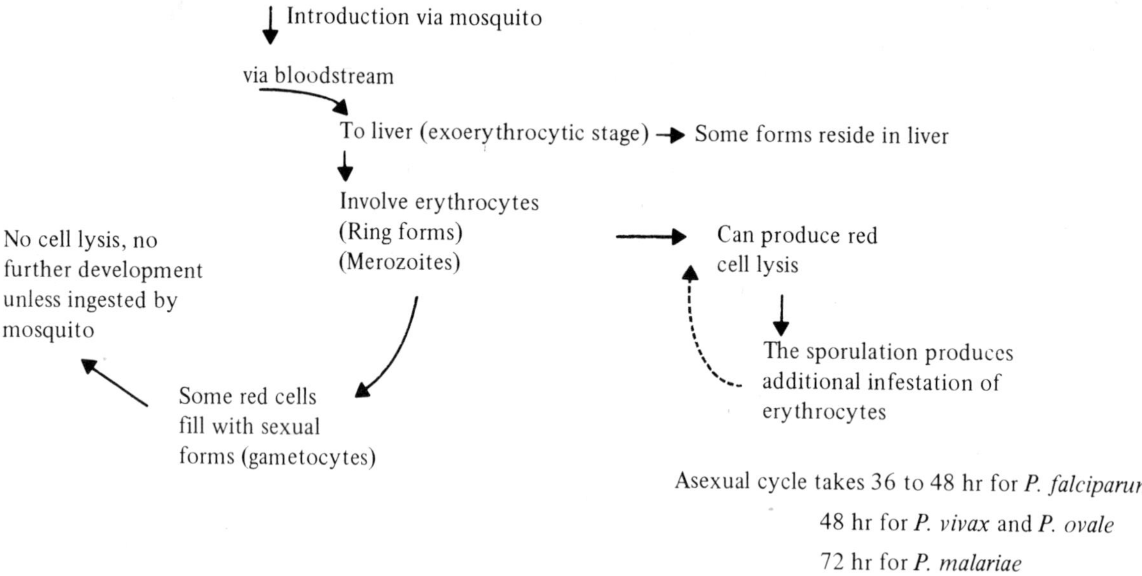

FIGURE 1. Cycle of the malaria parasites.

ring forms of the parasite in the erythrocytes are followed by daughter forms or merozoites. The process of "sporulation" (erythrocyte rupture with relase of parasites) frees organisms to infect other erythrocytes. Ability to parasitize red cells varies with the organism. *P. vivax* and *P. ovale* infest immature erythrocytes, while *P. malariae* apparently only attacks senescent red blood cells. These three malaria parasites hence only involve about 2% of the circulating erythrocytes (recall that in severe bartonellosis, nearly all erythrocytes may be attacked). The protozoan *P. falciparum* can attack erythrocytes, regardless of the age of the red cell. With *P. falciparum* infestation, the fraction of cells parasitized can reach high levels. At least with *P. vivax*, human platelets can be infested.[39]

Of great interest is the fact that hemoglobin S may limit the extent of parasitemia in malaria, and individuals with sickle cell trait may be relatively protected against the lethal effects of cerebral malaria and blackwater fever during childhood.[35] That is, erythrocytes containing hemoglobin S may be less susceptible to invasion by the genus *Plasmodium*. The specific role played by other hemoglobin variants has still to be defined. However, glucose-6-phosphate dehydrogenase deficiency and thalassemia have also been speculated to confer increased resistance to severe malaria. In a man with hereditary spherocytosis, vivax malaria was associated with severe anemia. After splenectomy, a relapse of the malaria did not have an accompanying marked anemia.[36] Perhaps in this instance, the effects of spherocytosis and malaria had been additive in producing the anemia (and the contribution of the spherocytosis was blunted by splenectomy).

In addition to erythrocyte destruction by the sporulation event ("intravascular hemolysis"), some infected red cells are removed from the circulation by phagocytosis in the liver and spleen ("erythrophagocytosis").[38] The spleen of monkeys with *P. knowlesi* malaria was capable of "pitting" (removing or plucking out) the parasite from red blood cells. Erythrocytes could be seen, on electron micrographs, which were seemingly split. Part of the cell, containing the malaria parasite, was trapped within the splenic pulp, while the other portion of the cell had passed into the sinusoid. These changes may be the basis for the presence of spherocytes in the circulatory system. Parasited red cells were also reported to be possibly hemolyzed extracellularly in the spleen. How the spleen recognizes infested erythrocytes is not known. Balcerzak and associates[26] noted that *P. falciparum*-infested red cells had surface defects, which may have been the "marker" to the spleen of cell damage. Other cells, without parasites, also had surface defects (suggesting that they previously held parasites).

The spleen can be quite large in malaria, and Gosio[7] has presented a detailed discussion of clinically outlining the organ. Verdon and co-workers[21] noted that in patients with malaria, the spleen accumulated a portion of intravenously injected radiocolloidal gold (^{198}Au). Spleen scans with radiocolloid can therefore presumably be used in following changes in the size of the organ in malaria. Some patients with malaria have leukopenia.[30] Whether the spleen is excessively trapping white blood cells is unclear.

Devakul and co-workers[8] studied male Thai patients with malaria. One of the tools employed was ^{59}Fe, which was administered intravenously. Surface counts were obtained over the liver, spleen, and bone marrow. In five of the ten cases, splenic radioactivity increased as soon as parasites were detected in circulating erythrocytes. In five cases, increased hepatic radioactivity occurred during the decrease in hemoglobin concentration (and three showed increased splenic radioactivity at this time). Radioactive organ counts, however, did not correlate with the degree of parasitemia.

Species-specific antibodies (IgG and IgM) occur in malaria, perhaps related to the hepatic involvement rather than as a response to the intraerythrocytic infestation. The general class of IgG antibodies can cross the placenta and might account for the paucity of cases of malaria in infants. Malarial infestation and immunoglobulins may also have a relationship to Burkitt lymphoma.[9] Other factors may also complicate the hematologic picture in malarial infestation. For example, folic acid deficiency can occur in malaria.[10]

Splenomegaly is frequent in tropical regions, and there are many causes of this (a discussion has been presented by Basu and Aikat).[11] A significant number of patients in the tropics, having chronic splenomegaly, but without well-identifiable causes ("tropical splenomegaly"), responded to antimalarial drugs.[12] The cases of tropical splenomegaly[13] or "big spleen disease"[14] are distributed in regions where malaria is endemic. The malarial antibody level is usually elevated, but circulating parasites cannot be found. In some cases, antimalarial therapy may have destroyed the parasites. In New Guinea, individuals with tropical splenomegaly had a low primary antibody response, perhaps related to the demands for antibody to malarial organisms.[28] The almost complete absence of the disease in Caucasians might be related to exposure rate or use of medications.[15] Sagoe has pointed out that patients with splenomegaly who did respond to an antimalarial (proguanil®) always had high levels of IgM before treatment, and the levels fell during treatment.[12] The relationship between IgM and spleen size is shown in Table 1. The responsive patients also had a normal response of their lymphocytes to the mitogen phytohemagglutinin. Patients not responding to proguanil had normal or low IgM values and low phytohemagglutin

TABLE 1

Relationship Between Spleen Size and the IgM Level

	Blood level of IgM, mg/100 ml	Estimated spleen length, cm*
Normal Nigerians (males)	189	–
Patients with no response to proguanil	81	–
Patients responding to proguanil	1,799	32
	553	22
	308	12

*Original values given by Sagoe[12] were as a percent of initially measured value. This was in terms of distance below the costal margin. Spleen sizes were reported as 10 to 30 cm (hence, a reasonable mean was 20 cm) below the ribs. The size of the spleen above the costal margin can be assumed to be about 12 cm, hence the figures in the last column. Normal subjects in the study did not have splenomegaly.

response. Perhaps this is related to the state of immunosuppression which can occur in malaria.[24] Part of the defect seems to be in antigen processing by macrophases, while uptake of ^{51}Cr-foreign red cells appears to be normal. Stiffel and coworkers[25] noted that plasmodium infection in nonvaccinated rats was worsened by splenectomy; liver macrophage activity was not affected by removal of the spleen.

Liver biopsy of individuals with tropical splenomegaly reveals infiltration of the sinusoids by lymphocytes. The spleen can be enormous, but there are no specific changes on the splenoportogram. The disease might represent a hyperimmune response to the malarial parasite (and the elevated immune globulins are perhaps consistent with this view). However, no generalized disorder of the reticuloendothelial systems has been noted in these patients, aside from a slight macroglobulinemia.[16] The basic stimulus to reticuloendothelial hypertrophy apparently persists (and splenomegaly can recur when patients who have been on antimalarials fail to take their medication).[40] Splenectomy in the tropical splenomegaly syndrome is followed by relief of the symptoms of hypersplenism. Despite this, Kupffer cell hyperplasia and hepatic sinusoidal infiltration by lymphocytes continue.[27]

The large size of the spleen in tropical splenomegaly and its progressive decrease that follows institution of antimalarial therapy allow approximations to be made as to the rate of change of splenic length or volume. Using literature data,[17] we have calculated that, in one series of cases, nearly 120 days were required to reduce the spleen to half of its original volume.[118]

BABESIOSIS

This disorder must be considered with bartonellosis and malaria since the parasites are also intraerythrocytic. There is a major difference, however. Of the four cases of *Babesia* infection reported in man, three occurred in individuals who had been splenectomized (and in the fourth patient, there was no splenomegaly).[19] *Babesia*, or piroplasmas, are protozoans which are transmitted by ticks. Like the *Plasmodiae*, the order to which Babesia belongs also alternates sexual and asexual cycles of development. Domestic animals and rodents can be infected by the organisms,[32] but man is a rare host. Within erythrocytes, *Babesia* resemble *P. falciparum* infestation. The number of infested red cells is about 1%; this is low as compared to some of the malarias. Within some involved erythrocytes, tetrad forms help to denote that the organisms are *Babesia*. Rodents and splenectomized monkeys can be used to grow the organisms from infested blood. In the one reported case (in a 59-year-old woman) without prior splenectomy, there was apparently repeated contact with ticks, brought in with rodents caught by a dog.[19] In this case, the spleen was reported to be of normal size by X-ray and to be functioning on a radioisotope scan[19] (but the scanning agent was not discussed, and no mention was made of whether Howell-Jolly bodies were present in circulating erythrocytes). The paucity of cases in man leaves many questions unanswered. Bovine infection with *Babesia major* has been studied,[20] and transmission through splenectomized calves has been reported to result in enhanced virulence of the organism.

Other intraerythrocytic parasites have also been reported in animals,[33] and the role of the spleen in removing these organisms has still to be determined.

REFERENCES

1. **Whitaker, J., Fort, E., Weinman, D., Tamastit, P., and Panas-Ampol, K.,** Acute febrile anemia associated with Bartonella-like erythrocytic structures, *Nature,* 212, 855, 1966.
2. **Schultz, M. G.,** Daniel Carrion's experiment, *N. Engl. J. Med.,* 278, 1323, 1968.
3. **Ricketts, W. E.,** Clinical manifestations of Carrion's disease, *Arch. Int. Med.,* 84, 751, 1949.
4. **Cuadra, M. and Takana, J.,** The relationship of *Bartonella bacilliformis* to the red blood cell as revealed by electron microscopy, *Blood,* 33, 708, 1969.
5. **Kreier, J. P. and Hall, L.,** The relationship of parasitemia to the life span of erythrocytes of rats infected with *Haemobartonella muris, J. Infect. Dis.,* 118, 443, 1968.
6. **Schnitzer, B., Sodeman, T., Mead, M. L., and Contacos, P. G.,** Pitting function of the spleen in malaria: ultrastructural observations, *Science,* 177, 175, 1972.

7. **Gosio, R.,** *La Milza Malarica,* edizione Italiane, Roma, Arti Grafiche Panetto & Petrelli, Spoletto, 1944, 502.
8. **Devakul, K., Harinasuta, T., and Kanakakorn, K.,** Erythrocyte destruction in *Plasmodium falciparum* malaria: an investigation of intravascular haemolysis, *Ann. Trop. Med. Parsitol.,* 63, 317, 1969.
9. Editorial, Burkitt lymphoma and malaria, *Lancet,* II, 300, 1970.
10. **Strickland, G. T. and Kostinas, J. E.,** Folic acid deficiency complicating malaria, *Am. J. Trop. Med.,* 19, 910, 1970.
11. **Basu, A. K. and Aikat, B. K.,** *Tropical Splenomegaly,* Butterworths, London, 1963, 195.
12. **Sagoe, A. S.,** Tropical splenomegaly syndrome: long term proguanil therapy correlated with spleen size, serum IgM, and lymphocyte transformation, *Br. Med. J.,* 3, 378, 1970.
13. **Marsden, P. D. and Hamilton, P. J. S.,** Splenomegaly in the tropics, *Br. Med. J.,* 1, 99, 1969.
14. **Gelfand, M.,** Big spleen disease: a probable case from Rhodesia, *J. Trop. Med. Hyg.,* 73, 71, 1972.
15. **Lowenthal, M. N. and Hutt, M. S. R.,** Tropical splenomegaly syndrome in a Caucasian in Africa, *Br. Med. J.,* 3, 262, 1970.
16. **Ziegler, J. L., Cohen, M. H., and Hutt, M. S. R.,** Immunological studies in tropical splenomegaly syndrome in Uganda, *Br. Med. J.,* 4, 15, 1969.
17. **Stuiver, P. C., Ziegler, J. L., Wood, J. B., Morrow, R. H., and Hutt, M. S. R.,** Clinical trial of malaria prophylaxis in tropical splenomegaly syndrome, *Br. Med. J.,* 1, 426, 1971.
18. **Spencer, R. P., Lange, R. C., Schwartz, A. D., and Pearson, H. A.,** Radioisotopic studies of changes in splenic size in response to epinephrine and other stimuli, *J. Nucl. Med.,* 13, 211, 1972.
19. **Western, K. A., Benson, G. D., Gleason, N. N., Healy, G. R., and Schultz, M. G.,** Babesiosis in a Massachusetts resident, *N. Engl. J. Med.,* 283, 854, 1970.
20. **Brocklesby, D. W., Purnell, R. E., and Sellwood, S. A.,** The effect of irradiation on intraerythrocytic stages of *Babesia major, Br. Vet. J.,* 128, iii, 1972.
21. **Verdon, T. A., Jr., Barrett, O., Jr., and Panettiere, F.,** Significance of spleen pickup of radioactive gold-198, *J. Nucl. Med.,* 8, 402, 1967.
22. **Blaustein, A.,** *The Spleen,* McGraw-Hill, New York, 1963, 51.
23. **Croft, D. N. and Dawson, J. L.,** Spontaneous subcapsular splenic haematoma in acute malaria, *Postgrad. Med. J.,* 38, 123, 1962.
24. **Loose, L. D., Cook, J. A., and DiLuzio, N. R.,** Role of macrophages in malaria induced immunosuppression, *Physiologist,* 15, 202, 1972.
25. **Stiffel, C., Mouton, D., Decreusefond, C., Bouthillier, Y., Biozzi, G., Pennachio, A. E., Bucci A., Verolini F., and Corradetti, A.,** Influence de la splenectomie sur l'immunite specifique et asepecifique (activite phagocytaire des macrophages) au cours de l'infection paludeene du rat par "Plasmodium berghei," *Ann. Inst. Pasteur,* 123, 55, 1972.
26. **Balcerzak, S. P., Arnold, J. D., and Martin, D. C.,** Anatomy of red cell damage by *Plasmodium falciparum* in man, *Blood,* 40, 98, 1972.
27. **Hamilton, P. J. S., Stuiver, P. C., and Ziegler, J. L.,** Splenectomy in tropical splenomegaly syndrome – a five year follow-up, *J. Trop. Med.,* 74, 230, 1971.
28. **Crane, G. G., Rowley, M. J., Warburton, M. F., and MacKay, I. R.,** Humoral immune responses in the tropical-splenomegaly syndrome in New Guinea, *Clin. Sci.,* 43, 869, 1972.
29. **Colwell, E. J., Legters, L. J., and Fife, E. H., Jr.,** Splenomegaly and malaria in the central highlands of South Vietnam, Am. J. Trop. Med., *Hygiene,* 19, 741, 1970.
30. **Reiley, C. G. and Barrett, O., Jr.,** Leukocyte response in acute malaria, *Am. J. Med. Sci.,* 262, 153, 1971.
31. **Crane, G. G. and Pryor, D. S.,** Malaria and the tropical splenomegaly syndrome in New Guinea, *Trans. R. Soc. Trop. Med. Hyg.,* 65, 315, 1971.
32. **Wright, I. G.,** Studies on the pathogenesis of *Babesia argentina* and *Babesia bigemina* infections in splenectomized calves, *Z. Parasitenk.,* 39, 85, 1972.
33. **Babudieri, B.,** Mycoplasma-like organism, parasite of red blood cells of an amphibian, Hydromantes (*Spelerpes fuscus*), *Infect. Immunol.,* 6, 77, 1972.
34. **Finch, S. C. and Jonas, A. M.,** Ethyl palmitate-induced Bartonellosis as an index of functional splenic ablation, *J. Reticuloendothel. Soc.,* 13, 20, 1973.
35. **Lehman, H. and Raper, A. B.,** Maintenance of high sickling rate in an African community. *Br. Med. J.,* 2, 333, 1956.
36. **Littman, E.,** Splenectomy in hereditary spherocytosis: effect on course of relapsing vivax malaria, *Am. J. Med. Sci.,* 267, 53, 1974.
37. **Galarza, A., Nieto, M., and Carriazo, D.,** Effect of splenectomy on circulating blood. II. Haemolytic anaemia produced by splenectomy, *Rev. Esp. Fisiol.,* 29, 5, 1973.
38. **Schnitzer, B., Sodeman, T. M., Mead, M. L., and Contacos, P. G.,** An ultrastructural study of the red pulp of the spleen in malaria, *Blood,* 41, 207, 1973.
39. **Fajardo, L. F. and Tallent, C.,** Malarial parasites within human platelets, *JAMA,* 229, 1205, 1974.
40. **David-West, A. S.,** Relapses after withdrawal of proguanil treatment in tropical splenomegaly syndrome, *Br. Med. J.,* 3, 499, 1974.

Chapter 7

SPLENIC VASCULAR SYSTEM AND PORTAL HYPERTENSION

VENOUS SYSTEM

Originating from several contributing vessels from the hilus of the spleen, the splenic vein courses close to and below the artery. The vein passes from the spleen to a few centimeters prior to the aorta. Here it joins the superior mesenteric vein to form the portal vein. The splenic vein itself has small contributions from the stomach (left gastroepiploic and short gastric veins) and from the gut (inferior mesenteric vein). These contributors can be of importance in the shunting of blood around an obstructed splenic vein.

Drainage of the splenic vein is, of course, into the portal system. Indeed, the portal vein begins at the point where the splenic and mesenteric veins meet. The quantity of blood contained in veins draining into the portal vein is quite large. In the dog, about 20% of the blood volume is in such a locale (Townsend and Kelso discuss methods for determining this value).[1] Disorders of the venous side must be considered in terms of both the splenic vein and the portal vein. Evaluation of venous drainage can be made by intrasplenic injection (the so-called splenoportogram).[2] Cannulation of the portal vein via the umbilical vein is another technique for delineating intrahepatic structure[3] but does not give details of the splenic vein in most cases.

Isolated thrombosis of the splenic vein is an uncommon entity. Sutton and co-workers[4] state that only 53 documented cases (plus their own) could be found in the English literature up to 1968. While isolated splenic vein obstruction is rare, the disorder occurs more often in conjunction with portal venous disease.[50] Associated with splenic vein occlusion are splenomegaly and gastrointestinal hemorrhage (in 64% of the cases). The "Banti syndrome" hematologic picture of leukopenia (with a relative lymphocytosis) occurred infrequently after splenic vein thrombosis, according to Sutton and associates. Yale and Crummy[47] reported on seven cases of bleeding esophegeal varices secondary to splenic vein thrombosis. Pancreatitis was the etiologic agent in five of the seven cases. Four of the five patients subjected to splenectomy were alive, without further hemorrages, 8 to 60 months after the operation. After obstruction of the splenic vein, the short gastric vessels, fundic plexus in the stomach, and, finally, the coronary vein form a venous pathway around the obstruction site.[48] Gastric varices and bleeding can occur. Nearly all authors have noted the limited role played by barium swallow radiographs (looking for varices) in establishing the diagnosis of splenic vein thrombosis; arteriography was the most useful tool.

We have carried out studies on acute splenic vein obstruction in the dog. With the animals anesthetized, ^{99m}Tc-sulfur colloid was administered intravenously, the abdomen opened, and a loose ligature placed around the splenic vein. The spleen was exteriorized (to separate it from the liver) and covered with warm saline pads. After visualization of the spleen under a gamma ray camera, the ligature around the vein was pulled tight. The spleen swelled in size as shown by the increased area of the scan (Figure 1) and by the greater separation of the radioactivity (that is, counts/area decreased). When viewed grossly, the spleen was swollen and congested.

The biological picture in gradual occlusion of the splenic vein may be quite different. We have studied a 69-year-old woman with angiographically documented splenic vein occlusion (on the basis of pancreatic carcinoma). The scan (Figure 2) revealed a spleen of normal size and with the ability to extract radiocolloid. The timing of the venous occlusion and the status of collateral vessels may be crucial factors in determining the ultimate size of the spleen.

Drainage of the splenic vein, into the portal, means that portal system obstruction produces an impediment to splenic out-flow. Again the timing of the event may be crucial in determining the extent of the development of collateral flow. Two cases of apparent chronic portal vein obstruction have been studied.[109]

1. *Case 70-485.* A 13-year-old girl with a long history of abdominal swelling and pancytopenia had angiographically demonstrated portal vein obstruction. The ^{99m}Tc-sulfur colloid scan showed the following interesting findings (Figure 3).

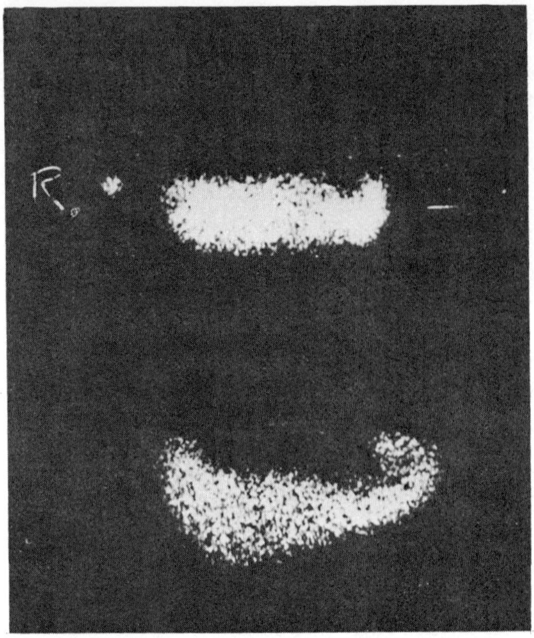

FIGURE 1. Anterior scintiphotos (organ exteriorized) in a dog injected with ^{99m}Tc-sulfur colloid. The top picture was the baseline view; the bottom picture was obtained after splenic vein ligation.

a. Small liver.

b. Uniform distribution of activity throughout the liver (tending to rule out a shrunken liver due to the late stages of cirrhosis).

c. Massive splenomegaly.

d. Only minimal shift of radiocolloid to the spleen.

e. Negligible uptake of radiocolloid in the bone marrow.

2. *Case 70-1908.* A 59-year-old man with intermittent hematemesis over several years (and without an ethanolic history) also had angiographically demonstrated portal vein obstruction. The ^{99m}Tc-sulfur colloid scan revealed findings nearly identical to the above case. A liver biopsy was interpreted as being normal.

We can speculate on the above two cases as follows. Reduction of blood flow to the liver might be a limiting factor in the growth of the organ. Hence, in chronic portal vein obstruction (beginning early in life) there may be a small liver. However, the hepatic tissue present is essentially normal. Splenomegaly can be viewed as the result

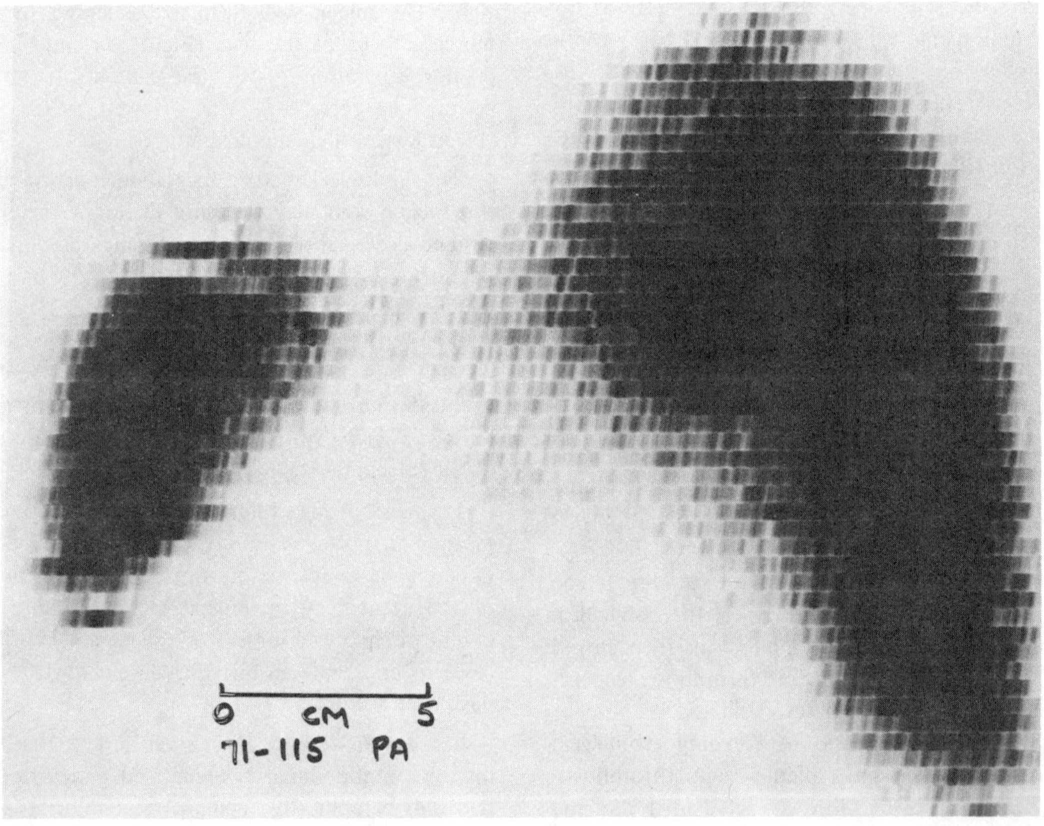

FIGURE 2. Posterior ^{99m}Tc-sulfur colloid scan in a 69-year-old woman with angiographically demonstrated splenic vein thrombosis. The spleen was not enlarged (11 cm) on either the angiogram or the scan. The normal spleen size and function were likely related to the presence of collateral vessels which carried blood from the organ. Case 71-115.

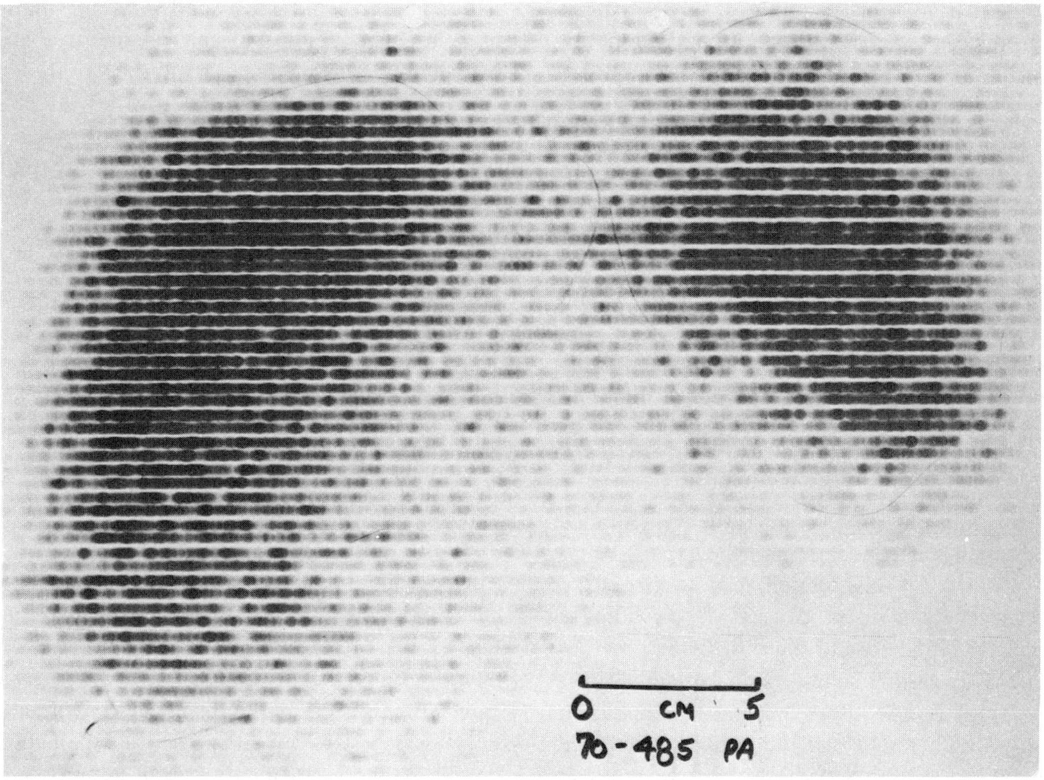

FIGURE 3. Posterior rectilinear scan (^{99m}Tc-sulfur colloid) demonstrating a small liver and massive spleen. The patient is a 13-year-old girl with portal vein obstruction. Case 70-485.

of difficulty in draining the splenic effluent. Sheldon and co-workers[5] reported that a case of portal vein thrombosis had a normal extraction (per passage) of colloidal heat-denatured serum album – ^{131}I. The total blood flow to the liver was low, but the flow/weight was presumably normal.

There have been a number of interesting studies on the splenic vein and effluent, including the following:

1. Splenorenal anastomosis (most often splenectomy, with anastomosis of the splenic vein to the left renal vein)[85] has been employed in the treatment of portal hypertension, particularly when there is hemorrhage from esophageal varices. There has been much comment on the procedure, and Riddell and co-workers[6] have reported a high degree of patency of the shunts.

2. Wilcox and associates[7] have developed animal models for taking the splenic effluent directly to the systemic circulation and by-passing the liver or the liver and lungs. In dogs, a splenic vein to pulmonary vein by-pass (by means of an autologous venous graft) has been described.[62]

3. In a general sense, any decompression of the portal vein results in decompression of the splenic vein (unless there is an obstruction between these vessels). Thus, portocaval, mesenteriocaval, and omphalocaval[8] shunts all aim at decompression of the portal bed and of the splenic effluent.

4. Molimard and Benozio[9] noted that in rats, splenectomy had no effect on compensatory liver hypertrophy. However, an increase in splenic weight followed partial hepatectomy. The nature of the humoral or other factors involved is unknown.

5. Hereditary pancreatitis has been described (transmitted as an autosomal dominant). Portal vein thrombosis and splenic vein thrombosis can occur in this condition.[49]

6. Cavernous malformation of the splenic vein can produce segmental portal hypertension.[51] The spleen itself can be involved by diffuse capillary hemangiomatosis, causing portal hypertension[52] (perhaps by acting as a shunt).

Hemangiomatous transformation of the spleen can also produce a chronic consumption coagulopathy and hemolysis.[53,54] In addition, a splenic angioma has been reported to occur along with hepatic adenoma.[55]

7. Cruveilhier-Baumgarten disease is an unusual entity, marked by patency of the umbilical vein, venous markings and a venous hum in the perumbilical area, portal hypertension, a liver that is not enlarged, but marked splenomegaly (and accompanying hematological changes).[56] The umbilical vein might open as the result of the increased portal pressure (that is, as the end product of the portal hypertension rather than its cause). Splenorenal shunting can result in a decrease in the portal hypertension.

8. Budd-Chiari syndrome is the term applied to the findings after occlusion of the hepatic veins. This posthepatic obstruction can yield portal hypertension. Treatment consists of providing a channel for blood around the obstructed point.[57] In a ^{99m}Tc-sulfur colloid scan obtained in a patient with Budd-Chiari syndrome,[59] Chaudhuri and co-workers noted that the findings resembled those seen in advanced cirrhosis. That is, the liver was poorly functioning, the spleen was enlarged, and there was a shift of radioactive colloid to the spleen and bone marrow.

SPLENIC ARTERIAL SYSTEM

The principal arterial supply of the spleen, the splenic artery, is a branch of the celiac. The abdominal aorta gives off a short vessel, referred to as the celiac axis or artery, which then divides into three branches for vascular supply of the stomach, duodenum, pancreas, liver, and gall bladder, as well as the spleen. The anatomic relations are of interest for at least two reasons. First, the celiac axis passes from the front of the aorta between the medial crura of the diaphragm slightly below its aortic opening. In this locale, the crura might compromise the celiac axis[60] (and celiac axis compression has also been reported as a cause of "visceral angina").[58] Second, the celiac artery (arising in the T-12 to L-1 region) gives off the splenic artery as its largest branch. The splenic artery then undergoes a tortuous path and passes along the upper border of the pancreas, where it can potentially be damaged in the course of pancreatic disorders. Near the kidneys, the splenic artery enters a ligament before passing into the hilus of the spleen. It then subdivides into multiple branches. The major anatomic relations are shown in Figure 4, in which are also illustrated the other two branches of the celiac axis (the left gastric and hepatic arteries). The lower curvature of the stomach is supplied by the right gastroepiploic artery, which is a branch of the right gastric (from the hepatic artery), also a division of the celiac. This vessel, on the underside of the stomach, anastomoses with the left gastroepiploic artery, which arises from the splenic. In segmental splenic artery disease, blood can still reach the spleen via the left gastroepiploic and likely by smaller vessels from other vascular channels (some of these may arise from connections with other branches of the splenic artery – the pancreatic, the vasa brevia, and the terminal vessels).

It is important to emphasize that blood vessels other than the splenic artery also supply the spleen. Because of this, the splenic artery can be ligated when necessary or used for other purposes (such as shunting) without gross splenic necrosis. Following ligation of the splenic artery, the spleen decreases in size, but in man[10] and perhaps the dog,[11] it does not undergo frank infarction. The resultant kinetics of the change in splenic size and function have not been well documented. An intriguing observation is that, in rabbits, partial ligation of the vessels in the splenic pedicle leads to hypertrophy of those areas where circulation remains intact.[63]

In two cases we have studied thus far, splenectomy could not be carried out in the face of hypersplenism and pancytopenia (in one instance, a Hodgkin's tumor mass bound the spleen to surrounding structures;[10] a second case, of myelofibrosis, had severe bleeding that did not permit a prolonged or extensive operation). Following splenic artery ligation, in each case there was prompt decrease in the size of the spleen and a return of the hematologic values toward normal limits. However, splenic artery ligation for hyperspenism and pancytopenia must be viewed as but a temporary (albeit life-saving) maneuver since the redevelopment of full splenic blood flow and function is possible. Figure 5 illustrates an additional case of splenic artery ligation.

Abrams has provided a good description of the arteriographic appearance of the splenic artery.[12] The average value for the diameter of the splenic artery at its origin in man was 8.2 mm. At the mid-portion it was 7.3 mm, while at the splenic

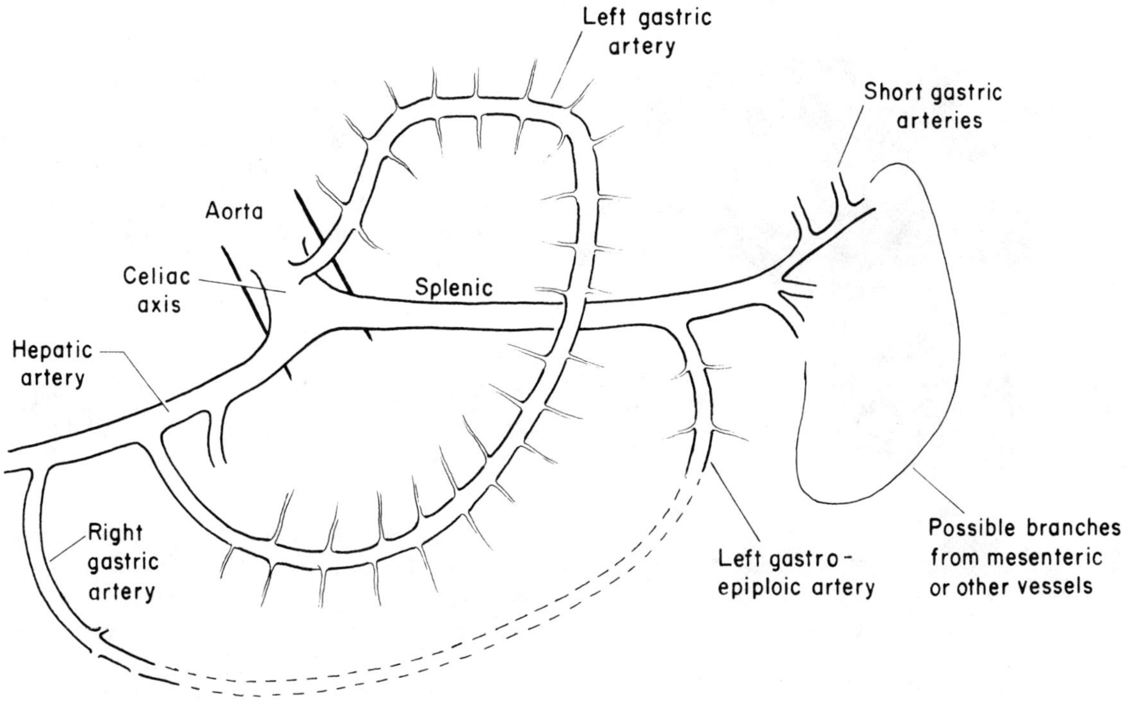

FIGURE 4. Diagrammatic representation of the arterial blood supply of the spleen.

hilum it was 6.5 mm (with the wide range of 3 to 10 mm). Variants of the splenic artery are illustrated by Abrams. In the course of cannulating the splenic artery, radionuclides can be injected into the artery, pressures can be obtained, and balloons can be introduced for splenic artery occlusion. Viamonte and associates[13] have discussed balloon occlusion of the splenic artery for 30 hr in a patient with hepatic cirrhosis, portal hypertension, and the "hyperkinetic circulatory syndrome." While the splenic artery was occluded, the wedged hepatic vein pressure initially fell. This suggested a major splenic flow contribution to the portal hypertension. A later rise in wedged hepatic vein pressure was consistent with the view that visceral arteriovenous shunts increased during occlusion of the splenic artery. Prolonged occlusion of the splenic artery apparently had no adverse effects on the organ.

The splenic artery may be the site of disease processes; calcification,[75] aneurysms, and fistulae can occur. While splenic arteriovenous fistulae are uncommon, their resection can provide therapy of the accompanying portal hypertension.[23] The characteristics of the murmur of a splenic arteriovenous fistula have been described.[61] A splenic artery aneurysm is rare, and arteriography is, of course, the diagnostic procedure of choice.[64] There have been a number of other studies on the splenic arterial blood supply.

1. Hyalinosis, an arteriolar degeneration, can affect splenic vessels.[65,82] The lesions contain the immunoglobulins IgG and IgM, complement, fibrin, and traces of other plasma components. Fibrin deposits in the splenic white pulp have been described as a common finding,[66] but the mechanism of their origin is uncertain (an analogy to the Shwartzman phenomenon was suggested). In microangiopathic hemolytic anemia (a hemolytic disorder associated with small blood vessel disease and the finding of fragmented or damaged erythrocytes in the circulation),[67] some of the peripheral erythrocytes are adherent and covered with a film, presumably fibrin.[68] Whether this activates the spleen to remove such cells is unknown at present.

2. Dumont and co-workers[69] commented on the finding of an enlarged splenic artery in patients with bleeding varices. The seven cases with an enlarged splenic artery did significantly better (splenic artery ligation and/or splenectomy) than five patients without such vessel enlargement.

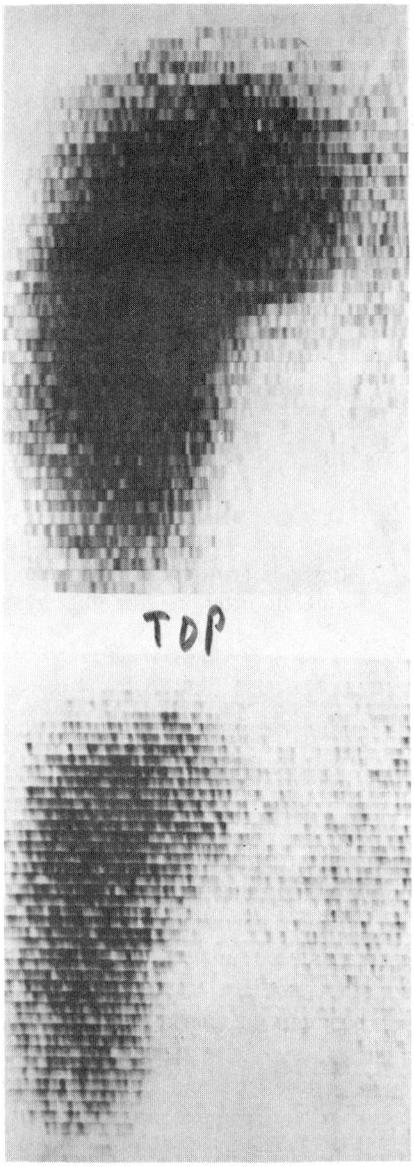

FIGURE 5. Two posterior rectilinear scans (^{99m}Tc-sulfur colloid) in a 75-year-old woman. The patient, with pancytopenia, had a spleen 20 cm in length on the initial picture. The splenic artery was ligated and the bottom scan obtained 7 days later. There was a reduction in the length of the organ to 16 cm. Case 71-650.

In the former group, splenic artery ligation and/or splenectomy appeared as a good alternative to portacaval shunting.

3. Groszmann and associates[70] injected ^{131}I-serum albumin into the splenic and superior mesenteric arteries in both normal subjects and those with portal hypertension. Radioisotope dilution curves were recorded from the right and left hepatic veins. No consistent pattern of hepatic distribution of portal blood flow was demonstrable in these studies. Gates and Dore,[112] however, noted streamline flow after microaggregate injection into the superior mesenteric vein.

4. Direct infusion of vasopressin into the splenic artery can be used to exclude the splenic circulation in the dog.[71] Both angiography and ^{99m}Tc-sulfur colloid scans were used to demonstrate the exclusion of the spleen. The effect of gastrointestinal hormones on the spleen has also been studied.[84]

5. Splenic vessels can be obtained which are suitable for characterization of proteins bound to the vascular wall (and this has been studied in lupus erythematosus).[72]

The precise role of splenic vessels in shock is uncertain. Under hypoxia (5% oxygen), the liver and spleen show ultrastructural changes which are reversible.[73] In hypoxic dogs, the splenic venous blood initially has a higher O_2 tension than arterial blood since the spleen adds erythrocytes to the circulation under these conditions.[81] Under different circumstances, the spleen of the dog can be noted to sequester erythrocytes during hypoxia.[83] Schildt[74] has summarized data showing that functioning of the reticuloendothelial system is depressed in shock. Possible factors in depressing reticuloendothelial function are as follows:

1. A paralysis of the microcirculation produced by endotoxin.
2. ACTH- and steroid-produced suppression of the reticuloendothelial system.
3. Decreased perfusion of organs with reticuloendothelial activity.
4. A paucity of factors in the plasma which promote phagocytosis.

Endotoxin shock has been studied in several species, but it is only recently that the roles of the liver and spleen have begun to emerge. In the dog, endotoxin shock produces mesenteric vasoconstriction and necrosis of the gut wall. However, the dog may not be a good model of the events in primate endotoxin shock. This is because findings in the baboon (that is, a fall in splenic arterial blood pressure during *E. coli* endotoxin shock, but no change in portal blood flow and pressure) suggest a different series of events.[76,77] Splenic blood flow paralleled the fall in arterial blood pressure in the baboon.[78] In the dog, a pronounced decrease in hepatic and splenic blood flows occurred along with an increase in the resistance across the vascular beds of these organs. *E. coli* toxin injected into the splenic artery of dogs has been stated to cause dilatation of the spleen, while when given intravenously, the spleen contracts.[80]

Both liver and spleen are sites of detoxification of *S. enteritidis* endotoxin in the mouse.[79] Homogenates from mice (rendered endotoxin tolerant) had increased ability to detoxify the endotoxin. This might indicate a varying role during the natural defense against endotoxin.

The splenic artery may be severed and used for other purposes (splenectomy may not be mandatory following this procedure). Goldsmith and Castillo[24] demonstrated that the splenic artery could be implanted in the kidney and used as a source of blood supply for that organ. The procedure has since been successfully used by several groups, particularly in an effort to overcome renal ischemia and hypertension.[25, 86-88] The splenic artery has also been anastomosed to the portal vein in order to bypass a block.[26]

Gardner and co-workers[27] stated that the splenic artery could be mobilized for at least 10 cm; they used the vessel for a splenic to distal hepatic artery anastomosis in order to by-pass an hepatic artery aneurysm. The splenic artery can also be used as the input for perfusing fluids,[28] and prolonged survival of the perfused pig spleen has been reported. Once within the spleen, the splenic vasculature may also be abnormal. For example, Rochmis[29] described splenic angioma with thrombocytopenia and reviewed the literature on microangiophathic thrombocytopenia. Yamamoto[30] reported that in the "Banti Syndrome," 10 to 20% of splenic arteriolar terminals opened directly into sinuses (an unusual finding, according to this author, in the normal spleen).

In dogs, Koyama[14] produced splenic ischemia by first freeing the spleen from all vessels except the splenic artery and vein and then clamping the splenic artery for 2 hr. Studies were carried out 50 to 55 days later. Also studied were seven patients (as controls) along with five with "Banti's Syndrome." Koyama found that in the dog's spleen previously rendered ischemic, blood flow was increased. Control human patients had a splenic blood flow of 300 ml/min, while the value was markedly elevated in "Banti's Syndrome" (however, the flow/gram was decreased since the spleens were of large size). While total oxygen consumption by the spleen in "Banti's Syndrome" was increased, the consumption per gram was depressed (and the spleens were concluded to be relatively anoxic).

Possible autoregulation of splenic blood flow has been discussed by Lutz and co-workers.[15] They also pointed out the presence of a venovasomotoric reaction in the splenic circulation of cats. Within the spleen, the exact pathway traversed by blood is still under debate. Knisely[16] has described a system of closed vessels in cat, mouse, and rat spleens with venous sinuses that were emptied by sphincterlike structures. Mackenzie and co-workers,[17] however, concluded that blood was carried through a mesh of pulp spaces which entered venous vessels. On the basis of isoproterenol increasing splenic blood flow without flushing out sequestered erythrocytes, Opdyke[22] concluded that neither of the above models was adequate to explain the findings. Burke and Simon[18] studied osmium tetroxide perfused rabbit spleens. They noted that there was no direct capillary to sinus or capillary to Billroth cord connections. However, they did note fenestrations in basement membranes throughout the red pulp's marginal zone and the periphery of the white pulp. These likely permitted movement of plasma and cells between sinuses and cords. Burke and Simon concluded that there was little significance to discussions of whether the splenic circulation was opened or closed.

Groom and Song[19] studied erythrocyte washout from the isolated spleens of cats. Examination of the cells and histologic study of the spleens allowed localization of the cells. Washout curves showed three components. The fast component (T½ = 30 sec) may have been from erythrocytes in vascular channels. The intermediate component (T½ = 8.4 min) was likely composed of cells stored in the red pulp. The slow component (T½ = 50 min) consisted of reticulocytes. The number of reticulocytes in the spleen was larger than the animal's daily production, suggesting residence in the spleen (attached to the sinus walls and reticulum fibers) and probably maturation in the organ.[89-93] How these observations fit with the hypothesized schemes of splenic blood flow[16,17] is unknown.

The volume of blood in the spleen is usually small. At autopsy, 12 cases contained a mean value of 20 ml of red blood cells[20] (mean spleen weight,

159 g; thus, erythrocytes constituted 20/159 or about 13% of the weight of the spleen). The value for red blood cells in the spleen is about 1 to 2% of the circulating quantity (and changes in splenomegaly are discussed in a different section). By use of radioactive carbon monoxide (^{11}CO) and scanning, Glass and associates[21] noted that in four normal adults, the red cell content of the spleen was 20 to 45 ml. In disease states, this value (and likely that for platelets in the spleen) can vary widely. The small erythrocyte component in the human spleen is in contrast to the dog, where the organ may contain a significant part of the erythrocyte pool.

QUANTITATIVE RELATIONSHIPS

A number of radioisotopic techniques have been, or could be, applied to quantifying splenic blood flow. The more important of these will be briefly reviewed.

Microsphere Technique

Following introduction of radioisotopically labeled microspheres (25 μm diameter) into the left side of the heart, distribution occurs in proportion to the blood flow to each organ. That is, if 20% of the cardiac output goes to a particular organ, then 20% of the microspheres will deposit in the organ. There are, of course, certain qualifications. The three principal ones are as follows: (1) Any organ having a dual influx, that is, from both the arterial and venous sides (such as the liver), will only have the arterial component or "first pass" component measured by this technique. The venous contribution to the liver can be measured by adding up the quantity of microspheres in those organs that would drain into the portal vein (spleen, stomach, small intestine, large intestine, pancreas, omentum, and mesentary). (2) The quantity of microspheres in an organ tells nothing of the pathway by which they entered. This is particularly important when an organ has more than one supplying artery. (3) The fact that the microspheres lodged in an organ means that they were larger than the diameter of the vessels. If smaller radiolabeled microspheres are used, some may "escape" via shunt pathways through the organ. These are paths that might not supply nutrition to the organ. This may have importance in the case of the spleen, where shunts might carry blood away from the sinusoids where reticuloendothelial activity is located.

Using the radiolabeled microspheres technique, Ohlsson and co-workers[31] found that in dogs 1.96 ± 0.70% of the cardiac output went to the spleen. Following common bile duct ligation, the fraction of the cardiac output going to the spleen rose to 4.47 ± 2.46% at 1 week after the operation and was 4.96 ± 3.28% 2 weeks postoperatively. In terms of ml/min/kg body weight, the values for the spleen at the three periods were 2.46 ± 0.81, 5.81 ± 3.99, and 5.98 ± 4.46. Returning to the results in terms of the fractionation of cardiac output, the flow to the dog's portal vein (that representing the contributions of spleen, stomach, small intestine, large intestine, pancreas, omentum, and mesentery) represented 15.46% of the cardiac output. The splenic component was 1.96/15.46 or nearly 13% of the total in dogs prior to common bile duct ligation. This value rose to 21% 1 week after ligation of the common bile duct and to 25% by the 2nd week. Why the spleen should make such a large contribution is as yet unknown. Incidently, the hepatic artery supplied 14% of total liver blood flow in control dogs and 22% 1 week after the duct ligation; the value was down to 15% by the 2nd week. The microsphere technique has also been used to measure cardiac output distribution to the spleen of unanesthetized monkeys. The spleen represented 0.2 ± 0.1% of body weight, had 1.9 ± 1.2% of cardiac output, and had a flow of 21 ± 12 ml/min (or 267 ± 124 ml/min · 100 g); resistance was also calculated.[44]

Inert Gas Clearance

By injecting a diffusible, soluble, and nonreactive gamma-emitting radiolabeled tracer into the arterial supply of an organ, the uptake and subsequent "washout" of the tracer can be monitored by external detection probes. Various inert radioactive gases such as ^{133}Xe (5.2 days half-life, 88 keV gamma emission) are assumed to reside in the organ principally in lipid-rich sites. The washout of ^{133}Xe is considered to be dependent on the blood flow from the organ. In such an instance, there is minimal recirculation of the tracer since it is blown off from the lungs upon arrival from the venous side. External collimation must include the true area of interest and has to exclude major afferent vessels. Use of the inert radioactive gas method for measuring blood flow was presaged by Kety and Schmidt[32] and developed by a number of investigators. A summary of the principles involved has been provided by Donato.[33]

Derivation of the relevant quantification has been given by several authors. The following discussion is based on the report of Thorburn and co-workers.[34]

The Fick principle states that the time rate of change of a material in a region depends on the product of the arterial flow and the arteriovenous concentration difference (if it is neither created nor destroyed). That is,

$$\frac{dQ}{dt} = F\,(C_A - C_V). \qquad (1)$$

We can check on the units involved by noting that dQ/dt must be expressed in terms of amount per time, such as moles/minute. Flow is in terms of milliliters/minute, while the concentration in the blood is expressed as moles/milliliter. The product of milliliters/minute × moles/milliliter is moles/minute, which is correct.

When recirculation of the radiotracer is negligible, the situation considerably simplifies. For inert gases such as ^{133}Xe or ^{85}Kr, recirculation is quite small since the gas is largely excreted via the lungs when it reaches the pulmonary circulation. Hence, if the radioactive inert gas is in an organ, and we suddenly remove the gas inflow (C_A set equal to zero), then,

$$\frac{dQ}{dt} = -F\,C_V. \qquad (2)$$

The minus sign indicates that under this circumstance of no further inflow, the quantity in the organ decreases with time. At this point we make the assumption that equilibration of the gas between blood and tissues is quite rapid and hence is not the rate-limiting step. Under this condition, desaturation of the tissue depends on the nutrient or capillary blood flow. We will define a partition coefficient as

$$\lambda = \frac{Cr}{C_V}. \qquad (3)$$

Here Cr is the concentration of the radioactive inert gas or other tracer in the region under study, and C_V is its concentration in the venous blood. We can also note that Cr (the concentration of the material in the region of interest) is given by:

$$Cr = \frac{Q}{V} \qquad (4)$$

where Q is the quantity of gas or tracer in the region, and V is the volume. Substituting Equations 3 and 4 into Equation 2 gives:

$$\frac{dQ}{dt} = -F\,\frac{Q}{V.\lambda}\ . \qquad (5)$$

This is rearranged

$$\frac{dQ}{Q} = \frac{-F}{V.\lambda}\,.dt \qquad (6)$$

and integrated to yield:

$$Q = Q_o e^{\frac{-F}{V.\lambda}\,.\,t} \qquad (7)$$

Hence, Q_o is the moles present at time zero (when the washout begins). Most commonly, we measure Q/Q_o, so that the units employed are immaterial (they cancel, whether counts or moles). If we plot Q/Q_o on a logarithmic scale, then the following graph emerges (Figure 6). The slope of the line (K) is given by:

$$K = \frac{F}{\lambda V} \qquad (8)$$

Hence, the flow *per unit volume* is given by:

$$\frac{F}{V} = K\,.\lambda. \qquad (9)$$

To be more precise, we should correct for the specific gravity (ρ) of the tissue. Hence, the equation often appears as:

$$F\ (\text{ml/g. min}) = \frac{K.\lambda}{\rho}\,. \qquad (10)$$

Another custom is to sometimes express the results in terms of flow per 100 g of tissue. In such an instance, the equation is

$$F\ (\text{ml/100 g . min}) = \frac{K.\lambda.100}{\rho}\,. \qquad (11)$$

Clear recognition must be given to the fact that flow is being expressed in terms of amount per unit of tissue. To obtain *total flow*, this value must be multiplied by the appropriate value of the organ volume.

There are two conditions necessary to obtain accurate values for splenic blood flow by the radioactive inert gas method.

1. The value of the partition coefficient

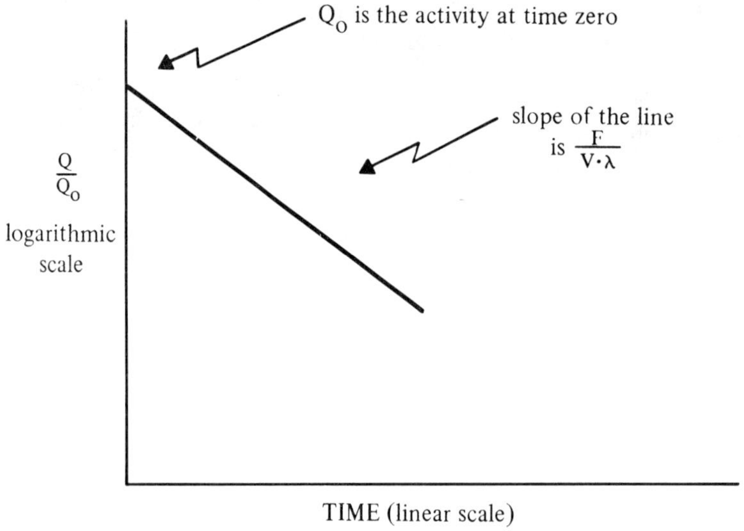

FIGURE 6. A plot of the results of a ^{133}Xe washout experiment.

must be known.[35] It should be determined for the normal and diseased spleen.

2. The washout curve must be carefully analyzed and the most accurate component utilized.[27]

Veall and Mallet[35] have discussed calculation of the partition coefficient. They noted that its value fell as the hematocrit of blood increased (a typical value for λ is about 0.85). Williams and co-workers[36] have noted that the proper value of K is the slope of the first exponential in the washout curve. Control patients gave a mean value of splenic blood flow of 95 ml/100 g · min (range of 60 to 145). In cirrhosis and portal vein thrombosis, this value was greater. In one patient with bleeding esophageal varices, vasopressin infusion resulted in a decrease in splenic blood flow.

In five dogs and an adult undergoing splenectomy, Blendis and co-workers[37] compared the ^{133}Xe clearance method with an electromagnetic flow meter determination of blood flow. A highly significant correlation was found between the two methods ($r = 0.89$, $P < 0.001$). Sandberg[38] measured blood flow to the spleen of guinea pigs by use of ^{133}Xe. He concluded that the flow per unit weight of the spleen slightly fell in larger animals. In addition, splenic blood flow increased following injection of pertussis vaccine (but not sheep erythrocytes). Blendis and associates[39] employed ^{133}Xe to measure splenic blood flow in patients with splenomegaly due to a variety of conditions.

Splenomegaly with blood dyscrasias or diseases of the reticulendothelial system may have an increased splenic blood flow. Gitlin and co-workers,[45] using the ^{133}Xe technique, noted that 31 of 36 patients with portocaval shunts had increased splenic blood flow (but that this flow contributed only slightly to the portal hypertension). Cotton and Richards have reported on the use of ^{133}Xe as a check on the local thermal dilution method for measuring splenic vein blood flow.[46]

As commonly performed, the radioactive inert gas method is carried out by delivering the gas via a catheter in the appropriate artery. A noninvasive variant has been described by Garnett et al.[40] The patient is connected to a respirometer, into which ^{133}Xe is injected. As the patient rebreathes from the closed system, the tissues slowly accumulate ^{133}Xe. After the process has gone on for about 5 to 15 min, the patient is disconnected from the closed system, and washout of ^{133}Xe from the spleen is monitored. In 19 patients with splenomegaly, splenic blood flow was 60 to 190 ml/100 g · min.

An interesting approach to use of the radioactive gas clearance method has been described by Jones and co-workers.[110] Denatured red cells are labeled with ^{81}Rb (a cyclotron produced radionuclide, with $T\frac{1}{2} = 4.5$ hr). As the ^{81}Rb decays, it forms the daughter radionuclide ^{81m}Kr. This daughter has a short half-life (13 sec). The rate of clearance of ^{81m}Kr depends on the blood flow through the organ. Hence, denatured red cells are tagged with ^{81}Rb and then injected intravenously. After the cells have accumulated in the spleen, a detector is used to measure the emissions from ^{81}Rb and ^{81m}Kr. The greater the blood flow, the more readily is ^{81m}Kr swept away. The technique is quite ingenious, but there are three problems. (1) The ^{81}Rb is cyclotron produced, short lived, and not readily available. (2) Quite sensitive detectors are needed in order to separate the emissions of ^{81}Rb and ^{81m}Kr (and a depth correction is needed). (3) The decrease in counts of ^{81m}Kr with blood flow is not striking.

Uptake from the Bloodstream

Following intravenous administration, if a material is quantitatively cleared by the spleen (that is taken up entirely by the spleen, with none accumulating elsewhere), splenic blood flow can be determined.

$$\text{splenic blood flow} = (\text{rate constant for clearance})(\text{volume of distribution}) \qquad 12$$

In practice, following intravenous administration of the substance, the bloodstream is sampled at several points in time and the curve extrapolated back to time zero (Figure 7). The counts per unit of blood at zero time, divided by the total dose injected, yields the volume of distribution. Then the product of the volume of distribution and the rate constant gives splenic blood flow. Again we must state that this is true only if the material is entirely cleared by the spleen on each passage and is not taken up by other sites. Wolf and Fischer[41] have reported that heat-denatured ^{51}Cr-labeled erythrocyted ("pyrospherocytes") are almost entirely cleared from the bloodstream by the spleen. Using "pyrospherocyte" clearance to measure splenic blood flow, the values obtained by Wolf and Fischer, on the order of 700 to 800 ml/min in the normal spleen, seem high (and confirmatory studies are necessary). These investigators reported that in very large spleens, blood flow values up to 1,400 ml/min were obtained. However, in some of these cases, the specific splenic blood flow (that is, blood flow per minute per unit weight of tissue) actually fell.

Fractional Distribution of Radiotracer

After an intravenous injection of ^{42}KCl or $^{86}RbCl$, Sapirstein[42] noted that a relatively steady concentration was reached in all organs (other than the brain) at 6 to 9 sec and that this persisted for over 60 sec. Organs with stable counts must have had extraction ratios equal to that of the whole body; hence, the technique could be used to measure organ blood flow. The fraction of the cardiac output in an organ was equal to the fraction of the administered radionuclide which was accumulated. In dogs, the spleen accumulated 1.3% of the administered ^{42}K.

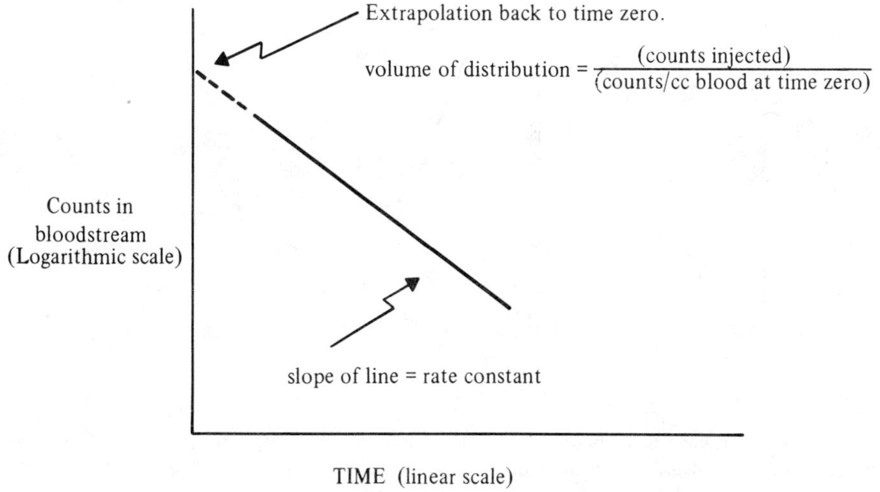

FIGURE 7. Technique for calculating organ blood flow when a material is entirely cleared by a single organ.

Mendell and Hollenberg[94] have shown that in the rat, the microsphere method gave higher results than did the rubidium technique. They pointed out that concepts of splenic function must deal with both limited capillary exchange and with the special anatomy of the microvasculature of the spleen.

Mean Transit Time Method

For most circulatory systems, the blood volume (V) in an organ and the blood flow (F) through the organ are related by

$$\bar{T} = \frac{V}{F} \qquad (13)$$

where $\bar{T}$ is the mean transit time (seconds), V is in milliliters, and F is measured in milliliters/second. A method for calculating the mean transit time, by use of a nondiffusible indicator, is shown in Figure 8. Zierler[95] has shown that the area under the curve, divided by the height of the curve, equals $\bar{T}$. Since $\bar{T}$ can be determined radioisotopically, F could be calculated if V was known. However, a very small bolus is needed, and approximations must be used in extrapolating the washout curve. A number of techniques for calculating the erythrocyte volume within the spleen have been described (including the use of ^{11}CO-erythrocytes[21] and ^{51}Cr-erythrocytes;[43] we can speculate that ^{99m}Tc-erythrocytes may be the radiolabel of choice in the future). A separate determination would have to be made of the plasma volume within the spleen.

Comments

The microsphere technique, as well as the radioisotope fractionation method, depends on counting of the organ in vitro; hence, these are not presently suited for clinical use. The inert radioactive gas clearance method, especially when used with xenon rebreathing (to avoid catheterization of the organ), appears to be a good approach to determining relative blood flow (flow/g · min) during life. The radionuclide accumulation technique depends on quantitative splenic clearance. A fully suitable material is not available for use at present, but there may be interesting future extensions. Once the splenic blood flow is determined, it can be used to calculate derived quantities. For example, the splenic vascular resistance (R) is described by

$$R = \frac{\Delta P}{F} \qquad (14)$$

where ΔP is the arteriovenous difference in pressure across the spleen. Again using the value for flow, splenic oxygen consumption (total O_2) is given by

$$\text{Total } O_2 = F(\Delta O_2) \qquad (15)$$

where ΔO_2 is the arteriovenous difference in

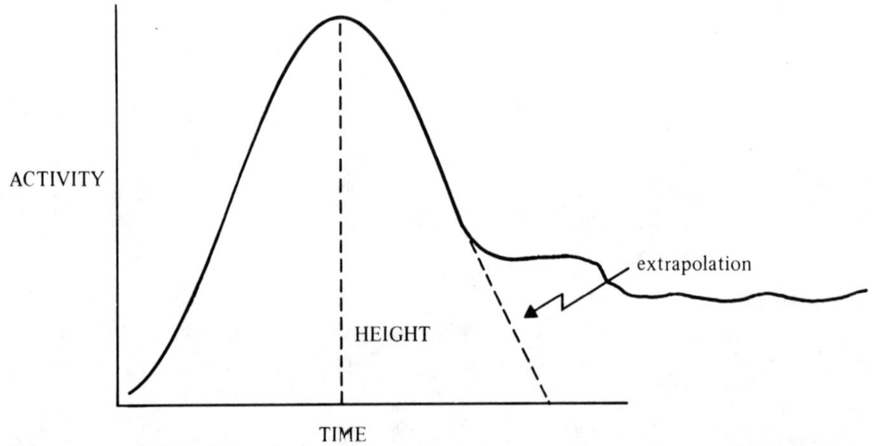

FIGURE 8. Idealized diagram of radioactivity detected over the spleen, following intravenous injection of a nondiffusible indicator. In reality, there is spread of the bolus and interference by overlying tissues. In the ideal case, the mean transit time is given by the area under the curve divided by the height of the peak. Use of the method by means of a small probe placed in an organ has also been described.[111]

oxygen content across the spleen. Koyama[14] has illustrated calculation of these quantities.

PORTAL HYPERTENSION

The normal human liver has a blood flow of approximately 1,500 cm^3/min, or 1 cm^3/min per gram of tissue. Perhaps two thirds of this flow is from the portal vein. Of the 1,000 cm^3/min coursing through the portal vein, about one sixth comes from the spleen. Indeed, the splenic blood flow/gram of tissue is about equal to that of the liver (1 cm^3/g).

A pressure in the portal vein of greater than 25 cm of saline is defined as portal hypertension. One approach to measuring this pressure, if the spleen is in communication with portal system, is to employ splenic pulp pressure measurements. The hypertension of the portal system likely results from an increased resistance to flow, along with a continued influx of blood without adequate collateral circulation. The obstruction can be in the portal vein, in the venous channels within the liver, or in the hepatic veins. As a consequence, collateral circuits tend to develop, and shunt blood around the block.

Banti (1882) described splenomegaly with leukopenia and occasional hemorrhages, in the absence of leukemia. The reticulum was thickened, and the alterations appeared to originate around the arterial supply to the follicles. Such changes are not specific, however, and result from any etiology that shows increased pressure in the portal venous tree (portal system obstruction, and rarely perhaps from cardiac failure). We recognize the blood changes as being most likely due to pooling in the spleen (which can be massively enlarged). The causes of the problem may dominate symptomatology until the pancytopenia (particularly thrombocytopenia) leads to bleeding from varices or in other locales.

Veda and co-workers[96] measured splenic blood flow by means of ^{85}Kr introduced via a catheter in the celiac artery. In control patients the splenic blood flow was 119 ± 29 ml/min/100 g, and total flow was 146 ± 87 ml/min. In idiopathic portal hypertension, splenic blood flow/gram was nearly normal, while total splenic flow was increased due to splenomegaly (537 ± 362 ml/min). In hepatic cirrhosis without gross splenomegaly, splenic blood flow per unit weight was reduced (64 ± 14 ml/min/100 g), while total splenic blood flow was about normal.

Groszmann and associates[97] investigated shunting through portasystemic collaterals by utilizing the area under radionuclide dilution curves recorded from the hepatic vein, following superior mesenteric or splenic artery injection, with that after hepatic artery injection.

Portal hypertension is one of the most common causes of splenomegaly. In North America, ethanolism ranks as a frequent causative agent. Perhaps 50% of cirrhotics have portal hypertension. Other etiologies (such as the sequelae of postnecrotic cirrhosis) must be considered. There are few simple quantitative guides for gauging the extent of portal hypertension or the effects of therapeutic measures. Therefore, the extent of accumulation of radiocolloids by various regions of the reticuloendothelial system has been proposed as an index of portal hypertension. We will not dwell on this topic at length but will simply point out the role of the spleen in proposed methods for quantifying portal hypertension.

It will be recalled that when ^{198}Au-colloid is used (particle size about 0.001 μm), little normally accumulates in the spleen. Thus, splenic uptake of radioactive gold colloid represents a departure from normal (but not necessarily portal) hypertension). Johnson and co-workers[98] performed ^{198}Au liver scans and used as indicators of "portal-systemic collateral circulation" the following: mottled appearance of the liver, splenic accumulation of radiocolloid, and bone marrow uptake of the radionuclide. Such findings were most common in hepatic cirrhosis, but some other disorders also gave a similar picture (perhaps on the basis of portal hypertension).

A slightly different perspective was taken by Fernandez and co-workers.[99] They studied patients with chronic diffuse liver disease. When significant spleen and/or vertebral bone marrow accumulation of ^{198}Au colloid was present on the scans (anterior view), each of the patients had an hepatic wedge catheterization pressure of 18 mm Hg or above. This is likely a highly significant finding since Joly and associates[100] noted that in compensated cirrhotics, there was a correlation between the presence of large varices and a portohepatic gradient of 10 mm Hg or greater. Esophageal varices, when associated with splenic vein thrombosis, are frequently benefited by splenectomy.[47] There have been inadequate radioisotopic studies of this entity. The ^{198}Au data have to be reinterpreted in the light of uneven particle size distributions and the fact that posterior scans were seldom obtained in older studies.

In patients with chronic liver disease, there can be a nearly linear relationship between extrahepatic uptake of ^{198}Au colloid and ammonia intolerance (which is a measure of portasystemic shunting).[101] However, despite the relationship of ammonia intolerance to portal hypertension and esophageal varices, the overall role of ^{198}Au scans in predicting varices is uncertain. Rogers and Feiss[102] found a 59% agreement between the radiogold scans and esophagoscopic findings. Obviously this is unacceptable since by guessing, one could end up with a 50% agreement. In addition, ^{198}Au is far from the ideal reticuloendothelial scanning agent and has been largely replaced by ^{99m}Tc-sulfur colloid (and, hopefully, better scanning agents are still to be developed). Gourgoutis and co-workers[103] reported on the spleen/liver uptake of ^{99m}Tc-sulfur colloid as an index of portal hypertension. Their report is difficult to interpret because tracings were made in the dynamic mode, while only equilibrium values are usually obtained clinically for the spleen/liver ratio. In addition, a 2-in. probe was utilized, instead of a focused collimator on a 3-in. or 5-in. scanner probe. However, there was an approximately linear relationship between the spleen/liver ratio of radionuclide and the wedged hepatic vein pressure. To a lesser extent, indices of the rate of trapping of radiocolloid have also been employed to estimate hepatic perfusion (and, hence, indirectly, portal-systemic shunting). For example, Rosenthall and associates[104] utilized a "liver trapping index," based on hepatic and mediastinal activities of ^{198}Au, 4.5 min after intravenous injection.

Our own approach to using ^{99m}Tc-sulfur colloid scans for estimating the degree of hepatic impairment, in portal hypertension, has been as follows. As hepatic disease progresses, the liver passes through a change in size. For example, during one stage of ethanolic cirrhosis, the liver suffers from fatty infiltration and can be quite large. During later stages of the disease, the liver begins contracting and can become shrunken. The spread of liver sizes (on scans) in adults seen at this medical center is approximately normally distributed. Only 5% of the patients have a liver over 21 cm in length. At the other extreme, only about 5% of the patients have a liver 13 cm in length or smaller.[108] Hence, as we will point out below, a change in the scan size of the liver can be a significant prognostic indicator.

During the progress of hepatic diseases, the liver's ability to trap radiocolloid is diminished (perhaps due to reduced blood flow and to Kupffer cell dysfunction). With a collimated 5- or 3-in. scanner probe, the maximal anterior liver/spleen count ratio per unit area usually ranges from 3:1 to 1:1. A shift of radiocolloid to the spleen likely means that splenic tissue is effectively trapping radiocolloid. This shows up only when the liver has been sufficiently damaged. When splenomegaly is combined with this splenic trapping, most of the injected radiocolloid can be found in the left upper quadrant. The bone marrow also functions as a depot of reticuloendothelial cells, and the vertebral bodies, sternum, and other bones can become significant sites of radiocolloid localization.

The following points have also been helpful to us:

1. Most useful have been serial studies. That is, serial scans can reveal marked changes in distribution of radiocolloid, with only minimal alterations in organ size. An example of this is shown in Figure 9. Over a period of 26 months the liver scans in this case revealed a diminished hepatic size, a decrease in hepatic trapping of radiocolloid, and a shift of radiocolloid to the spleen.

2. There are several signs of serious hepatic decompensation which can be shown by the scans. For example, the lungs possess some reticuloendothelial activity. When there is marked pulmonary uptake of radiocolloid, the heart is outlined as a "negative defect." This finding usually occurs in acute decompensation of chronic cirrhosis and is an indicator of a poor prognosis.

3. In the final stages of hepatic decompensation due to ethanolic cirrhosis, the liver can be contracted, and it shows poor accumulation of radiocolloid. The spleen may be enlarged, with massive uptake of the colloid. The vertebrae and ribs can be well defined (Figure 10). In some cases, the spleen/liver ratio of radiocolloid exceeds 10 to 1 (Figure 11).

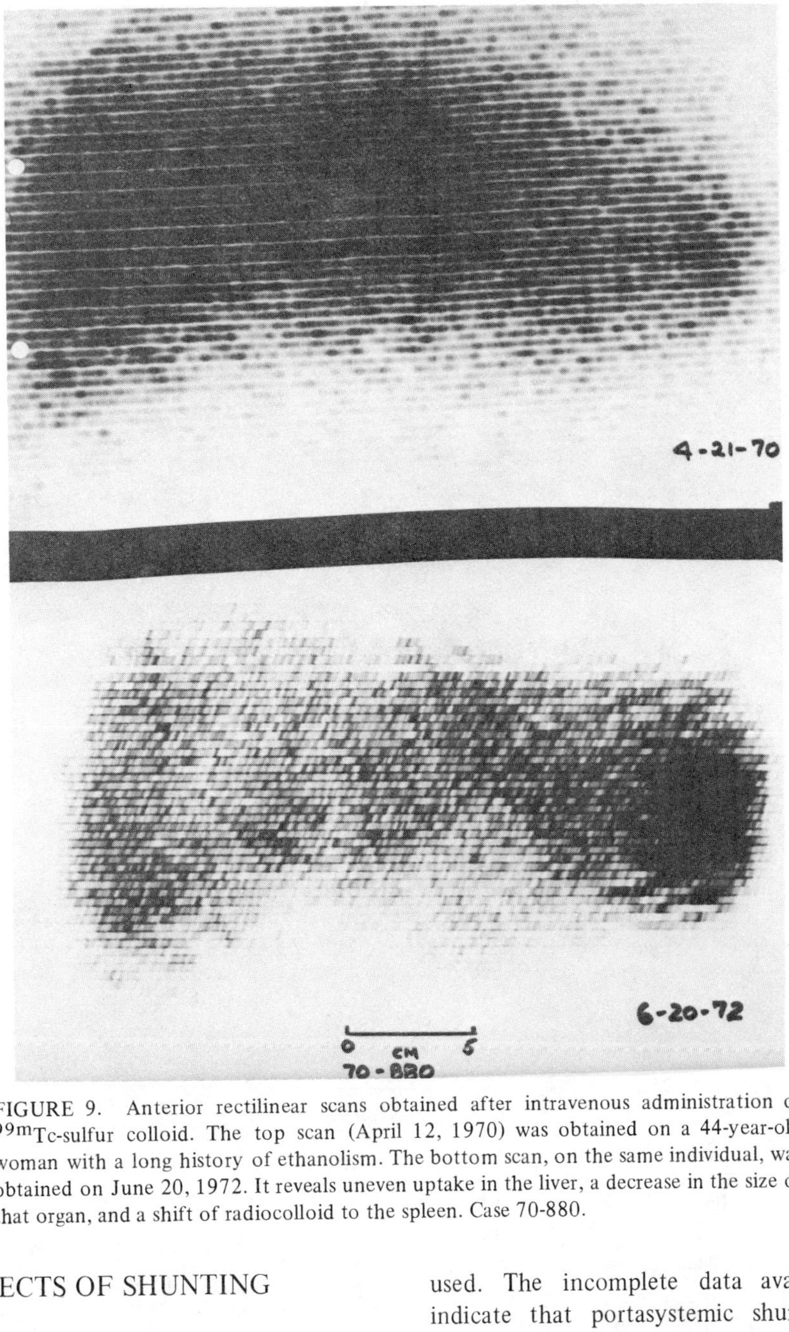

FIGURE 9. Anterior rectilinear scans obtained after intravenous administration of ^{99m}Tc-sulfur colloid. The top scan (April 12, 1970) was obtained on a 44-year-old woman with a long history of ethanolism. The bottom scan, on the same individual, was obtained on June 20, 1972. It reveals uneven uptake in the liver, a decrease in the size of that organ, and a shift of radiocolloid to the spleen. Case 70-880.

EFFECTS OF SHUNTING

The creation of artifical shunts (such as the portacaval anastomosis) has been used in the therapy of portal hypertension. Dumont and associates[69,105] pointed out that in hepatic cirrhosis with esophageal varices, patients who had splenomegaly tolerated portacaval shunting, while those without splenomegaly did not do as well.

Despite the variety of shunting procedures and the various techniques employed in obtaining follow-up data, spleen scans have not been widely used. The incomplete data available thus far indicate that portasystemic shunting has little effect on the spleen. Leger and co-workers,[106] after a radiological and pathological study, concluded that the spleen did not appreciably change in size in cirrhotic patients after portacaval anastomosis. Kyu and Cavanagh[107] produced portacaval shunts in rats. When operated rats were compared with controls (spleen weight/body weight), there was no difference in the findings.

We have had the opportunity to follow two interesting individuals who underwent portacaval shunts.

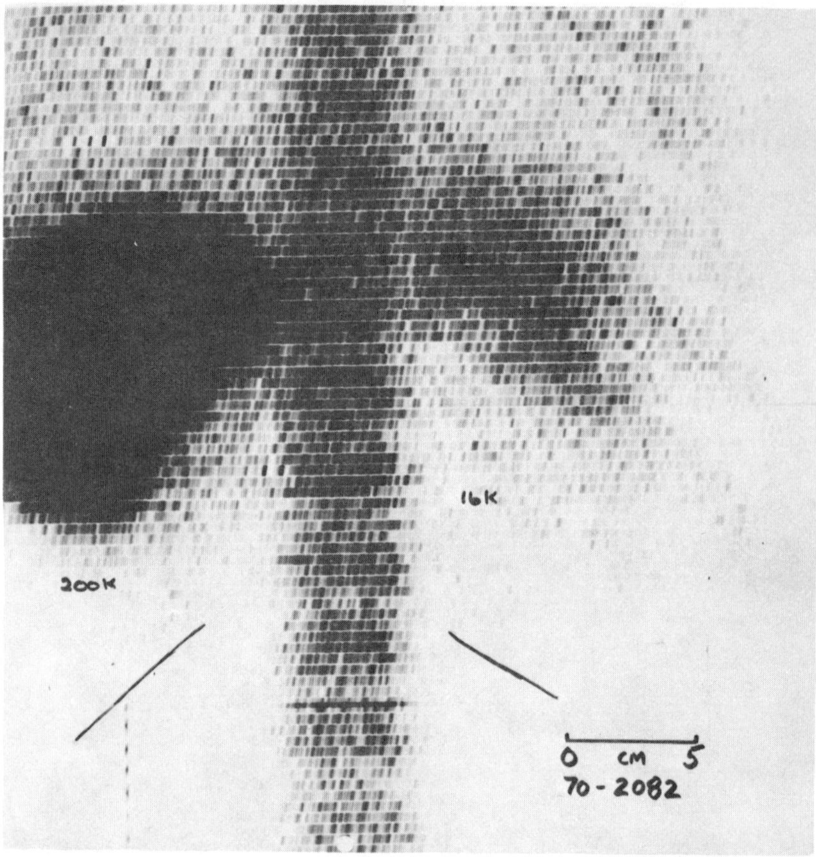

FIGURE 10. Posterior rectilinear scan obtained by use of ^{99m}Tc-sulfur colloid. The patient is a 73-year-old man with Laennec's cirrhosis, who noted dark urine and an increase in abdominal girth for several weeks prior to hospital admission. Splenomegaly with massive uptake of the radiocolloid, a contracted liver with poor uptake of colloid, and vertebral body and rib uptake can be noted. Case 70-2082.

1. *Case 68-108.* A 61-year-old male with a long history of ethanolism had a markedly abnormal ^{99m}Tc-sulfur colloid scan (spleen/liver ratio = 6:1), despite prior portacaval shunting. A repeat scan 19 months later showed the liver to be in a contracted or shrunken state. The spleen, however, changed but little in size (and the spleen/liver ratio had gone to 14:1).

2. *Case 70-1846.* A 7-year-old girl had previously undergone a mesocaval shunt because of polycystic disease of the liver and kidneys. When she showed little improvement, a portacaval shunt was performed about 18 months later. A repeat scan revealed no difference in the size or activity of the spleen.

There thus seems to be little change in splenic size after portacaval shunting. Although one might reason that release of splenic congestion, when the hypertension in the portal system is relieved, would lead to shrinkage of the organ, there is as yet no clear-cut evidence for this. Williams and co-workers[36] reported on the size of the spleen before and 3 months after portacaval anastomosis. They used radiographs to estimate splenic size and stated that in one case there was a 37% decrease, while a second case showed an 18% decrease in splenic size. Certainly further studies are warranted.

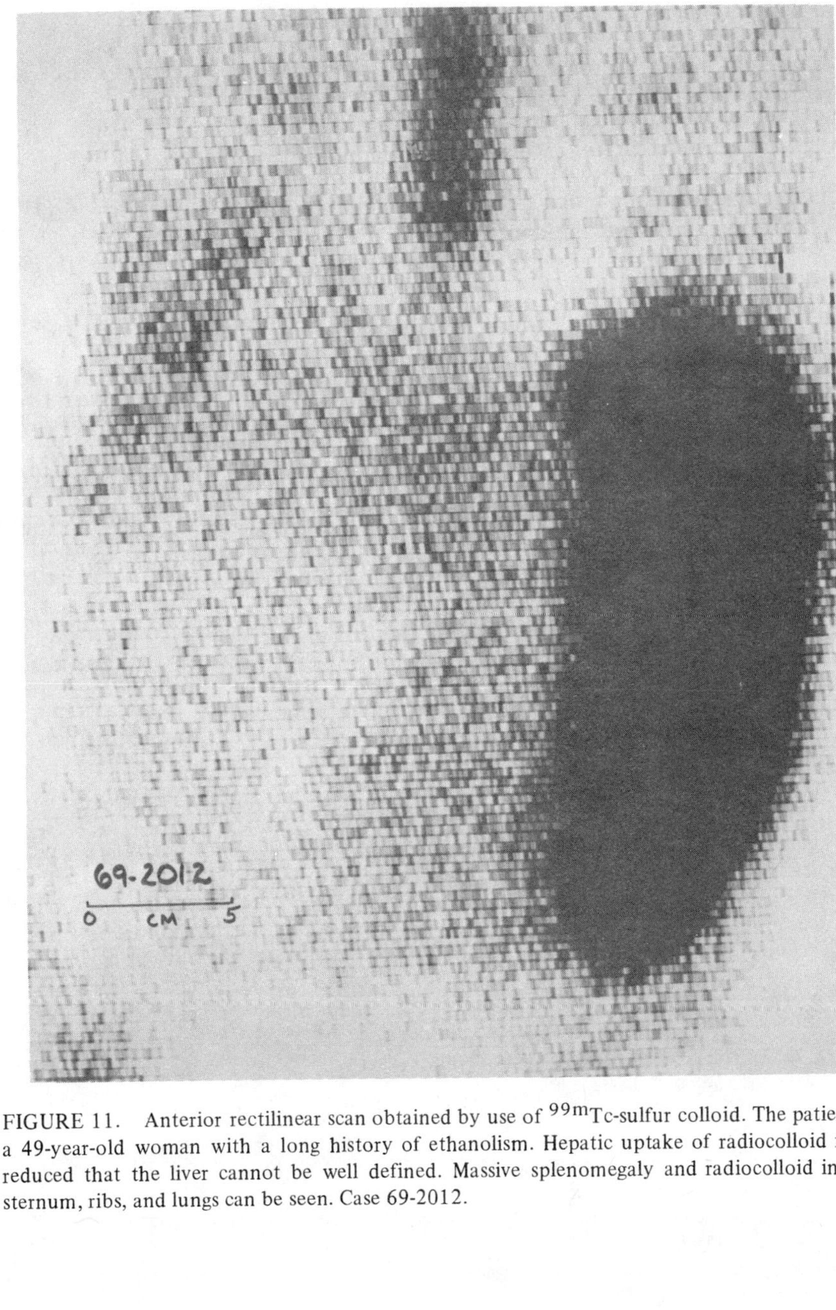

FIGURE 11. Anterior rectilinear scan obtained by use of ^{99m}Tc-sulfur colloid. The patient is a 49-year-old woman with a long history of ethanolism. Hepatic uptake of radiocolloid is so reduced that the liver cannot be well defined. Massive splenomegaly and radiocolloid in the sternum, ribs, and lungs can be seen. Case 69-2012.

REFERENCES

1. **Townsend, A. A. and Kelso, A. F.,** Influence of dual inflows on canine hepatic-circulation studies made with external scintillation detectors, *J. Nucl. Med.,* 9, 192, 1968.
2. **Baron, M. G. and Wolf, B. S.,** Splenoportography, *JAMA,* 206, 629, 1968.
3. **Braastad, F. W., Wukasach, D. C., and Jordan, P. H., Jr.,** The practicality of umbilical vein cannulation in patients with and without portal hypertension, *Arch. Surg.,* 101, 32, 1970.
4. **Sutton, J. P., Yarborough, D. Y., and Richards, J. T.,** Isolated splenic vein occlusion, *Arch. Surg.,* 100, 623, 1970.
5. **Sheldon, S. Chiandussi, L., Guevara, L., Caesar, J., and Sherlock, S.,** The estimation of hepatic blood flow and intrahepatic shunted blood flow by colloidal heat-denatured human serum albumin labeled with I^{131}, *J. Clin. Invest.,* 40, 1346, 1961.
6. **Riddell, A. G., Bloor, K., Hobbs, K. E. F., and Jacquet, N.,** Elective splenorenal anastomosis, *Br. Med. Jr.,* 1, 731, 1972.
7. **Wilcox, L. D., Gergely, N., Passi, R., Sales, J., Holder, D., and Moore, S.,** Spleen effluent manipulations: some biologic possibilities, *Am. J. Surg.,* 119, 269, 1970.
8. **Sobel, S., Kaplitt, M. J., Popowitz, L., Giradet, R. E., and Adamsons, R. J.,** Omphalocaval shunt: a new procedure for portal decompression, *Surgery,* 68, 456, 1970.
9. **Molimard, R. and Benozio, M.,** Étude de la rate au cours de la régénération hépatique après hépatectomie partielle, *Pathol. Biol.,* 18, 429, 1970.
10. **Nuland, S. B., Cornelius, E. A., and Spencer, R. P.,** Scan evidence of organ involution and improvement in Hodgkin's disease following splenic artery ligation, *J. Nucl. Med.,* 11, 693, 1970.
11. **Dalton, M. L. and West, R. L.,** Fate of dearterialized spleen, *Arch. Surg.,* 91, 541, 1965.
12. **Abrams, H. L.,** Splenic arteriography, in *Angiography,* Vol. II, 2nd ed., Abrams, H. L., Ed., Little, Brown & Co., Boston, 1971, 1003.
13. **Viamonte, M., Jr., Danner, P., Warren, W. D., and Fomon, J.,** A new technique for the assessment of hyperkinetic portal hypertension, *Radiology,* 96, 539, 1970.
14. **Koyama, K.,** Hemodynamics of the spleen in Banti's syndrome, *Tohoku J. Exp. Med.,* 93, 199, 1967.
15. **Lutz, J., Henrich, H., Peiper, U., and Bauereisen, E.,** Autoregulation and venovasomotorische Reaktion im Milzkreislauf, *Pflugers Arch.,* 313, 271, 1969.
16. **Knisely, M. H.,** Spleen studies. I. Microscopic observations of the circulatory system of living unstimulated spleens, *Anat. Rec.,* 65, 23, 1936.
17. **MacKenzie, D. W., Jr., Whipple, A. O., and Wintersteiner, M. P.,** Studies on the microscopic anatomy and physiology of living transilluminated mammalian spleens, *Am. J. Anat.,* 68, 397, 1941.
18. **Burke, J. S. and Simon, G. T.,** Electron microscopy of the spleen. I. Anatomy and microcirculation, *Am. J. Pathol.,* 58, 127, 1970.
19. **Groom, A. C. and Song, S. H.,** Washout kinetics correlated with morphological studies of red cells in the spleen, *Biophys. Soc. Abstr.,* 12, 1382, 1972.
20. **Motulsk, A. G., Casserd, F., Gillett, E. R., Broun, G. O., Jr., and Finch, C. A.,** Anemia and the spleen, *N. Engl. J. Med.,* 259, 1164, 1958.
21. **Glass, H. I., de Garreta, A. C., Lewis, P., Grammaticos, P., and Szur, L.,** Measurement of splenic red-blood cell mass with radioactive carbon monoxide, *Lancet,* 1, 669, 1968.
22. **Opdyke, D. F.,** Hemodynamics of blood flow through the spleen, *Am. J. Physiol.,* 219, 102, 1970.
23. **Stoppo, R., Pietri, J., Caron, M., Henry, X., and Abourachid, H. L.,** À propos d'un cas d'anevrisme arterio-veineux du pédicule splénique avec hypertension portale. *Ann. Chir.,* 24, 687, 1970.
24. **Goldsmith, H. S. and Castillo, J.,** A new method for kidney vascularization, *Arch. Surg.,* 97, 605, 1968.
25. **Beduhn, D. and Hallwachs, O.,** Selektive Nierenangiographie uber die implantierte Milzarterie, *Fortschr. Geb. Roentgenstr. Nuklearmed.,* 113, 133, 1970.
26. **Maillard, J. N., Benhamou, J. P., and Rueff, B.,** Arterialization of the liver with portacaval shunt in the treatment of portal hypertension due to intrahepatic block, *Surgery,* 67, 883, 1970.
27. **Gardner, W. J., Howe, R. F., and Olsen, D. O.,** Aneurysm of the hepatic artery treated by exclusion with splenic artery bypass, *Am. J. Surg.,* 118, 947, 1969.
28. **Atkins, R., Trimble, C., and Eiseman, B.,** A technique for prolonged splenic perfusion, *Surgery,* 67, 306, 1970.
29. **Rochmis, P. G.,** Splenic angioma with thrombocytopenia, *N. Y. State J. Med.,* 70, 70, 2133, 1970.
30. **Yamamoto, K.,** Histological studies on the terminals of the splenic artery in the normal and Banti spleens, *Tohoku J. Exp. Med.,* 101, 77, 1970.
31. **Ohlsson, E. G., Rutherford, R. B., Haalebos, M. M. P., Wagner, H. N., Jr., and Zuidema, G. D.,** The effect of bilary obstruction on hepatosplanchnic blood flow in dogs, *J. Surg. Res.,* 10, 201, 1970.
32. **Kety, S. S. and Schmidt, C. F.,** The nitrous oxide method for the quantitative determination of cerebral blood flow in man: theory, procedure and normal values, *J. Clin. Invest.,* 27, 476, 1948.
33. **Donato, L.,** The circulation principles, in *Principles of Nuclear Medicine,* Wagner, H. N., Jr., Ed., W. B. Saunders, Philadelphia, 1968, 531.

34. **Thorburn, G. D., Kopold, H. H., Herd, J. A., Hollenberg, M., O'Morchoe, C. C. C. and Barger, A. C.,** Intrarenal distribution of nutrient blood flow determined with Krypton 85 in the unanesthetized dog, *Circ. Res.,* 13, 290, 1963.
35. **Veall, N. and Mallet, B. L.,** The partition of trace amounts of xenon between human blood and brain tissues at 37°C, *Phys. Med. Biol.,* 10, 375, 1965.
36. **Williams, R., Condon, R. E., Williams, H. S., Blendis, L. M., and Kreel, L.,** Splenic blood flow in cirrhosis and portal hypertension, *Clin. Sci.,* 34, 441, 1968.
37. **Blendis, L. M., Roberts, V. C., Spiro, M., and Williams, R.,** The comparative measurement of splenic blood flow using ^{133}Xenon and an electromagnetic flow meter, *Cardiovasc. Res.,* 4, 44, 1970.
38. **Sandberg, G.,** Splenic blood flow in the guinea-pig measured with Xenon 133, and calculation of the venous output of lymphocytes from the spleen, *Acta Physiol. Scand.,* 84, 208, 1972.
39. **Blendis, L. M., Banks, D. C., Ramboer, C., and Williams, R.,** Spleen blood flow and splanchnic haemodynamics in blood dyscrasia and other splenomegalies, *Clin. Sci.,* 38, 73, 1970.
40. **Garnett, E. S., Goddard, B. A., Markby, D., and Webber, C. E.,** The spleen as an arteriovenous shunt, *Lancet,* 1, 386, 1969.
41. **Wolf, R. and Fischer, J.,** Estimation of splenic blood flow, *J. Nucl. Med.,* 7, 376, 1966.
42. **Sapirstein, L. A.,** Regional blood flow by fractional distribution of indicators, *Am. J. Physiol.,* 193, 161, 1958.
43. **Christensen, B. E.,** A new method for estimating splenic erythrocyte and plasma volume combined with quantitation of splenic iron incorporation, *Scand. J. Haematol.,* 8, 245, 1971.
44. **Forsyth, R. P., Nies, A. S., Wyler, F., Neutze, J., and Melmon, K. L.,** Normal distribution of cardiac output in the unanesthetized, restrained rhesus monkey, *J. Appl. Physiol.,* 25, 736, 1968.
45. **Gitlin, N., Grahame, G. R., Kreel, L., Williams, H. S., and Sherlock, S.,** Splenic blood flow and resistance in patients with cirrhosis before and after portocaval anantomoses, *Gastroenterology,* 59, 208, 1970.
46. **Cotton, L. T. and Richards, J.,** The measurement of venous blood flow by the method of local thermal dilution, in *Blood Flow Through Organs and Tissues,* Brain, W. H. and Harper, A. M., Eds., Williams & Wilkins, Baltimore, 1967, 11.
47. **Yale, C. E. and Crummy, A. B.,** Splenic vein thrombosis and bleeding esophageal varices, *JAMA,* 217, 317, 1971.
48. **Goldstein, G. B.,** Splenic vein thrombosis causing gastric varices and bleeding, *Am. J. Gastroenterol.,* 58, 319, 1972.
49. **McElroy, R. and Christiansen, P. A.,** Hereditary pancreatitis in a kinship associated with portal vein thrombosis, *Am. J. Med.,* 52, 228, 1972.
50. **Aronson, A. R. and Steinheber, F. U.,** Portal vein thrombosis in ulcerative colitis, *N.Y. State J. Med.,* 71–2, 2310, 1971.
51. **Ben-Ari, G., Mitty, H., Kark, A. E., and Rudick, J.,** Segmental portal hypertension due to congenital cavernous malformation of splenic vein, *Mt. Sinai J. Med.,* 39, 271, 1972.
52. **Tada, S., Shin, M., Takashima, T., Noguchi, M., Nishio, I., Miyake, A., and Matsubara, F.,** Diffuse capillary hemangiomatosis of the spleen as a cause of portal hypertension, *Radiology,* 104, 63, 1972.
53. **Shanberge, J. N., Tanaka, K., and Gruhl, M. C.,** Chronic consumption coagulopathy due to hemongiomatous transformation of the spleen, *Am. J. Clin. Pathol.,* 56, 723, 1971.
54. **Dufour, M., Hopfner, C., Potron, G., Lacour, F., and Miraucourt, G.,** Hemolytic anemia, defibrination syndrome in a case of splenic hemangioendothelia sarcoma, *Nouv. Presse Med.,* 1, 1347, 1972.
55. **Van Kemmel, M., Laurent, J. C., and Salembier, Y.,** Triple association (adenome hepatique, angiome splenique et lithiase du choledoque) compliquee simultanement d'hemoperitoine et d'angiocholite, *Sem. Hop. Paris,* 47, 2679, 1971.
56. **Ozsoylu, S., Hicsonmez, A., Olcay, E., and Kocak, N.,** Cruveilhier-Baumgarten disease, *Am. J. Dis. Child.,* 123, 492, 1972.
57. **Lataste, J. and Albou, J. C.,** Syndrome de Budd-Chiari, *Presse Med.,* 79, 1491, 1971.
58. **Jamieson, A. and Greig, J. H.,** Isolated celiac axis compression as a cause of visceral angina, *Can. Med. Assoc. J.,* 103, 374, 1970.
59. **Chaudhuri, Ta.K, Chandhuri, T. K., Suzuki, Y., and Christie, J. H.,** Liver scan in the Budd-Chiari syndrome, *JAMA,* 221, 506, 1972.
60. **Koikkalainen, K. and Kohler, P.,** Stenosis and occlusion in the coeliac and mesenteric arteries, *Ann. Chir. Gynaecol. Fenn.,* 60, 9, 1971.
61. **Hyman, A. L. and McDonald, C. D.,** Respiratory alterations in the intensity of the cautinuous murmur of splenic arteriovenous fistula, *Ann. Intern. Med.,* 74, 947, 1971.
62. **Gruenagel, H. H., Domres, B., Weber, V., and Baumann, S.,** Spleno-pulmonaler Shunt mit autologen Venentransplantat beim Hund, *Z. Ges. Exp. Med.,* 155, 128, 1971.
63. **Pietri, H., Assadourian, R., Bourde, J., and Varette, I.,** Compensatory hypertrophy of the rabbit spleen following partial ligation of its blood supply, *J. Surg. Res.,* 11, 594, 1971.
64. **Urca, I.,** Aneurysm of the splenic artery associated with primary carcinoma of the liver and splenomegaly, *Angiology,* 22, 470, 1971.
65. **Krawczynski, K.,** Immunohistochemical study of arteriolar (simple) hyalinosis in the spleen, *Am. J. Pathol.,* 62, 253, 1971.

66. **Stutte, H. J. and Schluter, E.,** Zur Atiologie von Fibrin pracipitaten in den Lymphfollikeln der menschlichen Milz, *Virchows Arch. Abt. A. Pathol. Anat.,* 356, 32, 1972.
67. **Brain, M. C., Dacie, J. V., and Hourihane, D. O.,** Microangiopathic haemolytic anaemia: the possible role of vascular lesions in pathogenesis, *Br. J. Haematol.,* 8, 358, 1962.
68. **Preston, F. E. and Christenhusz, R.,** Microangiopathic haemolytic anaemia: the phenomenon of red cell adherence, *J. Clin. Pathol.,* 23, 711, 1970.
69. **Dumont, A. E., Berman, I. R., Stahl, W. M., and Ring, S. M.,** Significance of an enlarged splenic artery in patients with bleeding varices, *Ann. Surg.,* 175, 466, 1972.
70. **Groszmann, R. J., Kostelanski, B, and Cohn, J. N.,** Hepatic lobar distribution of splenic and mesenteric blood flow in man, *Gastroenterology,* 60, 1047, 1971.
71. **Siegelman, S. S., Sprayregen, S., Bardfeld, P., and Boley, S. J.,** Vasopressin infusion of the splenic artery: splenic exclusion, *Invest. Radiol.,* 6, 341, 1971.
72. **Svec, K. H. and Allen, S. T.,** Antibody to nuclear material eluted from isolated spleen vessels in systemic lupus erythematosos, *Science,* 170, 550, 1970.
73. **Firket, H. and Beaumariage, M. L.,** Ultrastructural modifications of mitrochondria and encloplasmic reticulum of liver and spleen after a period of hypoxia, *Virchows Arch. Abt. B. Zellpathol.,* 8, 342, 1971.
74. **Schildt, B. E.,** The role of the RES in shock states, *Ann. Chir. Gynaecol. Fenn.,* 60, 165, 1971.
75. **Shuster, D. and Palayew, M. J.,** Accordion-like compression of a calcified splenic artery: a plain film roentgenographic sign of splenic enlargement, *Am. J. Roentgenol.,* 116, 423, 1972.
76. **Swan, K. G., Barton, R. W., and Reynolds, D. G.,** Mesenteric hemodynamics during endotoxemia in the baboon, *Gastroenterology,* 61, 872, 1971.
77. **Swan, K. G. and Reynolds, D. G.,** Blood flow to the liver and spleen during endotoxin shock in the baboon, *Surgery,* 72, 388, 1972.
78. **Swan, K. G., Evans, L. W., and Reynolds, D. G.,** Hepatic and splenic blood flows during endotoxic shock in baboons, *Physiologist,* 15, 280, 1972.
79. **Trejo, R. A. and DiLuzio, N. R.,** Enhanced endotoxin detoxification ability of liver and spleen during the state of endotoxin tolerance, *Physiologist,* 15, 289, 1972.
80. **Gunteroth, W. G. and Felsenfeld, A. J.,** Splenic constriction with endotoxin shock in the dog, *J. Appl. Physiol.,* 30, 517, 1971.
81. **Cherniak, N. S., Edelman, N. H., and Fishman, A. P.,** O_2 exchange across spleen during asphyxia, *Am. J. Physiol.,* 219, 1585, 1970.
82. **Gupta, R. K., Shuster, R., and Christian, W. D.,** A comparative immunohistochemical study of splenic arterial hyalinosis in health and disease, *Am. J. Pathol.,* 69, 79, 1972.
83. **Jones, E. F., Nelson, A. W., Erickson, H. H., and Stone, H. L.,** Regional blood flow during hypoxia, *Physiologist,* 15, 185, 1972.
84. **Chou, C. C., Hsieh, C. P., and Dabney, J. W.,** Local effects of G-I hormones on duodenal, jejunal, spleen, skin and muscle vascular resistance, *Physiologist,* 15, 107, 1972.
85. **Saubier, E. C., Brault, J. A., and Partensky, C.,** 57 Anastomoses spleno-renales pour hypertension protale, *Arch. Fr. Mal. Appar. Dig.,* 61, 161, 1972.
86. **Kille, J. F. and Hallwachs, O.,** Revascularization of the ischaemic kidney by implantation of the splenic artery and vein into the renal parenchyma. II. Reconstruction of arterio-arterial anastomoses by studies of histological serial sections, *Mikroskopie,* 28, 133, 1972.
87. **O'Grady, J. F., Bonakdarpour, A., Reichle, R. M., and Reichle, R. A.,** Effect of renal vascularization by splenic artery implantation on experimental renovascular hypertension, *J. Surg. Res.,* 2, 67, 1972.
88. **Manz, C. and Sako, Y.,** Splenic artery implantation in the kidney; effect on experimental renal hypertension, *Arch. Surg.,* 103, 242, 1971.
89. **Song, S. H. and Groom, A. C.,** Sequestration and possible maturation of reticulocytes in the normal spleen, *Can. J. Physiol. Pharmacol.,* 50, 400, 1972.
90. **Song, S. H. and Groom, A. C.,** The distribtution of red cells in the spleen, *Can. J. Physiol. Pharmacol.,* 49, 734, 1971.
91. **Song, S. H. and Groom, A. C.,** Immature and abnormal erythrocytes present in the normal, healthy spleen, *Scand. J. Haematol.,* 8, 487, 1971.
92. **Groom, A. C., Song, S. H., Linn, P., and Campling, B.,** Physical characteristics of red cells collected from the spleen, *Can. J. Physiol. Pharmacol.,* 49, 1092, 1971.
93. **Song, S. H. and Groom, A. C.,** Storage of blood cells in the spleen of the cat, *Am. J. Physiol.,* 220, 779, 1971.
94. **Mendell, P. L. and Hollenberg, N. K.,** Cardiac output distribution in the rat: comparison of rubidium and microsphere methods, *Am. J. Physiol.,* 221, 1617, 1971.
95. **Zierler, K. L.,** Equations for measuring flow by external monitoring of radioisotopes, *Circ. Res.,* 16, 309, 1965.

96. **Veda, H., Kitani, K., Kamedo, H., Takedo, T., Chiba, K., Nagatani, M., Yamada, H., and Iio, M.,** Splenic blood flow in idiopathic portal hypertension in Japan measured by ^{85}Kr clearance method, *Acta Hepato-Splenol.,* 18, 28, 1971.
97. **Groszmann, R., Kotelanski, B., Cohn, J. N., and Khatri, I. M.,** Quantitation of portasystemic shunting from the splenic and mesenteric beds in alcoholic liver disease, *Am. J. Med.,* 53, 715, 1972.
98. **Johnson, R. B., Castell, D. O., and Lukash, W. M.,** Liver scanning for detection of collateral circulation in liver disease, *JAMA,* 207, 528, 1969.
99. **Fernandez, J. P., O'Rourke, R. A., Cooper, J. N., Ewy, G. A., and Mullen, J. C.,** The extrahepatic uptake of ^{198}Au as an index of portal hypertension, *Am. J. Digest. Dis.,* 15, 883, 1970.
100. **Joly, J. G., Marleau, D., Legare, A., Lavoie, P., Bernier, J., and Viallet, A.,** Bleeding from esophageal varices in cirrhosis of the liver, *Can. Med. Assoc. J.,* 104, 576, 1971.
101. **Castell, D. O. and Johnson, R. B.,** The ^{198}Au liver scan: an index of portal systemic collateral circulation in chronic liver disease, *N. Eng. J. Med.,* 275, 188, 1966.
102. **Rogers, A. I. and Feiss, J. S.,** The application of liver scan to the diagnosis of esophageal varices, *South. Med. J.,* 63. 950, 1970.
103. **Gourgoutis, G. D., Das, G., and Lindsay, N.,** Splenic uptake of ^{99m}Technetium sulfur colloid as an index of portal hypertension, *Am. J. Gastroenterol.,* 57, 435, 1972.
104. **Rosenthall, L., Greyson, N. D., Lacourciere, Y., and Arzoumanian, A.,** A liver trapping index of radiocolloid as an estimation of perfusion, *Radiology,* 100, 363, 1971.
105. **Dumont, A. E., Amorosi, E., and Stahl, W. M.,** Significance of splenomegaly in patients with hepatic cirrhosis and bleeding esophageal varices, *Ann. Surg.,* 171, 522, 1970.
106. **Leger, L., Lemaigre, G., Lenriot, J. P., Gorin, J. P., Duclos, B., and Paulian, B.,** Le foie et la rate des cirrhotiques apres derivation porto-cave, *Presse Med.,* 79, 701, 1971.
107. **Kyu, M. H. and Cavanagh, J. B.,** Some effects of porto-caval anastomosis in the male rat, *Br. J. Exp. Pathol.,* 51, 217, 1970.
108. **Spencer, R. P. and Antar, M. A.,** Radionuclides in the investigaton of liver disease, in *Progess in Liver Disease,* Vol. IV, Popper, H. and Schaffner, F., Eds., Grune and Stratton, New York, 1972, 217.
109. **Spencer, R. P., Touloukian, R. J., Lange, R. C., Nuland, S. B., and Fischer, D. S.,** Effects of vascular lesions on hepato-splenic accumulation of radiocolloid, *J. Nucl. Med.,* 12, 397, 1971.
110. **Jones, T., Pettit, J. E., Rhodes, C. G., and Waters, S. L.,** Use of ^{81}Rb-^{81m}Kr ratio for the measurment of spleen blood flow, *J. Nucl. Med.,* 14, 414, 1973.
111. **Grangsjo, G., Ulfendahl, H. R., and Wolgast, M.,** Determination of regional blood flow by means of small semiconductor detectors and red cells tagged with phosphorus-32, *Nature,* 211, 1411, 1966.
112. **Gates, G. F. and Dore, E. K.,** Streamline flow in the human portal vein, *J. Nucl. Med.,* 14, 79, 1973.

Chapter 8

ECTOPIC SPLEEN, TRANSPOSITION, AND TRANSPLANTATION

Splenic transposition has been used as a tentative tool in the management of portal hypertension and as an experimental approach for studying splenic function. Surgically moving the spleen from the abdomen to the thorax, in an effort to create portal-systemic shunting, has been documented.[1] In the single case we have studied, the spleen could be noted (radiographically) to be present in the chest. However, it was not functioning some months after the surgery.[2] The lack of function was demonstrated by the presence of Howell-Jolly bodies, as well as inability to accumulate ^{99m}Tc-sulfur colloid. Subcutaneous transposition of the spleen has been tried in animals,[3,4] but this has no clearly demonstrated role in man at the moment. Williams[5] has reported on splenic autografts in the rabbit and so have Tavassoli and co-workers.[47]

Transplantation of the spleen, originally studied in animals, has now (to a limited degree) been extended to human subjects. Uses of splenic transplantation can be divided into three broad classes.

1. To study tissue mechanisms in transplantation and the effects of the spleen and of radiation on the transplanted tissue.
2. To provide immunocompetent lymphocytes (antitumor).
3. To supply an enzyme or factor otherwise lacking in the recipient.

Kountz and Cohn[6] studied the effect of the spleen on renal transplantation in dogs. Four groups were created.

1. Controls.
2. Splenectomized.
3. Splenic homograft.
4. Splenectomized plus splenic homograft.

In the last group, with the dog's own spleen removed and that of the donor surgically supplied, renal transplants from the donor survived for a longer period of time than in the other groups. The mechanism was thought to be the weakening of the recipient's immune mechanism by removal of the spleen and the presence of large amounts of donor antigen supplied by the donor spleen. Fiscus and co-workers[7] pursued this problem by utilizing three groups of dogs given whole body radiation.

I. Given 300 R.

II. Given 300 R after a splenic autograft (spleen shielded).

III. Given 300 R, 48 hr after splenic homograft.

Mortality rates in the groups were

Group I 17%
Group II 40%
Group III 86%

Irradiation likely affected lymphoid elements and immune competence. Giving an immunocompetent spleen resulted in a lowered survival, perhaps by tissue injury through the graft-versus-host reaction (GVHR). The spleen revealed erythrophagocytosis, consistent with GVHR. By an unknown mechanism (and unexpectedly), there is a report that heterotransplanted splenic tissue, placed in diffusion chambers within irradiated mice, was of benefit.[8] Woods and co-workers[9] studied patients having renal allografts. Leukopenia induced by azathioprine (Imuran®) was higher in nonsplenectomized patients than in those who were splenectomized before transplantation. Splenectomy after renal transplantation in two cases was followed by increased tolerance to azathioprine. One patient with a hepatoma had spleen and bone marrow transplants in an effort to help rejection of the tumor.[48] Upon injection of ^{99m}Tc-sulfur colloid, much accumulated in the lungs.

Immunocompetent lymphocytes of an animal will potentially attack foreign cells, including tumors. Starzl's group[10] injected homogenized tumor cells from a patient into the individual who was to be the donor of a spleen to the patient. Hence, the spleen was presumably presensitized to the tumor, but the recipient was not presensitized to the donor's tissues. Although the idea had merit, limited clinical trials did not demonstrate any beneficial effect (and other studies have also not been more encouraging).[19] Interestingly, ^{197}Hg-bromomercurihydroxypropane scans were used to demonstrate the transplanted spleens. Also of note was the fact that an A$^+$ recipient receiving a splenic transplant from an O$^+$ donor developed hypersplenism. This was documented by a shortened red cell survival (^{51}Cr survival T½ decreased from 25 days to 9 hr) and by a depressed platelet count and leukocyte count. However, there was no evidence of erythrophagocytosis in the (later removed) spleen. There has also been a note concerning a spleen graft from one man to his identical twin (who had lymphocytic sarcoma).[11] Again the rationale was that immunocompetent lymphocytes might attack the abnormal lymphoma cells. In the amphibian *Xenopus laevis*,[25] transplanted immunized spleens carry out immunological functions in tolerant animals, but the spleens themselves may be attacked in a host-versus-graft reaction.

A successfully transplanted spleen would conceivably function and supply materials not otherwise being produced by the recipient. Accordingly, splenic homotransplantation has been tried in a limited number of situations.[10,15]

Agammaglobulimemia[10] – There was no evidence of increased gamma globulin production following the transplant.

Hemophilia – Here the attempt was to introduce splenic tissue capable of producing factor VIII. However, there was no clear documentation that the desired effect was obtained in man[12] (and perhaps the spleen is a reservoir site and not the main region of production). However, techniques for preserving the spleen after removal have been described,[13] and in one case an infusion of spleen cells has been reported.[14] Interestingly, in heparinized dogs, spleen cells placed in the portal system can colonize in the liver.[24]

Gaucher's Disease – The spleen is an active site of the enzyme that cleaves glucocerebroside to glucose and ceramide. This enzyme is deficient in Gaucher's disease. In a case of splenic transplantation in Gaucher's disease, the spleen apparently functioned, as shown by a ^{99m}Tc-sulfur colloid scan.[16] After 40 days the spleen was rejected, and any transient improvement in the clinical picture was reversed.[18]

INTRASPLENIC TRANSPLANTS

The surgical placement of tissues in the spleen (intrasplenic transplants) has been investigated in animals, and there are also accompanying functional data. Mori has summarized the literature on intrasplenic testicular transplants in gonadectomized mice, rats, rabbits, and guinea pigs.[17] Tumors may arise in the intrasplenic ovarian or testicular grafts. The pathogenesis is thought to be related to hepatic inactivation of much of the sex hormones that enter via the portal system (since the intrasplenic gonadal graft drains via the splenic vein and portal vein). Gonadotrophins are then likely hypersecreted by the anterior hypophysis since the circulating peripheral levels of the target organ hormones would be low. The intrasplenic transplants appear to be functional in some cases[17,20,21] and may grow outward from the spleen. Indeed, a cystic ovary within the spleen can develop, likely in response to the gonadotrophic stimulation.[22] Thyroid tissue can also be implanted in the spleen. Dardik and co-workers[23] have reported on thyroid implants on the spleen and the shunting of the splenic effluent to avoid inactivation of hormones.

ECTOPIC AND ACCESSORY SPLENIC TISSUE

By accessory splenic tissue we mean that which occurs outside of the single spleen found in most of the population (an example is shown in Chapter 3). This accessory tissue has to be distinguished from the ectopic spleen (a single spleen "incorrectly" located) or the ptotic, wandering,[46] or migrating spleen (exaggerated mobility of the organ, Figure 1). The interesting condition of polysplenia was discussed in an earlier section.

An ectopic single spleen (occurring in an unusual place or location) is not common. Most reports may represent a migrating or "wandering" spleen,[26] likely due to an elongated pedicle.[30] We have seen a case (a 2-year-old boy) in which a low-lying spleen returned to a more normal position following gastric decompression.[27] The danger of an elongated splenic pedicle is that torsion can occur. Torsion has been reported in man[49] and the dog.[28] An ectopic spleen has also been reported to mimic a fundal lesion by indenting the stomach,[29] and, of course, the normal spleen can be adjacent to the stomach.

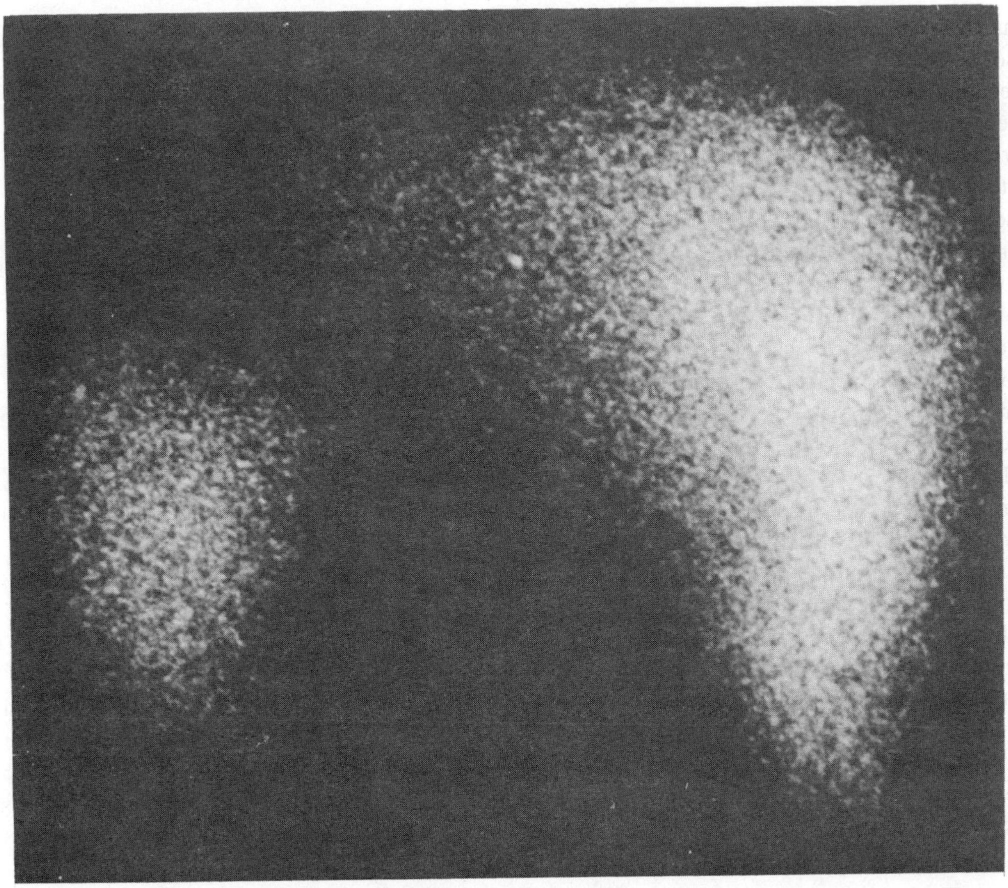

FIGURE 1. Posterior scintiphoto (^{99m}Tc-sulfur colloid) of the spleen and liver in a 2½-year-old girl. Anteriorly, the spleen could be palpated low in the abdomen. This likely qualifies as a case of wandering spleen.

Accessory splenic tissue in most instances causes no symptoms; the diagnosis is made at autopsy or operation. However, Settle[31] has pointed out that symptoms may be produced by: (1) mechanical interference, (2) inflammation, (3) neoplastic changes (especially the lymphomas), and (4) compensatory hypertrophy following primary splenectomy (this can also be shown in the chicken).[32] Settle[31] also quotes Schilling[33] as to the commonest locales of accessory splenic tissue. These are

1. Hilus of spleen.
2. Gastrosplenic ligament.
3. Splenocolic ligament.
4. Great omentum.
5. Pleurocolic ligament.
6. Peritoneal tissue along the splenic vessels.
7. Pancreas.

An interesting variant of ectopic splenic tissue is that which occurs in the testicular area. Mendez and Morrow[34] apparently reported the 54th case in the literature, all of which have been on the left side. Quoting B. M. Patten (*Human Embryology*, Blakiston, Philadelphia, 1946), Mendez and Morrow state that the coalescing tissue masses in the embryo, which are the progenitors of the spleen, push laterally into the coelomic cavity, coming close to the gonadal bud from the mesonephric ridge. Fusion may occur since a splenic or fibrous cord usually connects the primary spleen with the splenic tissue in the testicular area. These authors also refer to a fascinating case, reported by Talman,[35] in which the ectopic spleen in the testicular region grew and then decreased in size with intermittent attacks of malaria.

Cahalane and Kiesselbach[36] reviewed 945

post-mortem protocols in infants and children. An accessory spleen was reported in 10% of the females and 11% of the males. Their data on the number of spleens present are illustrated in Figure 2. Perhaps the most interesting value to emerge from this study was that 53% of the cases with an accessory spleen had a least one other congenital malformation. In the control group (single spleen), there was a 25% incidence of congenital malformations. When the malformations (in those with accessory spleens) were considered under individual organ systems, defects of the cardiovascular system were the commonest.

The occurrence of several small splenic "pieces" or spleniculi has been reported as a congenital malformation. This is often associated with cardiac abnormalities[37] (dextrocardia, artrial, and septal defects can be present; see discussion of Ivemark syndrome). It is interesting that this "polysplenia" may have accompanying cardiac defects, while congenital asplenia also has associated cardiac anomalies.

Cahalane and Kiesselbach[36] have provided a good review of the literature as to the occurrence of the accessory spleen and the blood supply of these organs.

Multiple peritoneal implants can occur in endometriosis, carcinomatosis, and other conditions. Buchbinder and Lipkoff[38] described such implants due to splenic tissue and termed the condition splenosis (earlier reports of the condition had appeared, but the term splenosis has gained wide acceptance). Splenosis likely arises from small implants of splenic tissue liberated by operation or trauma ("autotransplantation"). An extensive review of the literature, including animal experiments on splenic tissue implantation, has been provided by Widmann and Laubscher.[39]

The typical appearance of splenosis is that of small, dark red implants without muscle in their fibrous capsule. Such findings, in those with prior abdominal trauma or splenic surgery, likely establish the diagnosis. Jacobson and De Nardo[40] noted that such splenic autotransplants possess the ability to accumulate intravenously injected ^{99m}Tc-sulfur colloid. Another interesting point revolves about the blood picture in splenosis.[39,40] Following removal of the spleen, the typical post splenectomy blood picture develops, particularly Howell-Jolly bodies in erythrocytes. In some of the cases which develop postsplenectomy splenosis, there is apparently sufficient functional

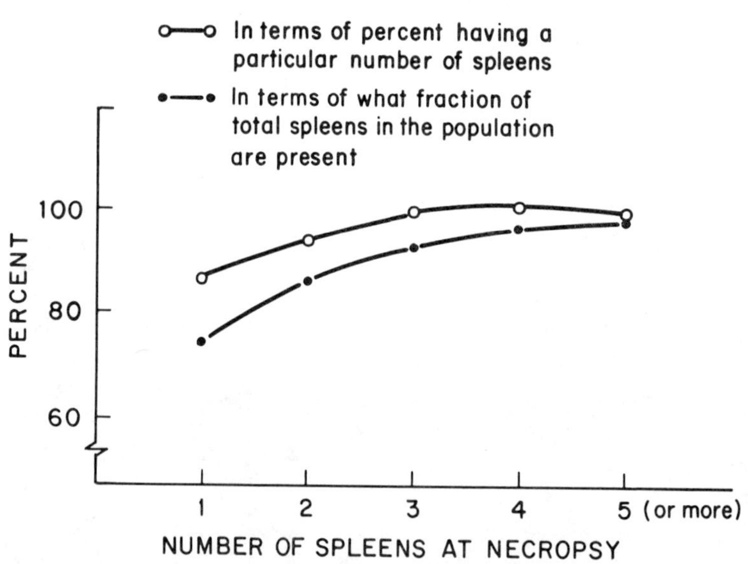

FIGURE 2. Data from Cahalane and Kiesselbach[36] on the number of spleens found in post-mortem examinations of infants and children. The top line represents the cumulative percent of examinations having a particular number of spleens. The bottom line represents the percent of the total spleens present in the population. For example 845 cases had one spleen (845 × 1 = 845), 61 cases had two spleens (61 × 2 = 122), 21 cases had three spleens (21 × 3 = 63), 10 cases had four spleens (10 × 4 = 40), and 8 cases had five or more spleens (assume 8 × 5 = 40). The total number of spleens was 1,110 in 945 cases or nearly 1.2 per case.

splenic tissue to clear the blood of Howell-Jolly bodies. Hence,

1. Splenosis or an accessory spleen should be suspected in an individual with prior abdominal trauma or splenectomy.

2. In a splenectomized person, absence of Howell-Jolly bodies from the peripheral blood may be diagnostic of remaining splenic tissue (but lesser degrees of splenosis may not clear all the Howell-Jolly bodies).[41]

3. The tissue implants in splenosis likely possess the ability to accumulate technetium sulfur colloid (and we can only speculate as to their ability to take up heat-denatured ^{51}Cr-erythrocytes and to make immunoglobulins.)

IDIOPATHIC THROMBOCYTOPENIC PURPURA (ITP) AND ACCESSORY SPLENIC TISSUE

Some conditions are markedly benefited by splenectomy. Included among these are a significant portion of the patients with idiopathic thrombocytopenic purpura (ITP). If the ITP is benefited by splenectomy, and symptoms later recur, serious thought must be given to the occurrence of hypertrophied functional accessory splenic tissue (and perhaps splenosis).

As yet, there is no ideal approach to the problem of detecting accessory splenic tissue. We would suggest proceeding as follows:

1. Blood smear should be carefully checked for the presence of Howell-Jolly bodies. Their absence means that a sufficient volume of functional splenic tissue is present to clear these intraerythrocytic inclusions.

2. In terms of minimal radiation exposure, ease of the technique, and general availability of the radionuclide, ^{99m}Tc-sulfur colloid scans are readily performed. Hence, this study should be carried out first (Figure 3). Clear demonstration of accessory functional tissue, in terms of ability to accumulate radiocolloid, answers the question. We have recently reported a case in which ITP was benefited by splenectomy; upon recurrence of the disease, an accessory spleen was shown on scan.[45] Sometimes, however, when using radiocolloids, a definitive answer cannot be obtained, even with angulated views. For example, the liver may extend across the midline, making interpretation

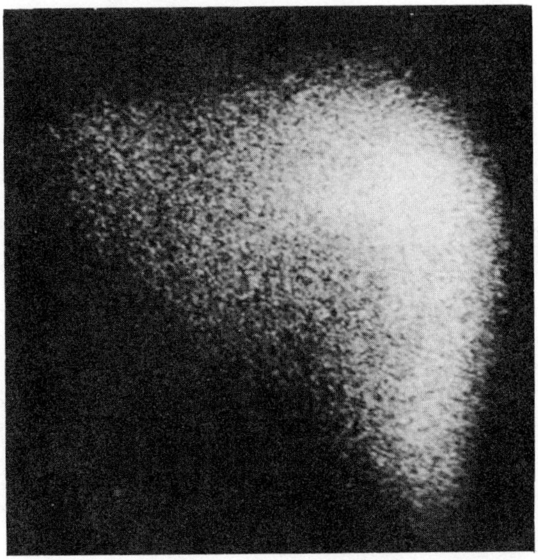

FIGURE 3. Posterior scintiphoto (^{99m}Tc-sulfur colloid) in a 7-year-old boy who had undergone splenectomy for idiopathic thrombocytopenic purpura. No splenic tissue is seen. Case 71-1478.

of activity on the left (posteriorly) quite difficult. In addition, the great activity in the liver may "shield" small quantities of splenic tissue.

3. A negative ^{99m}Tc-sulfur colloid scan, during a search for accessory splenic tissue, is an indication to proceed with studies utilizing labeled, denatured erythrocytes. There are at least three radiolabels available.

a. The technique with the longest use involves ^{51}Cr-erythrocytes, which have been heat denatured by heating to 50°C (Figure 4). Other methods for denaturing the tagged erythrocytes include treatment with antisera, or sulfhydryl inhibitors. Difficulties with this procedure are as follows: (1) The radiation dose from ^{51}Cr is much greater than that from ^{99m}Tc. (2) Even slight variations in technique may cause the tagged and denatured erythrocytes to be taken up entirely by the liver, instead of by splenic tissue. (3) Some erythrocytes (particularly those containing unstable hemoglobins or in cases of thalassemia with a probable excess of one type of hemoglobin chain) cannot tolerate the heating of 50°C. A lesser, or different, trauma might suffice but has yet to be quantified.

b. Wagner and co-workers[42] introduced radiomercury-labeled mercurihydroxy propane (MHP) as a compound for both labeling and denaturing erythrocytes. Mercury in the com-

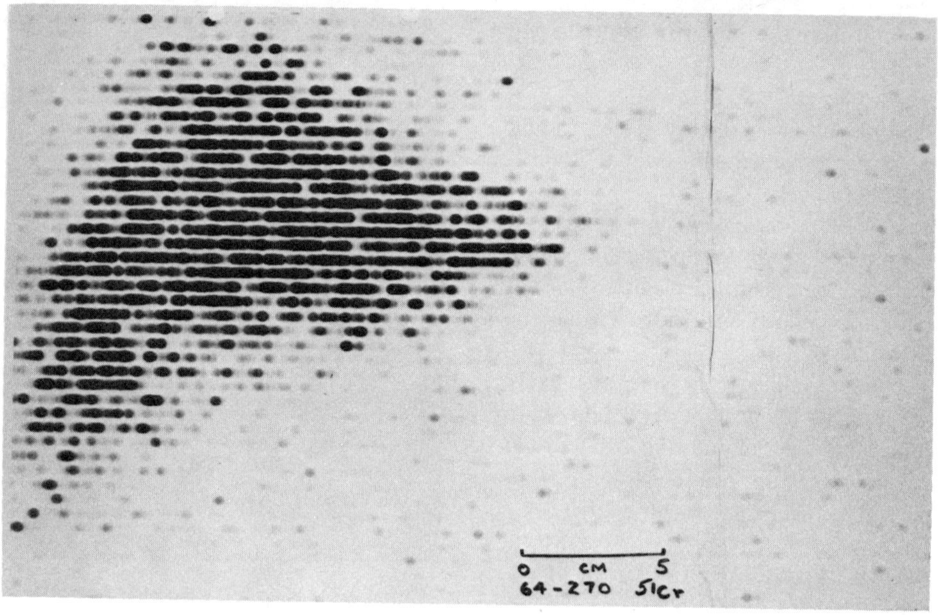

FIGURE 4. Anterior rectinilinear scan performed with ^{51}Cr-heat denatured erythrocytes. The patient is a 47-year-old man who had a splenectomy some years ago because of idiopathic thrombocytopenic purpura. No splenic tissue can be seen; the liver accumulates the radiolable. Case 64-270.

pound apparently binds to the erythrocytes (possibly through sulfhydryl groups), both providing a radiolabel and denaturation of the same step. With this agent there are also several problems. First, there are no ideal radionuclides of mercury available.

	T1/2	Emission	Problem
^{197}Hg	2.7 days	77 keV gamma ray	The low energy gamma ray is not very penetrating. Short half-life makes storage difficult.
^{203}Hg	46.7 days	279 keV gamma ray, 210 keV beta ray	High radiation dose due to the long physical half-life and the beta ray.

Wagner[43] has estimated that 100 μCi of ^{203}Hg-MHP delivers a radiation dose of 70 rd to the kidneys. Use of ^{197}Hg reduces the dose to about 7 rd. Second, mercury bound to the kidneys might obscure small amounts of functional splenic tissue. Third, although this is likely minor, the pharmacology of MHP has not been well described.

c. A number of techniques for labeling erythrocytes with ^{99m}Tc have been described. The group at Brookhaven[44] has reported success with use of $SnCl_2$, which apparently both aids in maintaining ^{99m}Tc within erythrocytes and in denaturing the cells so that they are accumulated by the spleen. Most of the ^{99m}Tc can be bound to erythrocytes in 15 min. Using this, the calculated radiation dose to the spleen was 0.43 rd/mCi, or about one tenth the dose received with ^{51}Cr. Development of ^{99m}Tc-Sn-citrate label for red cells by the Brookhaven group may make this technique widely available.

REFERENCES

1. **Strauch, G. O.**, Supradiaphragmatic splenic transposition, *Am. J. Surg.*, 119, 379, 1970.
2. **Spencer, R. P., Pearson, H. A., and Binder, H. J.**, Identification of cases of "acquired" functional asplenia, *J. Nucl. Med.*, 11, 763, 1970.
3. **Bengmark, S., Borjesson, B., Olin, T., Sakuma, S., and Vosmic, J.**, Subcutaneous transposition of the spleen: an experimental study in the rat, *Scand. J. Gastroenterol. Suppl.*, 7, 175, 1970.
4. **Blumgart, L. H., Leach, K. G., McLachlan, M. S. F., Seager, S., and Ryan, C. J.**, Portal venous injection in the rat, *Gut*, 12, 585, 1971.
5. **Williams, R. G.**, The microscopic structure and behavior of spleen autografts in rabbits, *Am. J. Anat.*, 87, 459, 1950.
6. **Kountz, S. L. and Cohn, R.**, Prolonged survival of a renal homograft by simultaneous splenectomy and splenic homotransplantation, *Surg. Forum*, 13, 59, 1962.
7. **Fiscus, W. G., Trentin, J. J., Collins, V. P., Fuller, D. G., and Jordan, G. L., Jr.**, Effect of spleen homotransplants in animals subjected to sublethal doses of total body irradiation, *Surg. Forum*, 14, 182, 1963.
8. **Spertzel, R. O. and Pollard, M.**, Heterotransplanted spleen tissues in diffusion chambers: therapeutic benefits to irradiated mice, *J. Reticuloendothel. Soc.*, 8, 1, 1970.
9. **Woods, J. E., DeWeerd, J. H., Johnson, W. J., and Anderson, C. F.**, Splenectomy in renal transplantation; influence on azathioprine sensitivity, *JAMA*, 218, 1430, 1971.
10. **Marchioro, T. L., Rowlands, D. T., Jr., Rifkind, D., Waddell, W. R., Starzl, T. E., and Fudenberg, H.**, Splenic homotransplantation, *Ann. N. Y. Acad. Sci.*, 120, 626, 1964.
11. **Anon.**, Spleen graft: theory and a life at stake, *Med. World News*, 11(11), 20, March 13, 1970.
12. **Russel, P. S. and Winn, H. J.**, Transplantation. III, *N. Engl. J. Med.*, 282, 896, 1970.
13. **Molokhia, F. A., Asimacopoulos, P. J., Pegg, C. A. S., and Norman, J. C.**, Simple method of 24 hour spleen preservation: further studies relating to hemophilia, *Transplant. Proc.*, 3, 654, 1971.
14. **Desai, R. G., Inami, K., Lavon, R., and Antoine, J.**, "Promising Results" Hemophilia treated with spleen cells, cited in Medical News Section, *JAMA*, 207, 1267, 1969.
15. **Hathaway, W. E., Mull, M. M., Githens, J. H., Groth, C. G., Marchioro, T. L., and Starzl, T. E.**, Attempt at spleen transplant in classical hemophilia, *Transplantation*, 7, 73, 1969.
16. **Groth, C. G., Hagenfeldt, L., Dreborg, S., Lofstron, B., Ockerman, P. A., Samuelsson, K., Svennerholm, L., Werner, B., and Westberg, G.**, Splenic transplantation in a case of Gaucher's disease, *Lancet*, I, 1260, 1971.
17. **Mori, T.**, Function of intrasplenic testicular transplants in ovariectomized mice, *Proc. Jap. Acad.*, 46, 434, 1970.
18. **Groth, C. G., Bergstrom, K., Collste, L., Egberg, N., Hogman, C., Holm, G., and Moller, E.**, Immunologic and plasma protein studies in a splenic homograft recipient, *Clin. Exp. Immunol.*, 10, 359, 1972.
19. **Starzl, T. E., Marchioro, T. L., Rifkind, D., Rowlands, D. T., Jr., and Waddell, W. R.**, Clinical experience with organ transplantation, *South. Med. J.*, 58, 131, 1965.
20. **Fels, E., Bosch, L. R., and Zurro, A. R.**, Die Lebensfähigkeit des in die Milz implantierten ovarium, *Endokrinologie*, 56, 213, 1970.
21. **Uhlarik, A. and Wiegand, H.**, Einfluss von Lynestrenol auf das in die Milz implantierte Ovar bei der Ratte, *Arch. Gynaekol.*, 212, 41, 1972.
22. **McGowan, L. and Dans, R. H.**, Intrasplenic ovarian grafts in Syrian hamsters and peritoneal fluid cellular distribution, *Proc. Soc. Exp. Biol. Med.*, 134, 507, 1970.
23. **Dardik, H., Dardik, I., Smith, R. B., Mitsudo, S., Sherman, A., and Gliedmann, M. L.**, Intrasplenic thyroid implantation with reverse splenocaval shunting: a morphologic and functional evaluation, *Surgery*, 70, 561, 1971.
24. **Pegg, C. A. S. and Norman, J. C.**, Intraportal spleen cell autotransplantation, *Surgery* 69, 433, 1971.
25. **Clark, J. C. and Newth, D. R.**, Immunological activity of transplanted spleens in *Xenopus laevis*, *Experientia*, 28, 951, 1972.
26. **Abell, I.**, Wandering spleen with torsion of pedicle, *Ann. Surg.*, 98, 722, 1933.
27. **Landgarten, S. and Spencer, R. P.**, Splenic displacement due to gastric dilatation, *J. Nucl. Med.*, 13, 223, 1971.
28. **Orman, M. E. and Lorenz, M. D.**, Torsion of the splenic pedicle in a dog, *J. Am. Vet. Med. Assoc.*, 160, 1099, 1972.
29. **Font, R. G., Sparks, R. D., and Herbert, G. A.**, Ectopic spleen mimicking an intrinsic fundal lesion of the stomach, *Am. J. Digest. Dis.*, 15, 49, 1970.
30. **Crossett, A. D., Jr., Nestler, W. B., and Cohen, S. J.**, Wandering spleen, *Johns Hopkins Med. J.*, 124, 28, 1969.
31. **Settle, E. B.**, The surgical importance of accessory spleens, with report of two cases, *Am. J. Surg.*, 50, 22, 1940.
32. **Glick, B.**, Hypertrophy of accessory spleens in splenectomized chickens, *Folia Biol.*, 16, 74, 1970.
33. **Schilling, K.**, Über einen Fall von multiplen Nebenmilzen, *Virchows Arch. Pathol. Anat.*, 188, 65, 1907.
34. **Mendez, R. and Morrow, J. W.**, Ectopic spleen simulating testicular tumor, *J. Urol.*, 102, 598, 1969.
35. **Talmann, I. M.**, Nebenmilze im Nebenhoden und Samenstrang, *Virchows Arch. Pathol. Anat.*, 259, 237, 1926.
36. **Cahalane, S. F. and Kiesselbach, N.**, The significance of the accessory spleen, *J. Pathol.*, 100, 139, 1970.
37. **Helwig, F. C.**, Multiple spleen combined with other cogenital anomalies: report of two cases, *Arch. Pathol.*, 8, 757, 1929.
38. **Buchbinder, J. H. and Lipkoff, C. J.**, Splenosis: multiple peritoneal splenic implants following abdominal injury, *Surgery*, 6, 927, 1939.

39. **Widman, W. D. and Laubscher, F. A.,** Splenosis: a disease or a beneficial condition? *Arch. Surg.,* 102, 152, 1971.
40. **Jacobson, S. J. and De Nardo, G. L.,** Splenosis demonstrated by splenic scan, *J. Nucl. Med.,* 12, 570, 1971.
41. **Widmann, W. D., Laubscher, F. A., Davidson, S. J., and Grenoble, R. A.,** Effect of splenectomy and splenosis on the blood and platelet count and red cell morphology, *Milit. Med.,* 136, 15, 1971.
42. **Wagner, H. N., Jr., Weiner, I. M., McAfee, J. G., and Martinez, J.,** 1-mercuri-2-hydroxypropane (MHP), *Arch. Intern. Med.,* 113, 696, 1964.
43. **Wagner, H. N., Jr., and Rhodes, B. A.,** The radiopharmaceutical, in *Principles of Nuclear Medicine,* Wagner, H. N., Jr., Ed., W. B. Saunders, Philadelphia, 1968, 288.
44. **Eckelman, W., Richards, P., Atkins, H. L., Hauser, W., and Klopper, J. F.,** Visualization of human spleen with ^{99m}Tc-labeled red blood cells, *J. Nucl. Med.,* 12, 354, 1971.
45. **Aspnes, G. T., Pearson, H. A., Spencer, R. P., and Pickett, L. K.,** Recurrent idiopathic thrombocytopenic purpura with "accessory" splenic tissue, *Pediatrics,* in 55, 131, 1975.
46. **Boshiak, M. A. and Byck, W.,** Wandering spleen diagnosed preoperatively by intravenous aortography, *Am. J. Roentgenol.,* 84, 898, 1960.
47. **Tavassoli, M., Ratzan, R. J., and Crosby, W. H.,** Studies on regeneration of heterotopic splenic autografts, *Blood,* 41, 701, 1973.
48. **Klingensmith, W. C., III and Ryerson, T. W.,** Lung uptake of ^{99m}Tc-sulfur colloid, *J. Nucl. Med.,* 14, 201, 1973.
49. **Cross, A. B.,** Diagnostic clue to acute splenic torsion in the tropics, *Br. Med. J.,* 3, 564, 1974.

Chapter 9

RELEASE OF OPSONINS AND OTHER MATERIALS

Our concern with the uptake of particulates by the reticuloendothelial system of the spleen has perhaps made us lose sight of the fact that the spleen also discharges materials. It is known that phagocytosis of bacteria or particles by leukocytes is an event associated with a burst of metabolic energy. We can assume, although this has been inadequately documented, that splenic uptake of colloids (and radiocolloids) requires the expenditure of energy and perhaps the release of degradation products. In addition to this, spleen cells and splenic products (such as prostaglandins)[1] are regularly discharged into the bloodstream (data on discharge of such materials into the pericapsular lymphatics are virtually nonexistent). Hence, we will briefly review some of the data on the discharge of spleen cells or spleen products.

1. Cells – By means of sampling of the splenic artery and vein, it can be shown that the spleen adds lymphocytes to the bloodstream of the guinea pig. The cells can be classified by the number of mitochondria present. There is an increase in the arteriovenous difference in the number of these cells with age in the guinea pig.[2] However, there is only a minimal change in the hematocrit, as blood passes through the spleen in this species (and Sandberg[2] has described the experimental techniques for sampling the arteriovenous difference).

The migration of spleen cells is of key importance in the survival of animals after whole body radiation, when the spleen is shielded (refer to the section on radiation effects on the spleen). The release of splenic lymphocytes, involved in the immune response in the guinea pig, can also be quantified by the arteriovenous sampling technique. When heterologous erythrocytes are used as antigens, they adhere to mononuclear cells which have the appropriate receptors (forming "rosettes" or "clusters," which have been used to identify splenic lymphocytes). Normal guinea pigs reveal no arteriovenous difference of rosette-forming cells across the spleen; that is, the normal spleen is not discharging such cells.[3] However, a small number of rosette-forming cells are released 3 weeks after injection of sheep red blood cells. A booster dose of sheep red cells increases the output of rosette-forming cells from the spleen. There is also an interesting dependence of the splenic output of large lymphocytes on an intact thymus in the guinea pig.[4] Platelets also appear to be stored in the spleen. Injection of epinephrine causes a 10 to 25% increase in the circulating platelet count in normal, but not in asplenic, individuals.[43,44]

Uptake of particulate antigens (such as red blood cells) by the spleen is likely the initial event in synthesis of certain antibodies. Suppression of the immune response occurs in some disorders. Loose and co-workers[5] found that intravascular clearance of sheep ^{51}Cr-erythrocytes was normal in malaria-infested mice. However, the malarial mice had a marked reduction in splenic plaque-forming cells. Malaria somehow impairs antigen processing (but whether it impairs the release of splenic cells into the bloodstream is presently unknown).

2. Protein output – a. It will be recalled that the spleen is responsible for certain proteins involved in the immune mechanism. A fragment of one of the proteins produced by the spleen, termed tuftsin, is involved as an opsonizing factor for leukocytes (see section on opsonins).

b. Uptake of materials by the reticuloendothelial system of the rat is associated with the release of "acute phase reactants," such as haptoglobin and seromucoid.[6] The same effect apparently occurs after injection of zymosan, which is a reticuloendothelial stimulant. Perhaps related to this is the observation by Gay and co-workers[7] that the C-reactive protein is an opsonizing factor for newly isolated leukocytes.

c. After exercise, platelet factor 3 in the blood increases, likely due to release of microparticulates from platelets.[35] Whether the spleen is involved in this release is not known.

d. There is also release of antihemophiliac globulin from the spleen (as well as platelets) after epinephrine administration.

e. The spleen may produce an antineoplastic factor,[40] although the evidence is sketchy. Release of a cytotoxic agent from the spleen, when there is a tumor allograft, has been noted.[42] The spleen may produce a factor or factors which reduce the platelet count in ITP.[41]

3. Release of phagocytized materials – An interesting point revolves around the ultimate fate of materials taken up by the reticuloendothelial system. The spleen does not have an excretory system similar to the biliary tract in the liver. Materials taken up by the splenic reticuloendothelial cells must (perhaps after processing) either be permanently retained or released to the blood or lymph. We have looked at this point by producing dual-labeled erythrocytes in the rat.[8] That is, rats were administered both ^{59}Fe and ^{75}Se-selenomethionine. The red cells being formed were cohort labeled with radioiron in the porphyrin ring of hemoglobin and with ^{75}Se in the globin moiety. The dual-labeled cells were then heat denatured and injected intravenously into recipient rats. As expected, the two radiolabels were taken up simultaneously as the denatured cells entered the spleen. Over a period of time, however, the two radiolabels left the spleen at different rates. The spleen likely degraded the labeled erythrocytes, and the components then underwent their individual metabolic transformations (but their exact chemical nature is unknown). A recent study is also consistent with this view.[39]

Whether the splenic degradative or release pathways are affected in various disease states is uncertain at present. Lipschitz and co-workers[9] followed the entry of heat-denatured ^{59}Fe-erythrocytes into the spleen of rats and noted the effects of the size of the erythrocyte load, chelating agents, and anemia. Some of the iron in the spleen was in the form of storage compounds. Haurani and O'Brien[10] pointed out that the injection of ^{59}Fe-sensitized erythrocytes intraperitoneally into mice resulted in a model that could be used to follow macrophage uptake of radioiron and its subsequent release.

Nilsson and Zilversmit[11] studied isolated Kupffer cells from the liver of rats, as well as spleen cells, which were obtained after the intravenous injection of radiolabeled cholesterol. The cells released little of the cholesterol but exchanged some with extracellular bathing proteins.

After the spleen phagocytizes ^{131}I-colloidal human serum albumin, the ultimate fate of the radiolabel is uncertain. The largest portion of this radiocolloid, when given intravenously, is accumulated by the liver. Following a period of time, ^{131}I (freed from the colloid) appears in the bloodstream. Hence, both a "phagocytic rate" and a "catabolic rate" can be calculated by the use of two tracers.[12,13] Careful monitoring of the liver and spleen might enable one to separate the contributions of these organs to the discharge of freed ^{131}I.

4. Release of materials by the damaged spleen – The spleen, damaged by trauma or other insults, undoubtedly releases materials to the bloodstream. The saturation of iron stores, following a major intrasplenic bleed, is well recognized (see section on splenic trauma). Maurice[14] has reported on the release of a factor into plasma after splenic irradiation in rabbits. The factor was identified as thymidine. Hence, thymidine release may be of value in following the effects of X-irradiation on the spleen, although the origin of the product is not clear.

OPSONINS AND THE SPLEEN

Stossel[15] has commented that the polymorphonuclear leukocytes are the first line of defense against bacteria, while monocytes and mononuclear phagocytes of internal organs are the second defense. Both the first and second lines utilize phagocytosis as a principal tool. The events that occur can be subdivided as follows:[15]

1. Phagocytes are produced by the bone marrow.
2. Phagocytes are attracted to the site of invasion of injury by factors from the bacteria or damaged cells.
3. Serum components (such as gamma globulin and third component of complement) act as opsonins, enhancing bacterial uptake by phagocytes (opsonin = enhancer of phagocytosis).
4. Within phagocytes, ingested bacteria are encased in vesicles.
5. The phagocytic vesicles join with cytoplasmic structures which contain hydrolytic enzymes. The contained enzymes enter the phagocytic vesicles ("degranulation").
6. Phagocytes also secrete hydrogen peroxide into the vesicles. This is likely a main component in killing bacteria.

We will look more closely at the third event above. There is much evidence, particularly obtained on infants under 2,000 g body weight, that one or more blood factors is necessary for the phagocytic event. In vitro phagocytosis of foreign particles (such as India ink and bacteria) by polymorphonuclear leukocytes of the small infant (bathed in their own serum) is deficient. Phagocytosis is returned to normal by addition of serum from adults (McCracken and Eichenwald[16] have reviewed some of the relevant literature). A measure of intracellular function, the reduction of nitro blue tetrazolium, by phagocytizing leukocytes from infants was also normal.[16] However, diluted serum from the smaller infants was deficient in opsonic activity for three bacterial species. There was a significant correlation between the level of the third component of complement (C 3) and opsonic activity for *Staphylococcus aureus* and *Pseudomonas aeruginosa*. Levels of both C 3 and total hemolytic component were related to the weight of the infant. We can likely conclude that in the small infant, a deficient serum component increases in activity with time. Winkelstein[38] has provided a review of some current concepts of opsonins.

Deficiency of various components of complement can result in the inability of phagocytes to take up bacteria. For example, deficiencies of C 3 or of C 5 can result in infections. Composite deficiencies are also known (and the topic has been summarized by Constantopoulos and coworkers[17]). In each instance, addition of the absent serum factor returns the phagocytic event toward normal. The absence of these factors is likely genetically determined (and a defective component may be produced in some cases, rather than total lack of production of a protein).[18] In many disorders with diminished phagocytosis, however, the etiology has not been clearly established.[19] In chronic granulomatous disease, an X-chromosome-linked recessive, there are frequent infections, hepatosplenomegaly, and hypergammaglobulinemia. The disorder appears to be caused by inadequate destruction of bacteria ingested by leukocytes. The oxidating step which goes along with phagocytosis is deficient, and the nitro blue tetrazolium test has been used to detect heterozygotes.[34] Uptake of radiocolloid by the spleen appears to be normal (Figure 1).

We have also been assuming that only one mechanism of opsonin activity is available. This may not be true. Conceptually, at least three simple interactions are possible. In the following, P is the material to be phagocytized and ϕ is the opsonin.

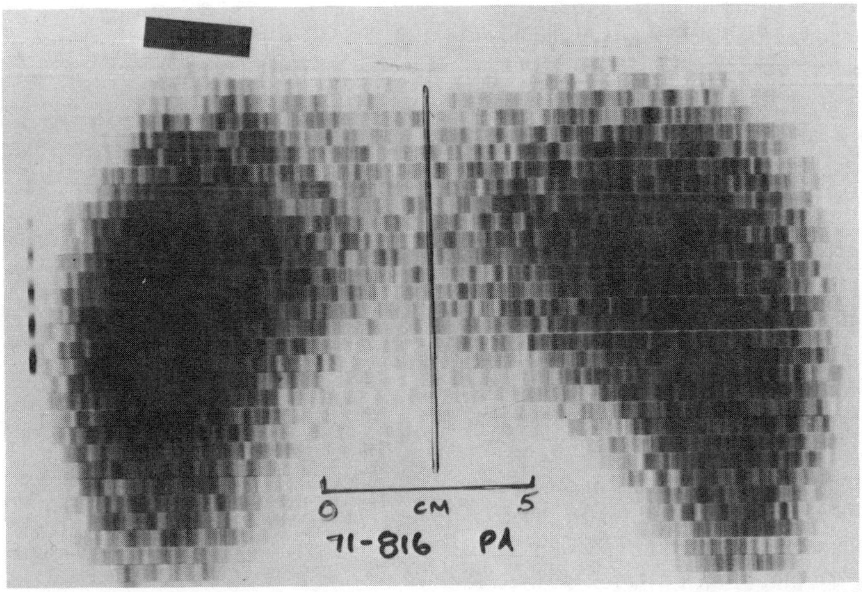

FIGURE 1. Posterior rectilinear scan (^{99m}Tc-sulfur colloid) obtained in a 4-year-old boy with chronic granulomatous disease. There was splenomegaly, but good accumulation of the radiocolloid. Case 71-816.

1. P + ϕ → Pϕ → uptake by phagocytes.
2. P + ϕ → Pϕ → uptake of P, release of ϕ.
3. ϕ → activation of phagocyte → uptake of P.

Additional data are needed before such schemes can be fully evaluated.

Najjar and co-workers[20] described the isolation of a γ-globulin that was bound to white blood cells. This leukophilic factor was present in fraction IV of γ-globulin and when bound to the leukocyte membrane was termed leukokinin. There were two additional interesting observations.

1. Following splenectomy, leukokinin activity was lost from the bloodstream.
2. Full activity of the leukokinin molecule was contained in a covalently bound peptide chain.[21] The fragment, named tuftsin (in honor of Tufts University), was cleaved from the larger molecule by an enzyme (leukokininase) present in leukocytes.

Tuftsin is a tetrapeptide: L-threonyl-L-lysyl-L-prolyl-L-arginine.[17] The positively charged tuftsin does not stimulate phagocytosis in neutrophils pretreated with neuraminidase (which cleaves negatively charged neuraminic acid from leukocytes). In addition to being decreased in amount in most splenectomized individuals[37] (the turnover rate of tuftsin is presently unknown), tuftsin has also been reported to be congenitally deficient in some families.[17,22]

To summarize the discussion thus far, tuftsin (as part of a larger molecule) originates from the spleen. While tuftsin stimulates leukocyte phagocytosis, there is no clear evidence at the moment that it also stimulates the fixed cells of the reticuloendothelial system. Other lines of evidence, however, point to serum factors as being involved in stimulating the fixed reticuloendothelial cells.

Saba and DiLuzio[23] studied tissue uptake of an emulsion consisting of ^{131}I-triolein, glycerol, and soybean lecithin (10:10:1 by weight, in 0.1% gelatin). From heparinized Krebs-Ringer solution, uptake of radioactivity by rat spleen, liver, and lung was stimulated by addition of serum. Shown in Figure 2 is a plot of their data for the liver. Rat serum contained one or more factors that stimulated uptake (reticuloendothelial function). While a straight line has been drawn in Figure 2, elucidation of the true shape of the curve awaits further data. Saba and DiLuzio[23] also stated that while 33% rat serum resulted in maximal hepatic uptake of the ^{131}I-triolein emulsion, 100% serum was needed to have maximal uptake of ^{198}Au-colloid. Hence, fixed phagocytic cells likely also respond to serum factors, but their chemical nature is as yet undefined.

DiLuzio and co-workers have provided additional data as to the possible opsonizing factors.

1. Whole body irradiation of rats was associated with impaired phagocytosis of ^{131}I-triolein emulsion.[24] Treatment of the emulsion with normal serum, prior to injection, improved the rate of clearance.
2. Following intravenous administration of ^{131}I-triolein emulsion, a temporary block occurred to uptake of more of the same material. However, opsonized emulsion was taken up normally during this period.[25]
3. Puromycin inhibited the recovery from reticuloendothelial blockade (produced by ^{131}I-triolein emulsion).[26]
4. More recently, Allen and associates[36] have greatly purified the heparin-dependent opsonically active protein from rat serum and noted that it is an α_2-globulin.

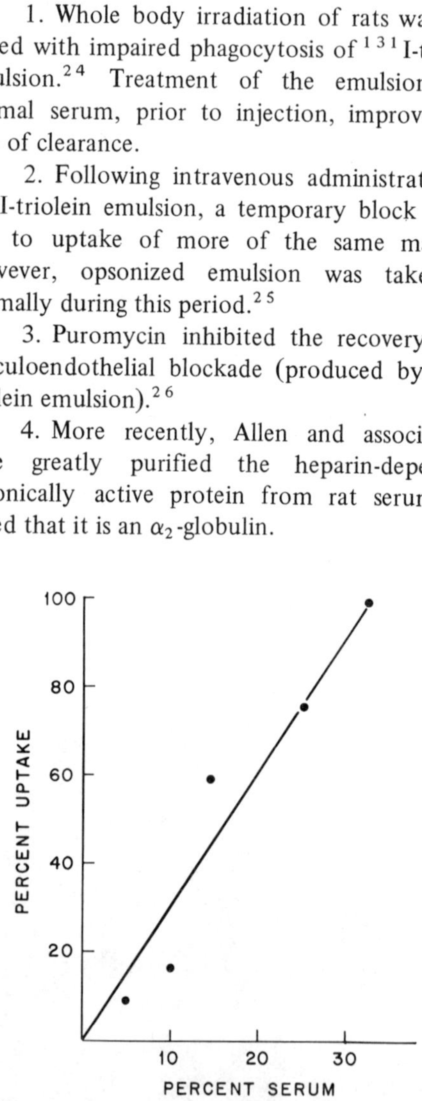

FIGURE 2. Stimulating effect of added serum on the uptake of radiolabeled emulsion by rat liver slices in vitro. Data were derived from Table 1 of Saba and DiLuzio[8] by subtracting out the small uptake that occurred in the absence of serum and then calling the maximum uptake 100%.

Despite this evidence, many aspects are still unclear. For example, why should "blockade" (temporary cessation of further uptake after a dose of emulsion) not affect uptake of other classes of colloids? There is always the possibility of multiple factors, each being class specific. Further, the studies with puromycin may have other interpretations since this medication has multiple effects.

In young individuals with homozygous hemoglobin S (sickle cell disease), the spleen is frequently nonfunctional, as judged by the inability to accumulate intravenously injected ^{99m}Tc-sulfur colloid. Following intravenous administration of fresh or fresh-frozen plasma, splenic ability to trap the colloid still does not reoccur.[27] However, transfusion of whole blood transiently restores the ability (in some cases) to trap ^{99m}Tc-sulfur colloid. Hence, mechanical blockade (and release by nonsickled cells) would appear to be an important factor. However, various opsonizing factors adherent to the transfused erythrocytes cannot be ruled out. Also, in sickle cell disease a deficiency of an alternate activating system has been demonstrated.[45]

Multiple areas still remain to be explored in connection with opsonins.

1. Most patients with neoplasms have been noted to show an increased rate of removal of intravenously administered ^{131}I-triolein emulsion.[28] Whether opsonins are involved in this altered state of the reticuloendothelial system is unknown.

2. "Opsonic adherence" (phagocytic cells making contact with molecules to be phagocytized), or a closely related phenomenon, apparently occurs with a number of tumor cells.[29]

3. During the uptake of foreign particles, a number of "acute phase reactant" proteins are released into the serum.[30] Whether these are involved in the blockade phenomenon or combine with or inactivate opsonins is presently unknown.

The immune responses not transferred by serum but by cells of the lymphoid series are referred to as "cell-mediated."[31] How (and whether) defects of cell-mediated immunity are manifest in the reticuloendothelial system of the spleen is presently not well understood. Studies on splenic uptake of radiocolloids have not been pursued on children with combined immunodeficiency (by combined immunodeficiency is meant that both the cell-mediated and serum systems are defective).[32] Such cases may be invaluable in studying serum factors which influence functioning of the reticuloendothelial system. The Wiskott-Aldrich syndrome is a genetically determined, sex-linked recessive disorder which shows a deficient cell-mediated immunity.[33] Recurrent infections, thrombocytopenia, and eczyma are marked. Transfer factor, which can be extracted from normal leukocytes, apparently causes regression of symptomatology in the Wiskott-Aldrich syndrome. The prominent splenomegaly in this syndrome (perhaps due to the repeated infections) apparently regresses after use of transfer factor. There does not appear to be any gross defect in the splenic uptake of radiocolloid in the Wiskott-Aldrich syndrome (Figure 3).

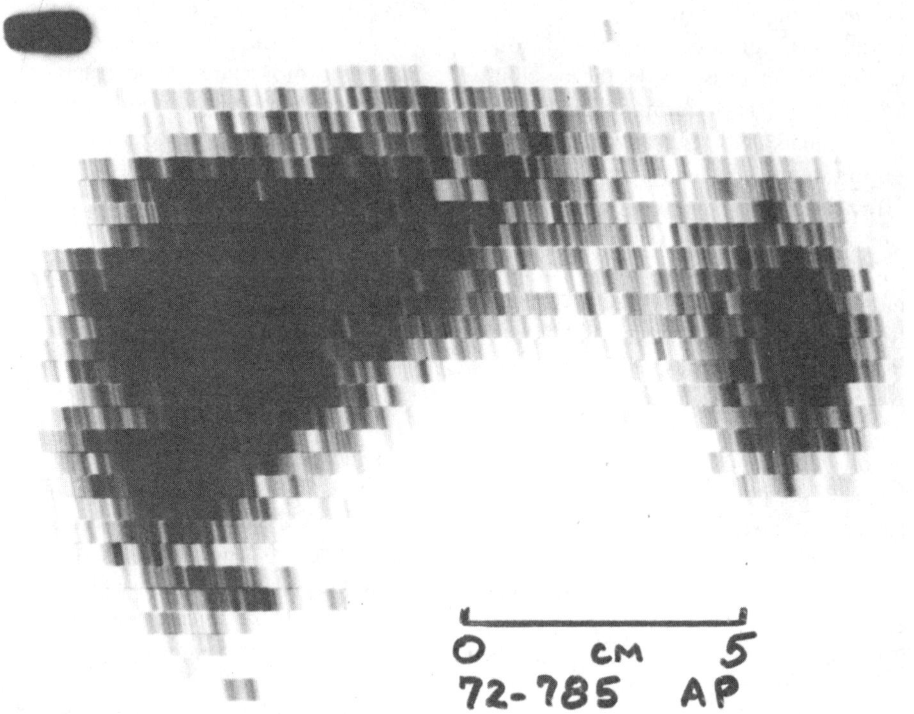

FIGURE 3. Anterior rectilinear scan (^{99m}Tc-sulfur colloid) in a 4-month-old boy with Wiskott-Aldrich syndrome. The spleen was functioning in terms of its ability to accumulate radiocolloid. Case 72-785.

REFERENCES

1. **Douglas, J. R., Jr., Johnson, E. M., Jr., Marshall, G. R., Jaffe, B. M., and Needleman, P.,** Stimulation of splenic prostaglandin release by angiotensin and specific inhibition by cysteine-AII, *Prostaglandin,* 3, 67, 1973.
2. **Sandberg, G.,** Release of splenic cells into the blood of guinea-pigs of different ages, *Scand. J. Haematol.,* 7, 104, 1970.
3. **Sandberg, G.,** Release of antigen-binding cells from the spleen into the blood, *Acta Pathol. Microbiol. Scand.,* 80, 477, 1972.
4. **Sandberg, G.,** Release of lymphocytes from the spleen in neonatally thymectomized guinea-pigs, *Scand. J. Haematol.,* 9, 52, 1972.
5. **Loose, L. D., Cook, J. A., and DiLuzio, N. R.,** Role of macrophages in malaria induced immunosuppression, *Physiologist,* 15, 202, 1972.
6. **Ohara, H., Nishio, H., Watanabe, K., and Wada, T.,** Regulation of the seromucoid and haptoglobin level in serum by the reticuloendothelial system, *J. Reticuloendothelial Soc.,* 11, 301, 1972.
7. **Gay, S., Michalski, H., Rosenkranz, M., and Geiler, G.,** In vitro- Untersuchungen zum Nachweis des C-reaktiven Proteins als "phagocytosis promoting factor," *Acta Histochem.,* 42, 273, 1972.
8. **Chaudhuri, T. K. and Spencer, R. P.,** Dual-labeling of erythrocytes: properties and splenic handling of ^{75}Se- and ^{59}Fe-labeled cells, *J. Nucl. Med.,* 10, 122, 1969.
9. **Lipschitz, D. A., Simon, M. O., Lynch, S. R., Dugard, J., Bothwell, T. H., and Charlton, R. W.,** Some factors affecting the release of iron from reticuloendothelial cells, *Br. J. Haematol.,* 21, 289, 1971.

10. **Haurani, F. I. and O'Brien, R.,** A model system for release of iron from the reticuloendothelial system, *J. Reticuloendothelial. Soc.,* 12, 29, 1972.
11. **Nilsson, A. and Zilversmit, D. B.,** Release of phagocytosed cholesterol by liver macrophages and spleen cells, *Biochim. Biophys. Acta,* 260, 479, 1972.
12. **Palmer, D. L., Rifkind, D., and Brown, D. W.,** ^{131}I-labeled colloidal human spleen albumin in the study of reticuloendothelial system function. II. Phagocytosis and catabolism of a test colloid in normal subjects, *J. Infect. Dis.,* 123, 457, 1971.
13. **Palmer, D. L., Rifkind, D., and Brown, D. W.,** ^{131}I-labeled colloidal human serum albumin in the study of reticuloendothelial system function. III. Phagocytosis and catabolism compared in normal, leukemic, and immunosuppressed human subjects, *J. Infect. Dis.,* 123, 465, 1971.
14. **Maurice, P. A.,** Release of thymidine from X-irradiated spleen in the rabbit as determined by a new bioassay, *Cancer Res.,* 32, 2799, 1972.
15. **Stossel, T. P.,** Phagocytosis: the department of defense, *N. Engl. J. Med.,* 286, 776, 1972.
16. **McCracken, G. H., Jr. and Eichenwald, H. F.,** Leukocyte function and the development of opsonic and complement activity in the neonate, *Am. J. Dis. Child.,* 121, 120, 1971.
17. **Constantopoulos, A., Najjar, V. A., and Smith, J. W.,** Tuftsin deficiency: a new syndrome with defective phagocytosis, *J. Pediatr.,* 80, 564, 1972.
18. **Jacobs, J. C. and Miller, M. E.,** Fatal familial Leiner's disease: a deficiency of the opsonic activity of serum complement, *Pediatrics,* 49, 225, 1972.
19. **Rawnsley, H. M. and Shelley, W. B.,** Diminished phagocytic function in patients with alopecia, *Acta Derm. Venereol.* (Stockh.), 51, 135, 1971.
20. **Najjar, V. A., Fidalgo, B. V., and Still, E.,** The physiological role of the lymphoid system. VII. The disappearance of leukokinin activity following splenectomy, *Biochemistry,* 7, 2376, 1968.
21. **Nishioka, K., Constantopoulos, A., Satoh, P. S., and Najjar, V. A.,** The characteristics, isolation and synthesis of the phagocytosis stimulating peptide tuftsin, *Biochem. Biophys. Res. Commun.,* 47, 172, 1972.
22. **Najjar, V. A. and Constantopoulos, A.,** A new phagocytosis-stimulating tetrapeptide hormone, tuftsin, and its role in disease, *J. Reticuloendothel. Soc.,* 12, 197, 1972.
23. **Saba, T. M. and DiLuzio, N. R.,** Comparative evaluation of the influence of opsonins on hepatic, splenic and pulmonary phagocytosis, *Proc. Soc. Exp. Biol. Med.,* 125, 630, 1967.
24. **Saba, T. M. and DiLuzio, N. R.,** Effect of X-irradiation on reticuloendothelial phagocytic function and serum opsonic activity, *Am. J. Physiol.,* 216, 910, 1969.
25. **Saba, T. M. and DiLuzio, N. R.,** Reticuloendothelial blockade and recovery as a function of opsonic activity, *Am. J. Physiol.,* 216, 197, 1969.
26. **Pisano, J. C., Patterson, J. T., and DiLuzio, N. R.,** Reticuloendothelial blockade: effect of puromycin on opsonin-dependent recovery, *Science,* 162, 565, 1968.
27. **Pearson, H. A., Cornelius, E. A., Schwartz, A. D., Zelson, J. H., Wolfson, S. L., and Spencer, R. P.,** Transfusion reversible functional asplenia in young children with sickle-cell anemia, *N. Engl. J. Med.,* 283, 334, 1970.
28. **Salky, N. K., DiLuzio, N. R., Levin, A. G., and Goldsmith, H. S.,** Phagocytic activity of the reticuloendothelial system in neoplastic disease, *J. Lab. Clin. Med.,* 70, 393, 1967.
29. **Cohen, D., Gurner, B. W., and Coombs, R. R. A.,** A phenomenon resembling opsonic adherence shown by disaggregated cells of the transmissible venereal tumor of the dog, *Br. J. Exp. Pathol.,* 52, 447, 1971.
30. **O'Hara, H., Nishio, H., Watanabe, K., and Wada, T.,** Regulation of the seromucoid and haptoglobin level in serum by the reticuloendothelial system, *J. Reticuloendothel. Soc.,* 11, 301, 1972.
31. **Gotoff, S. P.,** Cell mediated immune deficiency, *J. Pediatr.,* 78, 379, 1971.
32. **Montgomery, J. R., South, M. A., Barrett, F. F. and Williamson, A. P.,** Management of infections in severe combined immunodeficiency, *Fed. Proc.,* 30, 244, 1971.
33. **Levin, A. S., Spitter, L. E., Stites, D. P., and Fudenberg, H. H.,** Wiskott-Aldrich syndrome: a genetically determined cellular immunologic deficiency: clinical and laboratory responses to therapy with transfer factor, *Proc. Natl. Acad. Sci. U.S.A.,* 67, 821, 1970.
34. **Baehner, R. L. and Nathan, D. G.,** Quantitative nitroblue tetrazolium test in chronic granulomatous disease, *N. Engl. J. Med.,* 278, 971, 1968.
35. **Prentice, C. R. M., Hassanein, A. A., McNicol, G. P., and Douglas, A. S.,** Studies on blood coagulation, fibrinolysis and platelet function following exercise in normal and splenectomized people, *Br. J. Haematol.,* 23, 541, 1972.
36. **Allen, C., Saba, T. M., and Molnar, J.,** Isolation, purification and characterization of opsonic protein, *J. Reticuloendothel. Soc.,* 13, 410, 1973.
37. **Constantopoulos, A., Najjar, V. A., Wish, J. B., Necheles, T. H., and Stolbach, L. L.,** Defective phagocytosis due to tuftsin deficiency in splenectomized subjects, *Am. J. Dis. Child.,* 125, 663, 1973.
38. **Winkelstein, J. A.,** Opsonins: their function, identity, and clinical significance, *J. Pediatr.,* 82, 747, 1973.
39. **Iyengar, B. and Chandra, K.,** Iron release in the reticuloendothelial cells of the spleen after red cell damage, *Acta Haematol.,* 48, 354, 1972.
40. **Janes, J. M., Higgins, G. M., and Herrick, J. F.,** The influence of splenectomy on the induction of osteogenic sarcoma in rabbits, *J. Bone Joint Surg.,* 38A, 809, 1956.

41. **McMillan, R., Longmire, R. L., Yelenosky, R., Smith, R. S., and Craddock, C. G.,** Immunoglobulin synthesis in vitro by splenic tissue in idiopathic thrombocytopenic purpura, *N. Engl. J. Med.,* 286, 681, 1972.
42. **Vaillier, D., Dunner, M., and Burg, C.,** Release of a cytotoxic factor by murine spleen cells in the presence of a tumor allograft, *Experientia,* 28, 1352, 1972.
43. **Aster, R. H.,** Pooling of platelets in the spleen: role in the pathogenesis of "hypersplenic" thrombocytopenia, *J. Clin. Invest.,* 45, 645, 1966.
44. **Penny, R., Roxenberg, M. C., and Firkin, B. G.,** The splenic platelet pool, *Blood,* 27, 1, 1966.
45. **Johnston, R. B., Jr., Newman, S. L., and Struth, A. G.,** An abnormality of the alternative pathway of complement activation in sickle-cell disease, *N. Engl. J. Med.,* 288, 803, 1973.

Chapter 10

POLYCYTHEMIA VERA: A COMPARISON WITH DISORDERS HAVING EXTRAMEDULLARY HEMATOPOIESIS

The spleen is normally a hematopoietic organ only during fetal life. However, as a response to appropriate stimuli, splenic production of formed blood elements may continue or resume in extrauterine life. Some disorders in which this may occur are thalassemia major, myeloid metaplasia, and osteopetrosis. A study of myeloid metaplasia and osteopetrosis points out a number of contrasts with polycythemia vera; hence, these entities are considered in the same chapter.

POLYCYTHEMIA

Polycythemia denotes an increased number of circulating red blood cells. In some cases the polycythemia is relative, that is, without an increase in the red cell mass,[1] because the plasma volume is decreased. This "stress polycythemia" can be associated with hypertension or cardiovascular problems and may improve as the hypertension is treated.[37,38] In absolute polycythemia, the total red cell mass is elevated. When this absolute increase occurs in relationship to an identifiable stimulus, the designation erythrocytosis is used. An elevation in the red cell mass in a disease of uncertain etiology (polycythemia rubra vera) is referred to as erythemia. Polycythemia rubra vera is closely related to a number of aspects of splenic function.

However, a few words must first be devoted to erythrocytosis. Likely the most common cause is diminished saturation of blood with oxygen. This can be due to a number of entities, including reduced atmospheric pressure (such as living at high altitudes), pulmonary disease with impaired ventilation, right-to-left shunts, or the presence of an abnormal hemoglobin which does not readily give up oxygen.[2] In cases caused by the hemoglobinopathies (such as hemoglobin M), the erythrocytosis may be familial because of the genetic determination of the unusual hemoglobin. Erythrocytosis may also occur with hereditary methemoglobinemia or when there is a deficiency of intraerythrocytic enzymes (such as the NADPH diaphorase). These causes of erythrocytosis are usually not associated with splenic disorders (Figure 1). An exception occurs when right-to-left shunting occurs with cardiac defects which are part of the asplenia or polysplenia syndromes. Miscellaneous causes of erythrocytosis, such as that in the presence of renal or other tumors or the use of cobalt or adrenocortical hormones in animals, are also usually not associated with specific splenic problems. There is also no discrete splenic pathology found in cases of stress polycythemia.

Polycythemia rubra vera (referred to in the remainder of this section as polycythemia vera or erythremia) can usually be diagnosed on the basis of the following criteria:

1. Specific causes of erythrocytosis are absent. Most germaine, the blood is not unsaturated with oxygen, and urinary erythropoietin excretion is decreased.
2. Not only is the hematocrit high, but the red cell mass is also increased. By the ^{51}Cr-erythrocyte labeling technique, values above 36 ml/kg body weight are often found. The hemoglobin concentration is increased unless recent phlebotomy has been performed.
3. Hyperplasia of other blood elements, such as a leukocytosis (granulocytosis) and thrombocytosis, is also present. This suggests a possible relationship to myeloproliferative diseases, such as chronic myelocytic leukemia, but the leukocyte alkaline phosphatase is usually normal or high, whereas in the chronic leukemias it is low. Occasional nucleated erythrocytes, or early leukocyte forms, appear in the circulation and serve as reminders of the hyperplastic bone marrow.
4. Splenomegaly is present in about two thirds of the cases (Figure 2). Berg and coworkers[29] reported that needle aspirates of the spleen in polycythemia vera revealed no abnormalities other than a high number of platelets.

The immediate threat to the patient in polycythemia vera is the likelihood of a vascular accident due to the high specific viscosity of the blood. The long-term threat is the development of one of the other myeloproliferative diseases, such as leukemia. The relationship between the specific viscosity of blood and the hematocrit is not a

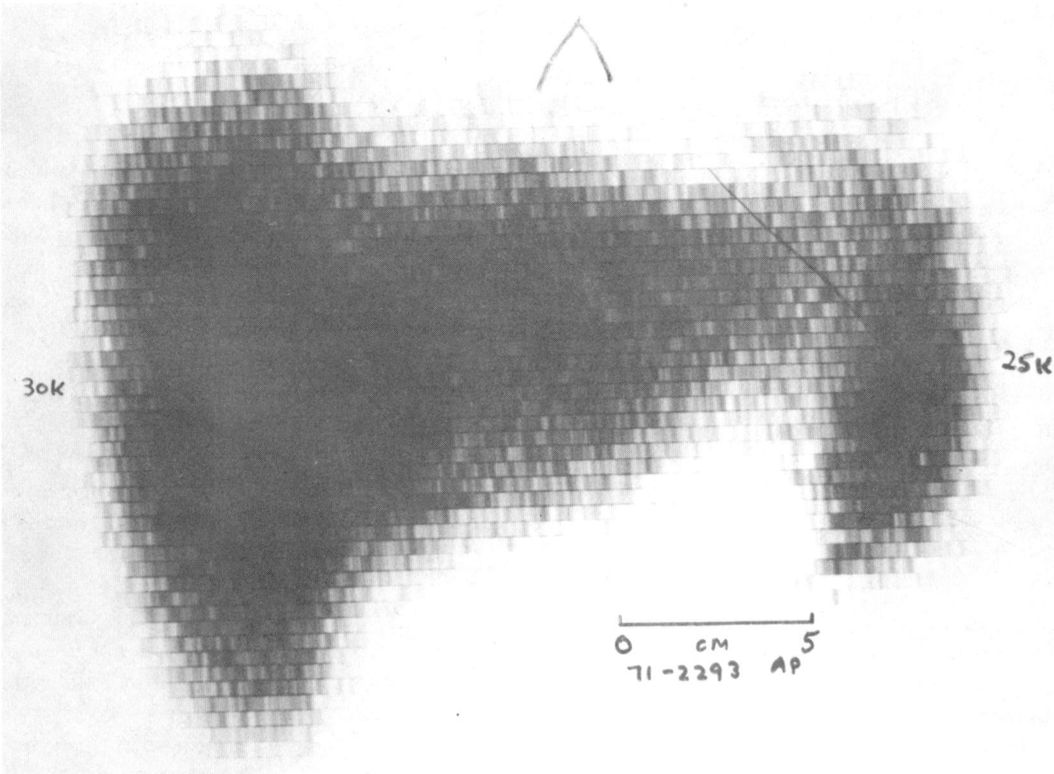

FIGURE 1. Anterior rectilinear scan obtained by use of ^{99m}Tc-sulfur colloid. The patient is a 20-year-old man with cyanotic heart disease (tricuspid atresia with a Pott's procedure). The hematocrit was 77 and the blood volume 5.5 l (123 ml/kg body weight). The red cell mass was 90 ml/kg (quite elevated). There was no splenomegaly. Case 71-2293.

linear one.[3] Up to a hematocrit of about 60, the specific viscosity rises slowly as the hematocrit goes up. However, an abrupt upward change in the curve occurs above this, so that the slope is about eight times steeper. The practical implication is that with hematocrits above 60, the specific viscosity might be high enough to imperil circulation, with resultant vascular accidents. Most of the symptoms of the disease can likely be explained on the basis of the increased red cell mass and the splenomegaly (the reason for the high incidence of duodenal ulceration in these patients is uncertain).

Polycythemia vera occurs, in the white U.S. population, in about 1.8 cases per 100,000.[4] While the etiology of the disorder is unknown, there have been reports of chromosomal abnormalities in some affected adults, perhaps in part related to therapy (and Wasserman has summarized the literature).[5] The rare finding of polycythemia vera in childhood and the report of an abnormality of an E-group chromosome in an affected individual who had the onset of the disease in childhood[6] may serve to stimulate studies in this area. A familial history of polycythemia vera or related disorders can sometimes be obtained (Figure 3).

Bowdler[7] noted that in 23 patients with polycythemia vera, the mean ratio of whole body hematocrit (determined by use of ^{51}Cr-erythrocytes and ^{131}I-human serum albumin) to that of the peripheral hematocrit was 0.92; this value was indistinguishable from controls. Thus, the spleen was not significantly trapping red cells above the concentration in the general circulation (and this can be contrasted with the situation in splenomegaly due to other disorders, which is discussed in Chapter 4).

In 15 of 23 cases of polycythemia vera, Bowdler was able to palpate the spleen;[7] however,

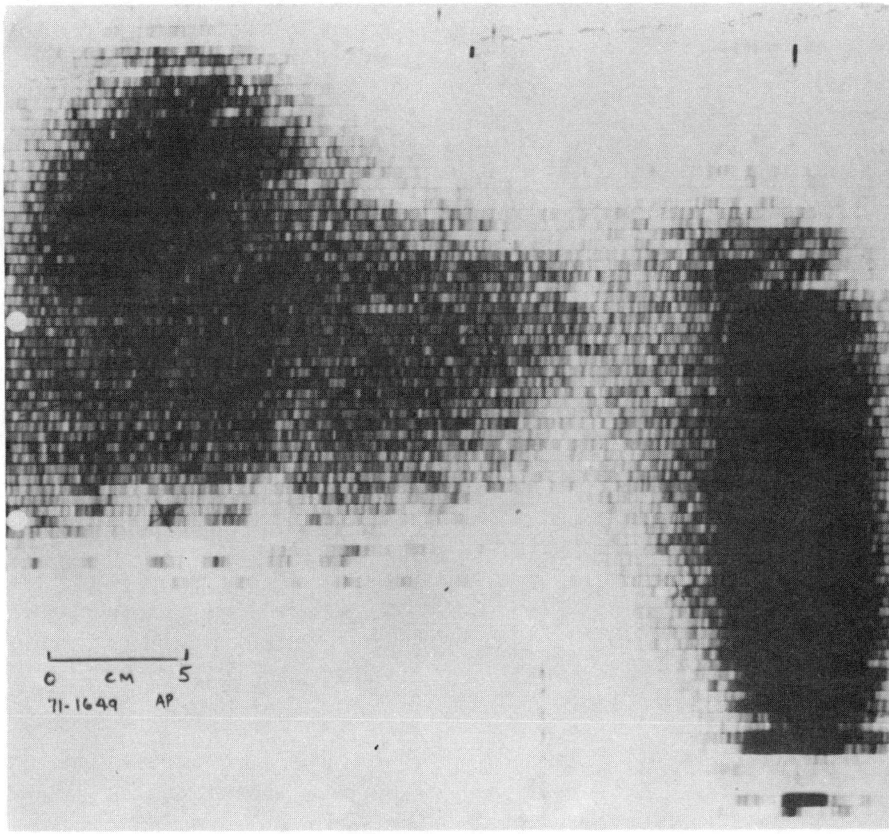

FIGURE 2. Anterior rectilinear scan obtained with ^{99m}Tc-sulfur colloid. The patient is a 63-year-old man with a hematocrit of 52. The blood volume was 8.6 l, or 82 ml/kg body weight. These findings, the lack of oxygen unsaturation and the marked splenomegaly, are consistent with polycythemia rubra vera. There is also a shift of radioactive colloid to the spleen in this case. Case 71-1649.

some had previously been treated with ^{32}P. Of the 15 patients with a palpable spleen, 8 also had a palpable liver. The size of these organs, as determined by radioisotopic scans, was not reported. Westin and co-workers[8] did obtain ^{99m}Tc-sulfur colloid scans on patients with polycythemia vera, as well as roentgenograms of the abdomen. A plot of the posterior spleen scan area in polycythemia vera as a function of the lateral spleen scan area showed deviation toward the latter. That is, the spleen did not seem to enlarge symmetrically, and with larger spleens, there was more enlargement laterally than posteriorly. The mean spleen scan area (from the view giving the largest result) was 57 ± 12 cm^2 in controls. In untreated polycythemia vera, the figure was 136 ± 49. This was identical to that of polycythemia vera in relapse (135 ±, 31 cm^2). In remission, the spleen in polycythemia vera had a largest mean scan area of 89 ± 22 cm^2. Roux and co-workers[9] reported that using ^{51}Cr-heat-denatured erythrocytes, 96% of 50 patients with polycythemia vera had an estimated spleen weight of over 300 g. In 48 cases of secondary polycythemia, 93% had estimated spleen weights below 300 g. Kutti and Weinfeld[10] studied ten patients with polycythemia vera in an active phase. Twelve of these (60%) were stated to have splenomegaly (but scan data were not presented). When ^{51}Cr-platelets were injected into the polycythemic patients, platelet recovery was lower in the splenomegalic individuals than in those who did not have splenomegaly. Hence, while the spleen in polycythemia vera does not excessively trap erythrocytes, there may be platelet trapping. Enlargement of the spleen in erythremia is due to a hyperplastic pulp and blood distention. Both infarcts and sites of extramedullary hematopoiesis are observed in this disease. In some cases of polycythemia, the spleen is not enlarged, but there

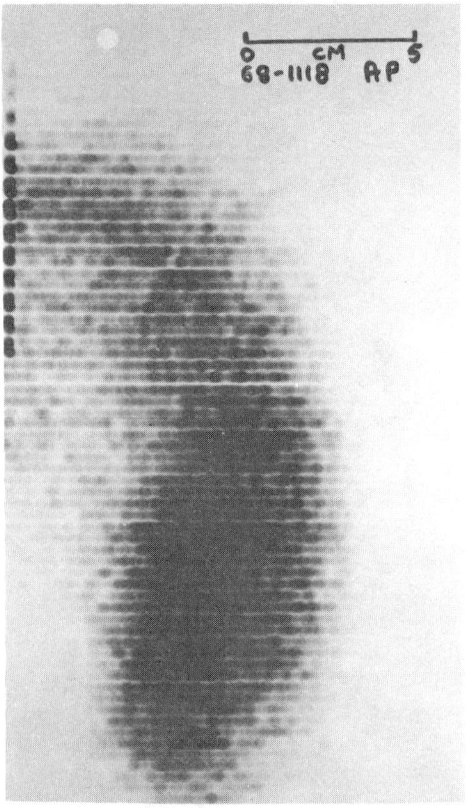

FIGURE 3. Anterior rectilinear scan of the spleen (^{99m}Tc-sulfur colloid) in a 27-year-old male. There was a strong family history of polycythemia. This patient had a series of vascular accidents. Case 68-1118.

is a shift of radioactive colloid to the organ, suggesting reticuloendothelial hyperfunction (Figure 4).

It is of interest that there are models of polycythemia. The Friend leukemia virus apparently transforms otherwise erythropoietin-responsive stem cells so that they develop into erythroblasts without erythropoietin.[11] The spleen does not have to be present for the polycythemia to develop.[33] The compound virazole (1-β-D-ribofuranosyl-1,2,4-triazole-3-carboxyamide) has been reported to inhibit splenomegaly and hepatomegaly produced by the Friend leukemia virus.[12] The differences between embryonal and adult hematopoiesis, and possible factors controlling polycythemia, have been discussed.[13] The applicability to human polycythemia vera has still to be determined.

We will try to bring together some of the areas in which nuclear medicine can help in diagnosing or managing polycythemia vera.

1. The diagnosis rests upon the establishment of an elevated red cell mass (^{51}Cr-labeled erythrocytes).

2. Diagnosis of polycythemia vera is strengthened by the finding of scan-documented splenomegaly, as well as reticuloendothelial scans

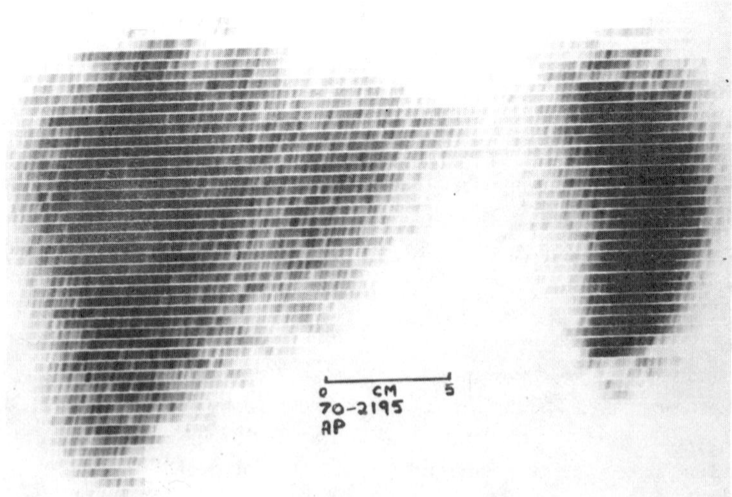

FIGURE 4. Anterior rectilinear liver and spleen scan (^{99m}Tc-sulfur colloid) in a 60-year-old man. The patient, with documented polycythemia, had a borderline enlarged spleen, but a shift of radiocolloid to the organ. Case 70-2195.

showing hyperplasia of the central marrow and peripheral extension of marrow.[11]

3. While there is no excessive splenic trapping of erythrocytes in this disorder, platelet sequestration may occur.[10,32]

4. Radionuclides, more particularly ^{32}P, may have a role to play in the therapy of polycythemia vera, and extensive reviews have appeared.

The classical treatment of polycythemia vera has been venesection (with or without return of plasma to the patient, in order to reduce the blood viscosity). In an effort to reduce overproduction of erythrocytes and other blood elements, induced iron deficiency (through repeated phlebotomies) or suppression of bone marrow can be attempted (chemical agents or external or internal radiation). A voluminous literature has grown up around the use of ^{32}P as an internally administered agent for radiating the bone marrow. Whether ^{32}P therapy leads to a higher incidence of myeloid metaplasia or acute leukemia is still uncertain. Splenomegaly can regress with the institution of ^{32}P treatment for erythremia. From the study of Sharma and co-workers,[13] we can note that in the case of a 68-year-old-woman, use of 7 mCi of ^{32}P was followed by the shrinkage of the spleen to two thirds of its original length.

MYELOID METAPLASIA

This disorder, or perhaps collection of disorders, is of great interest since it provides a challenge to the diagnostic techniques of hematology and nuclear medicine. Essential features of myeloid metaplasia are as follows:

1. Splenomegaly (often massive).
2. Myelofibrosis or osteosclerosis occurs in some 49% of cases. Trephine biopsy reveals lack of active marrow.
3. Extramedullary hematopoiesis occurs, particularly (but not exclusively) in the spleen. In some cases this extramedullary hematopoiesis may be "agressive" with tumor formation.[34]

A discussion of myeloid metaplasia must refer to the work of Jackson and co-workers[14] (in which the term agnogenic myeloid metaplasia was used). Block and Jacobson[15] have reviewed the differences between myeloid metaplasia and leukemia and pointed out the significance of potential sites of extramedullary hematopoiesis. Ward and Block[16] have provided an extensive review of the literature on myeloid metaplasia and pointed out that at least 37 different terms have been used as synonyms (for example, myelofibrosis and chronic nonleukemic myelosis). The disorder can be idiopathic or occasionally can precede or follow apparent chronic myelocytic leukemia, or polycythemia vera. The term myeloproliferative disorder has been used to suggest that these diseases (and myeloid metaplasia) are the result of the overgrowth of one or more of the cell types that usually occur in the bone marrow. The initiating stimuli have still to be identified. Studies on immunoglobulin levels have pointed out both similarities and differences between polycythemia vera and myelofibrosis.[17]

The often long and variable course of myeloid metaplasia makes specific observations difficult to evaluate in the overall picture. However, the following information is available on the spleen in this disorder.

1. The spleen was palpable below the left costal margin in 100% of Ward and Block's 45 cases of myeloid metaplasia.[16] In 84% of the patients, the spleen was 8 or more cm below the costal margin.

2. The size of the spleen progressively increases in the course of the disorder.[16] A composite plot of spleen extension (S) below the costal margin (in cm) as a function of the years (Y) of observation in 16 cases was approximated by:

$$S = 0.9\ Y$$

There was, however, much scatter to the plot. Short bursts of rapid increase of spleen size can apparently occur in this disorder. Over 35 years ago, Hickling[18] provided drawings of the change in spleen size as a function of time in myeloid metaplasia. From these, rates of change can also be calculated. Pain in the splenic area occurred in over one fourth of the patients with myeloid metaplasia having massive splenomegaly,[16] perhaps related to traction or infarction.

3. The histologic pattern observed in the bone marrow in myeloid metaplasia roughly correlates with the size of the spleen.[16] That is, as the marrow progresses from panhyperplasia to myeloid atrophy and, finally, to myelofibrosis and

osteosclerosis, the spleen increases in size (likely as increased splenic hematopoiesis occurs). As a corollary, the fraction of the splenic red pulp involved in myeloid metaplasia increases with the length of time the disease has been present. Unlike the spleen in chronic granulocytic leukemia, the splenic follicles are preserved (but the splenic white pulp is apparently not involved in extramedullary hematopoiesis). Tavassoli[31] has noted distinct ultrastructural changes in the spleen in myeloid metaplasia with myelosclerosis.

4. The massively enlarged spleen can be a problem because of the mechanical effects. It is clear that the spleen could not be surgically removed if it was the only site of extramedullary hematopoiesis.[18] However, the following observations are pertinent.

a. In myeloid metaplasia, multiple areas other than the spleen can be involved in extramedullary hematopoiesis (for example, liver, lymph nodes, gastrointestinal tract, and other sites).[16]

b. Although the initial view was that splenectomy was contraindicated in myeloid metaplasia, more recently many patients have survived the operation. The suggestion has even been made that splenectomy be performed when myeloid metaplasia is diagnosed.[19] Recent studies have discussed the indications for splenectomy in myeloid metaplasia, the subsequent course of the patients,[20,21] and the use of radionuclides as diagnostic aids.[22] While surgical complications of splenectomy in this disorder have been reduced, and other organs may assume the hematologic burden, one complication has been distressing. This has been the postoperative abdominal infections which follow splenectomy for myeloid metaplasia. The infections might be due to general debility. However, loss of the "filtering" function of the spleen and the removal of the spleen as a source of opsonizing factors such as tuftsin might also be contributory.

5. In addition to its function in hematopoiesis, the spleen may also be playing a role in removal of formed blood elements in myeloid metaplasia. ^{51}Cr-erythrocyte survival and ^{59}Fe-iron disappearance and organ uptake studies in myeloid metaplasia indicate that the anemia is due primarily to depressed hematopoiesis. In about one third of the cases, there is increased erythrocyte destruction.[22,23] A typical scan in this disorder, performed with a radioactive colloid, reveals hypoplasia of the marrow, as well as splenomegaly.[24] In rare cases of myeloid metaplasia, hypersplenism can be marked (Figure 5). The spleen in myeloid metaplasia retains the ability to accumulate ^{51}Cr-heat-denatured erythrocytes (Figure 6).

6. Pancytopenia, related to splenic trapping of all blood elements, can occur in myeloid metaplasia. The hypersplenism does not respond well to external beam radiation therapy.[16] Ward and Block reported on a limited experience with ^{32}P therapy in myeloid metaplasia; this did not appear to be the treatment of choice. Chemotherapy has been utilized in many cases of myeloid metaplasia since the original observations of Dameshek and co-workers.[25] When Myleran® is utilized, the spleen often shrinks in size.[26] The principal indication for myelosuppressive therapy may be thrombocythemia since pancytopenia may be worsened by suppressives and there is no clear evidence that the medication ameliorates hypersplenism. Androgens may have a role to play in therapy of myeloid metaplasia, but experiences with androgens or corticosteroids in this disorder have not been impressive.[16]

We have seen a man (a patient followed by Dr. David S. Fischer) who had the diagnosis of myeloid metaplasia established at age 60 in 1968. At that time, the spleen was 3 cm below the left costal margin, and there was extensive sclerosis of the bones of the pelvis and spine. Hemoglobin was 13.6 g%. One year later, the spleen had considerably enlarged. A trephine bone biopsy did not reveal any marrow. The hemoglobin had decreased to 12.2 g%. The ^{51}Cr-erythrocyte spleen-to-liver ratio was 2:1, while the erythrocyte survival T½ was shortened to 15 days. He was given Myleran on a decreasing dose schedule, but the medication was discontinued when the hematocrit and white cell count both fell precipitously. An androgen was administered, as well as steroids and several transfusions of packed erythrocytes. The hematocrit stayed at 15 and was brought to a value of 22 only by erythrocyte transfusions. There was pancytopenia, with the white count 2,500 (including 41 segmented forms, 14 bands, 25 lymphs, 3 monocytes, 7 myelocytes, and 10 metamyelocytes). The platelet count was 24,000. Because of the prior reaction to a myelosuppressive and the failure to respond to androgen therapy after multiple transfusions, the splenic

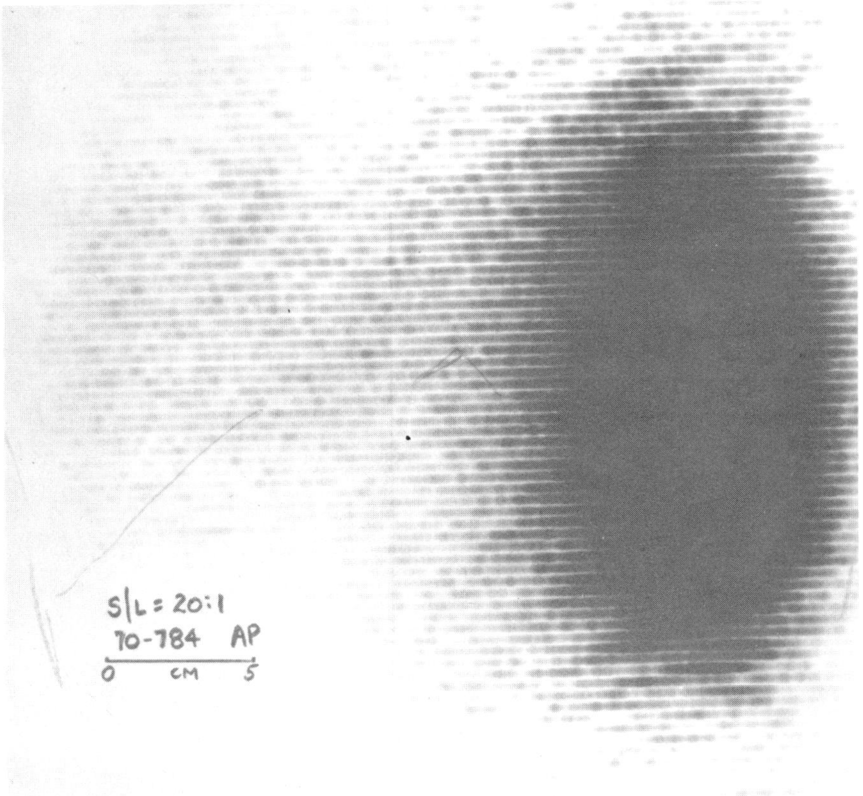

FIGURE 5. Anterior rectilinear scan obtained after intravenous injection of ^{99m}Tc-sulfur colloid. The patient is a 60-year-old man, with the diagnosis of myeloid metaplasia. The spleen-to-liver ratio of uptake of the radiocolloid, per unit area, was 20 to 1. No accumulation was noted in the bone marrow. The ^{59}Fe plasma disappearance half-time was 78 min (normal). Case 70-784.

artery was ligated by Dr. Sherwin Nuland. This was based on the experience with a prior individual who had Hodgkin's disease and whose hypersplenism was ameliorated by splenic artery ligation.[27] The patient did relatively well for 7 months with the white count remaining above 5,000 and the hematocrit about 40 without additional transfusions. He expired after a bout of infection. At autopsy, there was bilateral pneumonia and septic infarcts in the spleen. Two additional interesting aspects of this case were as follows:

1. The leukocyte alkaline phosphase on three separate occasions was reported as 7, 10, and 7 units (low, and consistent with chronic myelocytic leukemia).

2. A leukoagglutination test revealed the patient to have leukocyte antibodies against all donors tested.

To summarize, the procedures of scanning the reticuloendothelial system with a radioactive colloid can document the extent of spleen and liver size in myeloid metaplasia, as well as the location of any bone marrow which still remains active. ^{51}Cr-erythroctye studies likely have a role to play in demonstrating hemolysis and hypersplenism. ^{59}Fe studies have a more limited role to play in determining which sites are carrying out erythropoiesis in myeloid metaplasia (and ^{111}In may also have a role insofar as it mimics iron metabolism). There has been a report of increased bone blood flow in myelofibrosis,[28] studied by means of ^{18}F. Whether this will prove of value in following the course of the disease is uncertain. Of

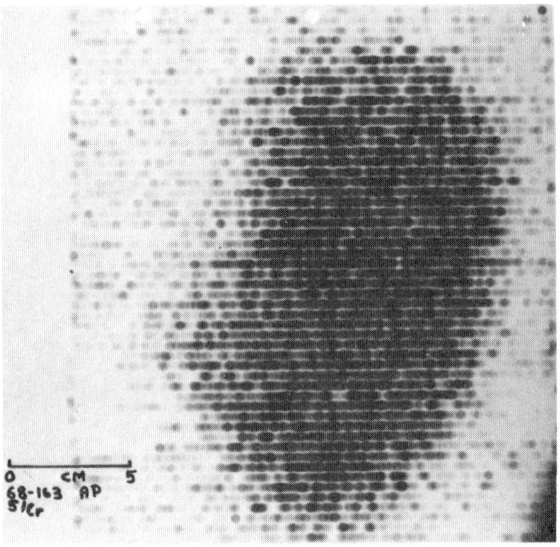

FIGURE 6. Anterior rectilinear spleen scan obtained by use of ^{51}Cr-heat-denatured erythrocytes. The patient is a 54-year-old man with myeloid metaplasia marked by myelofibrosis and hepatosplenomegaly. Case 68-163.

particular interest is the report by Szur and co-workers,[30] who studied the spleen in three individuals who had myelosclerosis and evidence of splenic erythropoiesis. After splenic irradiation (1,000 to 2,000 R), the accumulation of radioiron by the spleen was suppressed, while the ability to take up radiocolloid was not affected. Myeloid metaplasia and its accompanying bone changes must be distinguished from other causes of myelofibrosis (some of which may be reversible).[35]

A discussion of the role of the spleen in assuming hematopoietic function must include mention of osteopetrosis (also referred to as marble bone disease, or Albers-Schonberg disease, after the radiologist who first recognized it in 1904). The bones are unusually dense, with apparent obliteration of the marrow cavity. In addition to the anemia due to marrow replacement, there is likely a hemolytic component. There are two forms of the disease – a malignant childhood disorder which is transmitted as a recessive and a more benign adult form which is transmitted as a dominant.[36] In the malignant form of osteopetrosis, 62% of 50 cases had splenomegaly. Splenectomy may be indicated in osteopetrosis when there is a significant splenic contribution to hemolysis.

In many diseases associated with hemolysis, splenic hematopoiesis may be evident at birth. Most striking is the spleen in erythroblastosis fetalis due to Rh incompatibility. The large spleen in this disorder may rupture at birth. In later life, exuberant splenic hematopoiesis is seen in thalassemia major. We have presented preliminary scan data that transfusions may suppress this activity in the spleen.[39]

REFERENCES

1. **Campbell, A., Emery, E. W., Godlec, J. N., and Prankerd, T. A. J.,** Diagnosis and treatment of primary polycythemia, *Lancet.* I. 1074, 1970.
2. **Fairbanks, V. F., Maldonado, J. E., Charache, S., and Boyer, S. H.,** Familial erythrocytosis due to electrophoretically undetectable hemoglobin with impaired oxygen dissociation (hemoglobin Malmo, α_2 β_2 ^{97}gln), *Mayo Clin. Proc.,* 46, 721, 1971.
3. **Rudolph, A. M., Nadas, A. S., and Borges, W. H.,** Hematologic adjustments to cyanotic congenital heart disease, *Pediatrics,* 11, 454, 1953.
4. **Silverstein, M. N. and Lanier, A. P.,** Polycythemia vera, 1935–1969. An epidemiologic survey in Rochester, Minnesota, *Mayo Clin. Proc.,* 46, 751, 1971.
5. **Wasserman, L. R.,** The management of polycythemia vera, *Br. J. Haematol.,* 21, 371, 1971.
6. **Natelson, E. A., Lynch, E. C., Britton, H. A., and Alfrey, C. P., Jr.,** Polycythemia vera in childhood, *Am. J. Dis. Child.,* 122, 241, 1971.
7. **Bowdler, A. J.,** Plasma volume and splenomegaly in polycythemia vera, *Br. J. Haematol.,* 22, 331, 1972.
8. **Westin, J., Lanner, L. O., Larsson, A., and Weinfeld, A.,** Spleen size in polycythemia. A clinical and scintigraphic study, *Acta Med. Scand.,* 191, 263, 1972.

9. **Roux, A., Fischer, J., Leon, A., and Ruberg, R.**, Weight and function of the spleen in primary and secondary polycythemia, in *Die Milz.* Lennert, K. and Harms, D., Eds., Springer-Verlag, Berlin, 1970, 270.
10. **Kutti, T. and Weinfeld, A.**, Platelet production and platelet survival in polycythemia vera with special reference to the spleen size, *Scand. J. Haematol.*, 9, 97, 1972.
11. **Dibos, P. E., Judisch, J. M., Spaulding, M. B., Wagner, H. N., Jr., and McIntyre, P. A.**, Scanning the reticuloendothelial system (RES) in hematological diseases, *Johns Hopkins Med. J.*, 130, 68, 1972.
12. **Sidwell, R. W., Huffman, J. H., Khare, G. P., Allen, L. B., Witkowski, J. T., and Robins, R. K.**, Broad-spectrum antiviral activity of virazole: 1-β-D-ribofuranosyl-1,2,4-triazole-3-carboxamide, *Science,* 177, 705, 1972.
13. **Sharma, S. M., Patel, M. C., Ramanathan, P., and Ganatra, R. D.**, Role of spleen scanning in planning the treatment and assessment of splenic response in blood dyscrasias, *Am. J. Roentgenol.*, 101, 656, 1967.
14. **Jackson, H., Jr., Parker, F., Jr., and Lemon, H. M.**, Agnogenic myeloid metaplasia of the spleen, *N. Engl. J. Med.*, 222, 985, 1940.
15. **Block, M. and Jacobson, L. O.**, Myeloid metaplasia, *JAMA*, 143, 1390, 1950.
16. **Ward, H. P. and Block, M. H.**, The natural history of agnogenic myeloid metaplasia (AMM) and a critical evaluation of its relationship with the myeloproliferative syndrome, *Medicine,* 50, 357, 1971.
17. **Meytes, D., Shacked, N., Padeh, B., Czerniak, P., Pinkhas, J., and Ramot, B.**, Immunoglobulin levels in polycythemia vera, erythrocytosis, secondary polycythemia and myelofibrosis, *Isr. J. Med. Sci.,* 8, 925, 1972.
18. **Hickling, R. A.**, Chronic non-leukaemic myelosis, *Q. J. Med.*, 6, 253, 1937.
19. **Crosby, W. H.**, Indications for splenectomy, *Hosp. Pract.*, 2, 28, 1967.
20. **Dechavanne, M., Viola, J. J., Barbier, Y., and Revol, L.**, Indications for splenectomy in the anemic forms of myelofibrosis with myeloid metaplasia of the spleen, *Sem. Hop. Paris,* 48, 1187, 1972.
21. **Morgenstern, L.**, Splenectomy for massive splenomegaly due to myeloid metaplasia, *Am. J. Surg.*, 122, 288, 1971.
22. **Viala, J. J., Dechavanne, M., and Barbier, Y.**, Étude radioisotopique de l'erythropoiese et de l'hemolyse dans la myelofibrose avec metaplasie myeloide de la rate son interet dans les indications de la splenectomie, *Lyon Med.*, 228, 237, 1972.
23. **Bowdler, A. J.**, Radioisotope investigations in primary myeloid metaplasia, *J. Clin. Pathol.*, 14, 595, 1961.
24. **Dibos, P. E., Judisch, J. M., Spaulding, M. B., Wagner, H. N., Jr., and McIntyre, P. A.**, Scanning the reticuloendothelial system (RES) in hematological diseases, *Johns Hopkins Med. J.*, 130, 68, 1972.
25. **Dameshek, W., Granville, N. B., and Rubie, F., Jr.**, Therapy of the myeloproliferative disorders with Myleran, *Ann. N.Y. Acad. Sci.*, 68, 1001, 1958.
26. **Bouroncle, B. A. and Doan, C. A.**, Myelofibrosis. Clinical, hematological and pathologic study of 110 patients, *Am. J. Med. Sci.*, 243, 697, 1962.
27. **Nuland, S. B., Cornelius, E. A., and Spencer, R. P.**, Scan evidence of organ involution and improvement of hypersplenism in Hodgkin's disease following splenic artery ligation, *J. Nucl. Med.*, 11, 693, 1970.
28. **Van Dyke, D., Anger, H. O., Parker, H., McRae, J., Dobson, E. L., Yano, D. Y., Naets, J. P., and Linfoot, J.**, Markedly increased bone blood flow in myelofibrosis, *J. Nucl. Med.*, 12, 506, 1971.
29. **Berg, B., Stahl, E., and Soderstrom, N.**, The cytology of spleen aspiration in uncomplicated polycythemia vera, *Scand. J. Haematol.*, 10, 59, 1973.
30. **Szur, L., Pettit, J. E., Lewis, S. M., Bruce-Tagoe, A. A., and Short, M. D.**, The effect of radiation on splenic function in myelosclerosis: studies with ^{52}Fe and ^{99}Tc^{m}, *Br. J. Radiol.*, 46, 295, 1973.
31. **Tavassoli, M.**, Splenic white pulp in myeloid metaplasia, *Arch. Pathol.*, 95, 419, 1973.
32. **Kutti, J., Weinfeld, A., and Westin, J.**, The relationship between splenic platelet pool and spleen size, *Scand. J. Haematol.*, 9, 351, 1972.
33. **McGarry, M. P. and Mirand, E. A.**, Influence of Friend virus-induced polycythemia in splenectomized mice, *Proc. Soc. Exp. Biol. Med.*, 142, 539, 1973.
34. **Glew, R. H., Haese, W. H., and McIntyre, P. A.**, Myeloid metaplasia with myelofibrosis – the clinical spectrum of extramedullary hematopoiesis and tumor formation, *Johns Hopkins Med. J.*, 132, 253, 1973.
35. **Viola, M. V., Kovi, J., and Nukhopadhyay, M.**, Reversal of myelofibrosis in Hodgkin's disease, *JAMA*, 223, 1145, 1973.
36. **Johnston, C. C., Jr., Lavy, N., Lord, T., Vellios, F., Merritt, A. D., and Deiss, W. P., Jr.**, Osteopetrosis: a clinical, genetic, metabolic and morphologic study of the dominantly inherited, benign form, *Medicine,* 47, 149, 1968.
37. **Emery, A. C., Jr., Whitcomb, W. H., and Frohlich, E. D.**, "Stress" polycythemia and hypertension, *JAMA,* 229, 159, 1974.
38. **Gaisböck, F.**, Die Bedeutung der Blutdruck messung für die Praxis, *Dtsch. Arch. Klin. Med.*, 83, 363, 1905.
39. **O'Brien, R. T., Pearson, H. A., and Spencer, R. P.**, Transfusion-induced decrease in spleen size in thalassemia major: documentation by radioisotopic scan, *J. Pediatr.*, 81, 105, 1972.

Chapter 11

LYMPHOMAS AND LEUKEMIAS: SARCOIDOSIS, AMYLOIDOSIS, AND EOSINOPHILS

The word lymphoma has been used as a general one to include traditionally at least four disorders.

	Percent
Hodgkin's disease	42.6
Lymphosarcoma	34.7
Reticulum cell sarcoma	16.2
Giant follicular lymphoma	6.5

These percentages indicate the relative frequency in five series of cases reviewed by Moss and Brand.[1] The lymphomas have many similar features, despite some controversy on the multicentricity of their origin, and are usually clinically staged in a similar manner (described below).

Hodgkin's disease variously constitutes about 30 to 50% of the cases of lymphoma. Although individuals of any age can be affected, the disorder is most common in young adults. However, no age is exempt. Strum and Rappaport[2] have studied 35 children with Hodgkin's disease occurring in the first decade of life. In these juvenile cases, there was a preponderance of males.

Within the past several years, it has been recognized that patients who have Hodgkin's disease limited to the lymphatic system can often be cured by radiation therapy. In general, prognosis can be related to three factors.

1. Histology – particularly numbers of lymphocytes, histiocytes, and Reed-Sternberg cells.
2. Anatomic staging.
3. Systemic symptoms – specifically fever, night sweats, significant weight loss.

A relationship between survival and the histology of Hodgkin's disease was noted first by Rosenthal[3] and further illuminated by Jackson and Parker.[4] The histopathological classification in current use was put forth by Lukes in 1963.[5] The four major classifications are as follows:

1. Lymphocyte predominance (proliferation of lymphocytes) with few Reed-Sternberg cells.
2. Nodular sclerosis (collagen bands separate nodules of lymphoid tissue).
3. Mixed type (lymphocytes, histiocytes, and a fibrillar pattern).
4. Lymphocyte depletion (few lymphocytes, disordered fibrosis, many Reed-Sternberg cells).

The lymphocyte predominance type usually carries the best prognosis. In addition, one specific pathologic feature, vascular invasion, has been recognized as having a particularly serious outlook on ultimate survival.[9]

In addition to the histology, the lymphomas are usually described by:

Clinical Staging	(CS)
Pathological Staging	(PS)
Symptoms	(A or B)

By clinical staging is meant the following,[10] which is an outgrowth of the suggestions of earlier workers[6,7] and the Rye classification of 1956 (this is actually defined for Hodgkin's disease but is often extended to all the lymphomas).

Clinical Staging:

I. Single lymph node region or extralymphatic site involved.

II. Two or more lymph node groups on same side of diaphragm are involved or localized extralymphatic and one or more lymph nodes.

III. Lymph nodes on both sides of the diaphragm are involved. There may be localized extralymphatic or splenic involvement.

IV. Diffuse or disseminated disease.

The pathological staging (PS) describes whether there is involvement (+) or no involvement (−) of lymph nodes, liver, spleen, lung, marrow, pleura, osseous, and skin tissues. Symptoms are "B" (defined, generalized) if there is over 10% body weight loss, unexplained fever over 38°C, or night sweats. In these classifications, lymphatic structures are taken to include the lymph nodes, spleen, thymus, Waldeyer's ring, appendix, and Peyer's patches.

The type of therapy used in Hodgkin's disease

depends on the clinical staging of the particular case. Most patients in Stages I and II (and some in Stage III A) are treated and many can be cured by megavoltage radiotherapy.[8] The clinical staging is thus of great importance. Many diagnostic aids are used in making the assessment. The following diagnostic procedures may be employed:

1. Chest x-ray.
2. Lymph node biopsy.
3. Bone marrow biopsy.
4. Liver scan.
5. Lymphangiogram.
6. Lymph node scans with ^{67}Ga, ^{198}Au, or other agents.
7. Spleen scan.
8. Bone scan.
9. Laparotomy with splenectomy and biopsy of abdominal and paraaortic nodes and liver biopsy.

It is apparent that the finding of widespread extralymphatic involvement immediately changes the staging of the disease, and hence the therapy (but localized extralymphatic involvement can respond to radiotherapy). Liver scans have a role in staging Hodgkin's disease.[11] In addition, reticuloendothelial scans of the bone marrow may have a limited usefulness.[12]

Since the spleen is considered part of the subdiaphragmatic lymphatics for staging purposes, adequate evaluation of the organ is essential. Even as sophisticated a technique as splenic arteriography may not provide a definitive answer. Castellino ánd co-workers[13] at Stanford point out that the spleen is pathologically involved in 35% of consecutive untreated patients with Hodgkin's disease and that spleen size is an inadequate indicator of the presence of the disease. Further, they observed that splenic arteriography, prior to splenectomy for staging, showed no correlation with the presence or absence of Hodgkin's disease in the spleen (except for filling defects on tomographs obtained in conjunction with arteriography).

What role do spleen scans have in the staging of Hodgkin's disease? Silverman and associates[14] reported on 42 patients with Hodgkin's disease who had spleen scintigrams and subsequent splenectomy. The scintigrams were evaluated in terms of splenic size, concentration of radionuclide, eveness of uptake, and presence or absence of focal defects. Marked splenomegaly and focal defects indicated the presence of Hodgkin's disease in the spleen; however, these two findings were often not present (focal defects were observed in only two cases and massive splenomegaly in three). It would appear then that a focal splenic defect (Figures 1 and 2) or massive splenomegaly (Figure 3) in Hodgkin's disease carries a high assurance of the presence of the disorder in the spleen. However, the disease can be present without these findings, and histological examination of the organ is needed in such instances. Recall, again, that focal defects are nonspecific and may have many causes.

There are a number of other reports on spleen scanning in Hodgkin's disease, and we will review some of them. Fischer and Wolf[15] studied 62 cases of Hodgkin's disease by means of spleen scans utilizing ^{51}Cr-heat-treated erythrocytes. Only 4 of the patients had clinically detectable splenomegaly (6.4%), but 38 had splenomegaly on the scan (61.3%). Thus, only 4/38 or 10.5% of the instances of splenomegaly were detected clinically. Wagner and Verdon[16] noted that spleen scans revealed 5 out of 13 cases of Hodgkin's disease to have splenomegaly that was not appreciated clinically (^{99m}Tc-sulfur colloid). Milder and co-workers found that all the spleen scans showing an organ over 15 cm in length in Hodgkin's disease revealed

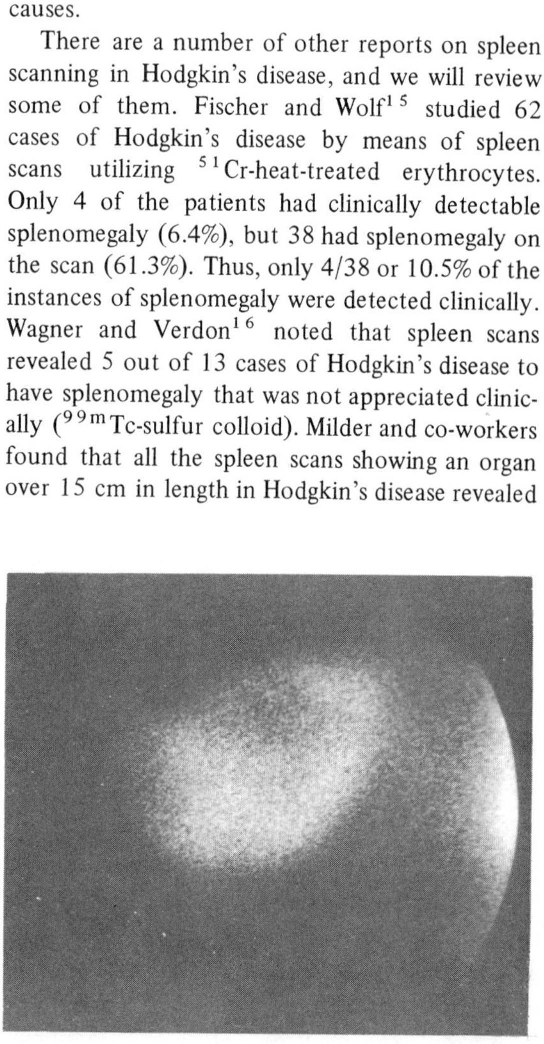

FIGURE 1. Posterior scintiphoto of the spleen (^{99m}Tc-sulfur colloid) in a 55-year-old man who had Hodgkin's disease first diagnosed 20 years ago. There was recurrent disease as shown on a lymphangiogram. The defects noted here are unusual in Hodgkin's disease involving the spleen and clearly show intrasplenic pathology. Case 72-2013.

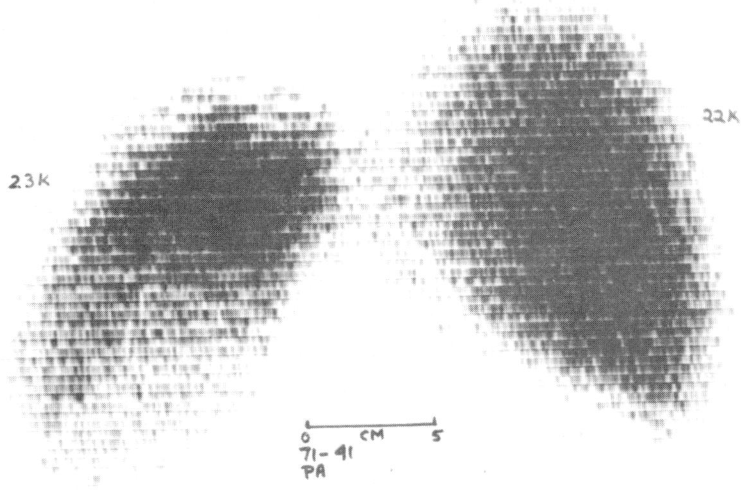

FIGURE 2. Posterior rectilinear scan (^{99m}Tc-sulfur colloid) in a 45-year-old woman who presented with a left inguinal node. Biopsy revealed Hodgkin's disease. Lymphangiography showed the presence of enlarged paraaortic nodes. The spleen scan reveals an enlarged organ (over 16 cm in length) with an area of diminished activity at the lower, mesial portion. Case 71-41.

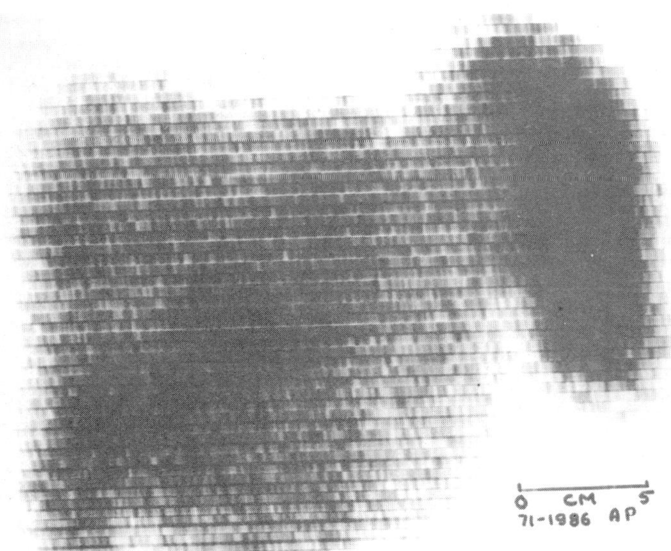

FIGURE 3. Anterior rectilinear scan (^{99m}Tc-sulfur colloid) in a 58-year-old woman with Hodgkin's disease and abnormal liver function tests. The presence of hepatomegaly and liver defects stages the disease as IV. In this case the minimal splenomegaly (about 14 cm in length) may be related to Hodgkin's disease in the spleen and/or the presence of portal hypertension resulting from the liver involvement. There is a shift of radioactive colloid to the spleen. Case 71-1886.

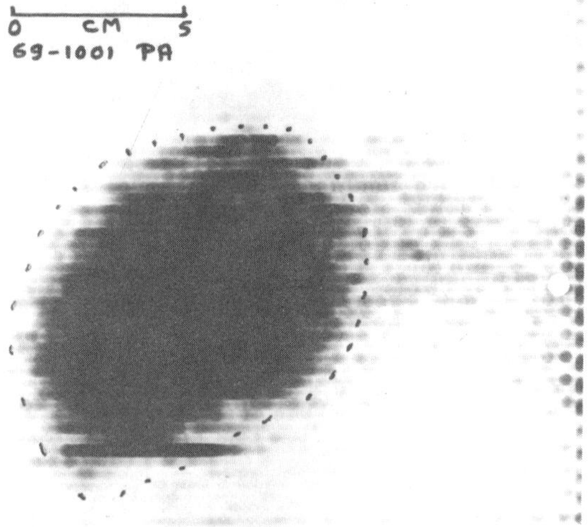

FIGURE 4. Posterior spleen scan (^{99m}Tc-sulfur colloid) in a 42-year-old male with Hodgkin's disease. Using the scan, the spleen was outlined on the skin surface (as shown by the dots) prior to radiation therapy. Case 69-1001.

tumor involvement.[44] The duration of Hodgkin's disease is not an indication of the likelihood of splenic involvement.[17] Also, there may not be correlation between the lymphangiogram and splenic involvement on scan.[19] Filling defects and heterogeneity of uptake on the spleen scan in Hodgkin's disease may be related to tumor masses or to the confluence of micronodules.[18] A number of cases of Hodgkin's disease reveal granulomas in the spleen of uncertain origin.[14,25] Pettit and co-workers[20] noted that in Hodgkin's disease the spleen may have a larger size than normal and may contain a larger red cell volume than normal. Sharma and associates stressed the role of spleen scans in planning the therapy of Hodgkin's disease and other disorders.[21]

Laparotomy and splenectomy have been playing an increasingly important role in the staging of Hodgkin's disease,[22] even though the view has been expressed that the disorder may be multifocal in origin.[23] When operation is contraindicated, the spleen can be irradiated through external ports. Spleen scans can be useful in outlining the organ prior to radiation and hence in reducing the radiation exposure of surrounding tissues (Figure 4). There are few findings in nuclear medicine which are pathognomonic. However, one scan in Hodgkin's disease begins to come close. This is a radioactive colloid scan, following splenectomy for Hodgkin's disease and irradiation of paraaortic nodes. The picture is one of an absent spleen and a sharp cutoff of the liver (due to radiation damage to the hepatic cells of the left lobe). An example is shown in Figure 5. At time of operation for diagnostic removal of the spleen, it may be difficult or impossible to mobilize the organ, due to adherent tumor. We have had experience with one such case of Hodgkin's disease, in which there was dramatic transient improvement of accompanying hypersplenism, following splenic artery ligation.[24]

Microfoci of Hodgkin's disease in the spleen will, of course, escape detection by splenic scans. Other parameters do not offer much help at present in detecting such cases. Some reports have noted a shift of ^{99m}Tc-sulfur colloid to the spleen in Hodgkin's disease,[14] but this has yet to be correlated with intrasplenic disease (Figure 6). When ^{198}Au-colloid is used, increased splenic uptake in Hodgkin's disease has been noted in some cases,[26] but again there has been inadequate correlation with the presence or absence of disease in the spleen. It will be recalled that ^{198}Au-colloid has a particle size on the order of 0.001 to 0.01 μm, while ^{99m}Tc-sulfur colloid has a diameter of 0.1 to 1.0 μm. In Hodgkin's disease, there is accelerated clearance of ^{125}I-aggregated albumin from the bloodstream,[27] and this approximately parallels the extent of the disease. What relationships these different clearances have to the nature or the progression of Hodgkin's disease is uncertain. Recently Chaudhuri and associates[55] noted the accumulation of ^{87m}Sr in a spleen affected by Hodgkin's disease; the mechanism is unknown.

Abrahamsen[28] tagged autologous platelets with ^{51}Cr and followed their recovery after infusion into patients with Hodgkin's disease. Platelet recovery increased dramatically after splenectomy, indicating a pooling of platelets in the spleen. The quantity of platelets pooled was related to spleen size and could be approximated by:

$$R = 62 - 0.054S$$

where R is platelet recovery in percent, and S is splenic weight in grams. Splenectomy did not significantly affect platelet survival in these patients with Hodgkin's disease.

Splenectomy in Hodgkin's disease may not be innocuous, however. Ravry and co-workers[29] noted serious infections in 2 of 47 patients within the first year after splenectomy for Hodgkin's

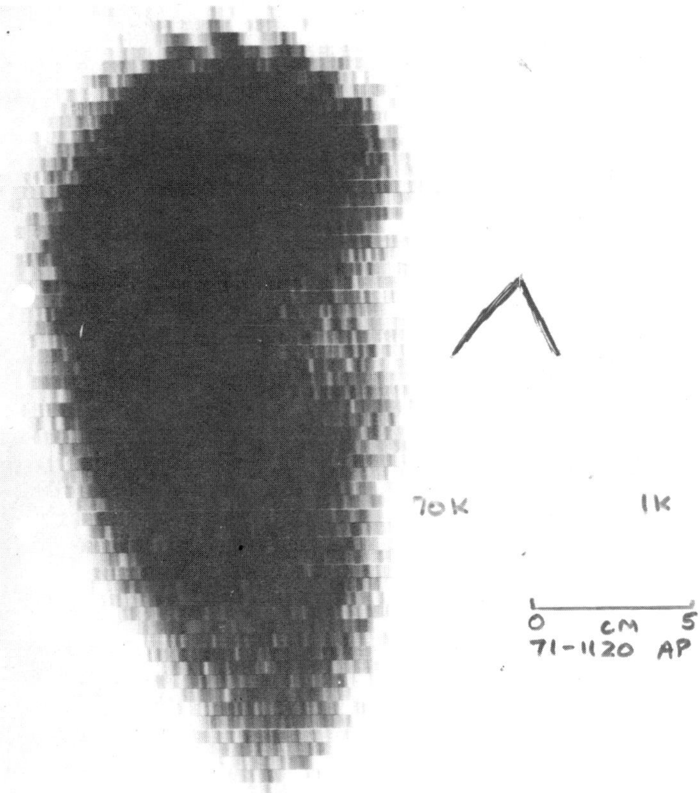

FIGURE 5. Anterior scan of the abdomen (^{99m}Tc-sulfur colloid) in a 21-year-old woman with Hodgkin's disease. The spleen had been removed surgically for staging. There is a medial cutoff of hepatic activity, corresponding to the portal employed in irradiation of paraaortic nodes. Case 71-1120.

disease. Both individuals had meningitis, related to *D. pneumoniae* in one case and *H. influenzae* type B in the other. In the second case, septicemia due to *D. pneumoniae* later developed. It is likely that these kinds of infections will be more frequent when splenectomy is done on young children (see Chapter 4).

There is at least one reticuloendothelial tumor in animals that is Hodgkin's-like[30] and transplantable from generation to generation. Despite evidence for a tumor-associated antigen in Hodgkin's disease[31] and studies on leukocyte phenotypes,[32-34] there is still no clear indication of the etiology of the disease (although a virus of low virulence has been suggested).[35] Localized "epidemics" of the disorder have been reported. Of interest has been the frequent occurrence of infections in patients with Hodgkin's disease. A number of these patients are anergic (no reaction to multiple skin tests and increased tolerance to skin homografts).[36,37] Anergy, however (at least in the one case we have seen), did not interfere with uptake of ^{99m}Tc-sulfur colloid.

An interesting development has been the use of radioactive gallium in the study of Hodgkin's disease. The radionuclide ^{67}Ga has a half-life of 3.2 days and emits a series of Zn x-rays (93, 184, 296 keV, principally). The observation by Edwards and Hayes[38] that ^{67}Ga concentrates in some human tumors has precipitated much work to define the conditions necessary for its uptake. The normal pattern of distribution of ^{67}Ga has been studied.[40] Uptake of ^{67}Ga by the normal liver and spleen makes for difficulty in detecting lesions in these organs.[41] The small bowel must be cleansed before paraaortic nodes can be identified. The spleen can have the highest concentration of ^{67}Ga following intravenous administration,[42] but

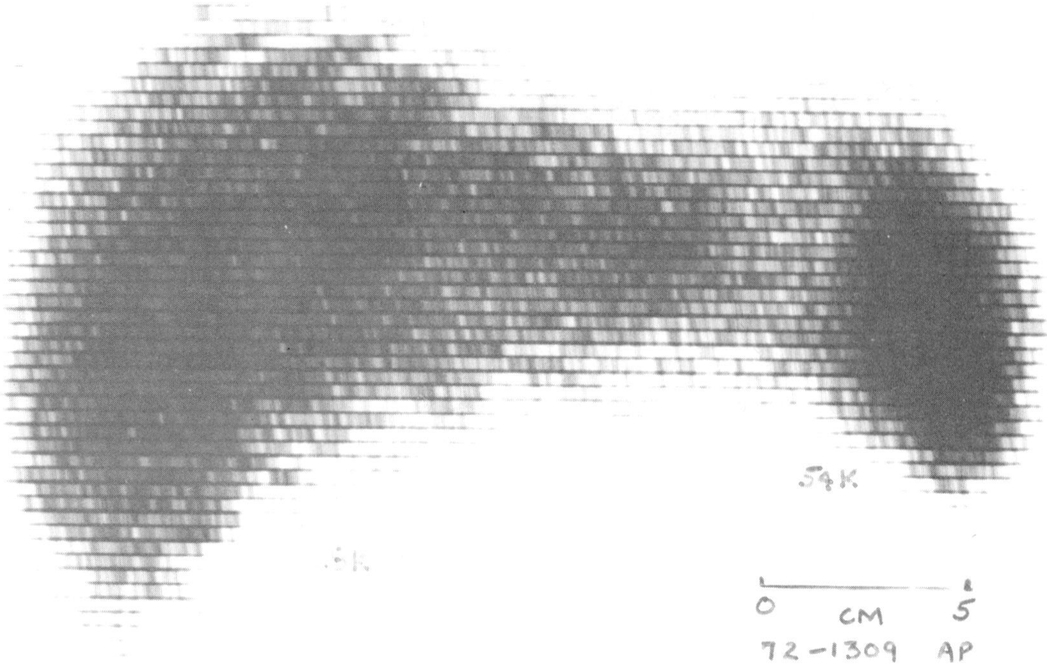

FIGURE 6. Anterior rectilinear scan (^{99m}Tc-sulfur colloid) performed on a 20-year-old woman. The patient had stage IV B Hodgkin's disease (positive bone marrow). There was no hepatomegaly or splenomegaly, but a shift of radiocolloid to the spleen is apparent. Case 72-1309.

the relationship to the presence or absence of disease or to the rate of discharge of radionuclide has not been defined. In one study, ^{67}Ga was noted to concentrate in lesions in 14 of 17 patients with Hodgkin's disease.[39] Despite much promise,[43,58] there are not yet definitive data on the role to be played by ^{67}Ga in staging Hodgkin's disease. The use of radioindium (^{111}In) in detecting tumors has also been proposed, but additional data are required. The radiolabeled amino acid ^{75}Se-selenomethionine has been used for detecting lymphomas.[53,54,56] However, the high radiation dose and uptake in surrounding tissues makes it difficult to use. ^{198}Au has been used to search for thoracic lymph node accumulation of radiocolloid in lymphomas.[57] Again, there is a high radiation dose. Radiocolloids of other materials may offer a better approach.

THE OTHER LYMPHOMATOUS DISEASES

Lymphomas can involve the spleen either as part of a generalized process or as the principal organ affected. Skarin and co-workers[45] described 11 patients with primary lymphosarcoma of the spleen. All had splenomegaly, and spleen weights varied from 550 to 4,500 g. They believed that splenectomy was beneficial, although some patients went on to develop a leukemic blood picture.

There has been much discussion of staging the other lymphomas in a manner similar to that of Hodgkin's disease[46] (that is, by use of laparotomy and splenectomy). While this controversy has not been resolved, there appears to be some merit to such attempts since the results of radiation therapy (in an older series) appear related to the clinical staging.[47] It must also be recognized that while the lymphomas are usually considered together, there are very real differences. For example, a considerably larger fraction of patients with reticulum cell sarcoma respond to vincristine therapy than do patients with Hodgkin's disease.[48] Newell and Friedman[49] pointed out that the clinical behavior of reticulum cell sarcoma was "disorderly," i.e., different from that of Hodgkin's disease, and made planning of treatment difficult.

Fuzy and associates[50] utilized denatured ^{51}Cr-erythrocytes for visualizing the spleen in 102 patients with malignant lymphomas. They remarked on the usefulness of the procedure in detecting splenomegaly or infiltrates of the spleen, and hence the value of scanning in the staging of the disease. While massive splenomegaly (Figure 7) and filling defects (Figure 8) certainly indicate the presence of abnormality, again it should be emphasized that the presence of a spleen of normal size does not exclude the possibility of lymphomatous involvement. The scan may have some use in following the progression of the size of the spleen in lymphoma or its response to therapy.[50]

There are a number of animal models of the lymphomas. For example, a reticulum cell sarcoma affects Japanese quails,[51] and there can be marked splenomegaly. The likely relationship between continued stimulation of the lymphoid tissue and lymphoid neoplasia has been discussed.[52] Whether radionuclide studies of the spleen have anything to offer in following splenic changes during such malignant transformation is unknown.

LEUKEMIA

An abnormal increase in the number of leukocytes, without demonstration of a specific cause, is referred to as leukemia. One classification is based on the type of leukocyte involved and its degree of maturity. It is of interest that even before blood-staining procedures were developed, it was recognized that white blood cells were involved and that two forms of the disorder were identifiable: a lymphatic and a splenic (now referred to as myelocytic). While clinical features aid in distinguishing the leukemic forms, definitive diagnosis depends on microscopic examination of blood and bone marrow. Involvement of two or more cell lines ("myelomonocytic leukemia")

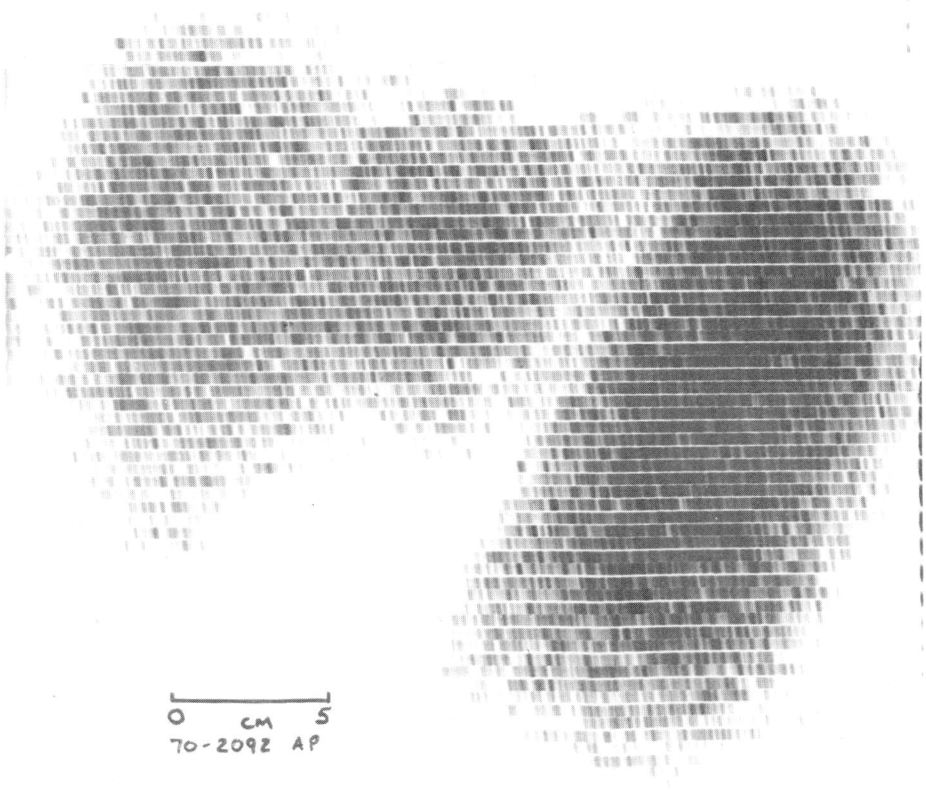

FIGURE 7. Anterior rectilinear scan (^{99m}Tc-sulfur colloid) in a 41-year-old man with widespread lymphoblastic lymphoma. Marked splenomegaly is evident. Case 70-2092.

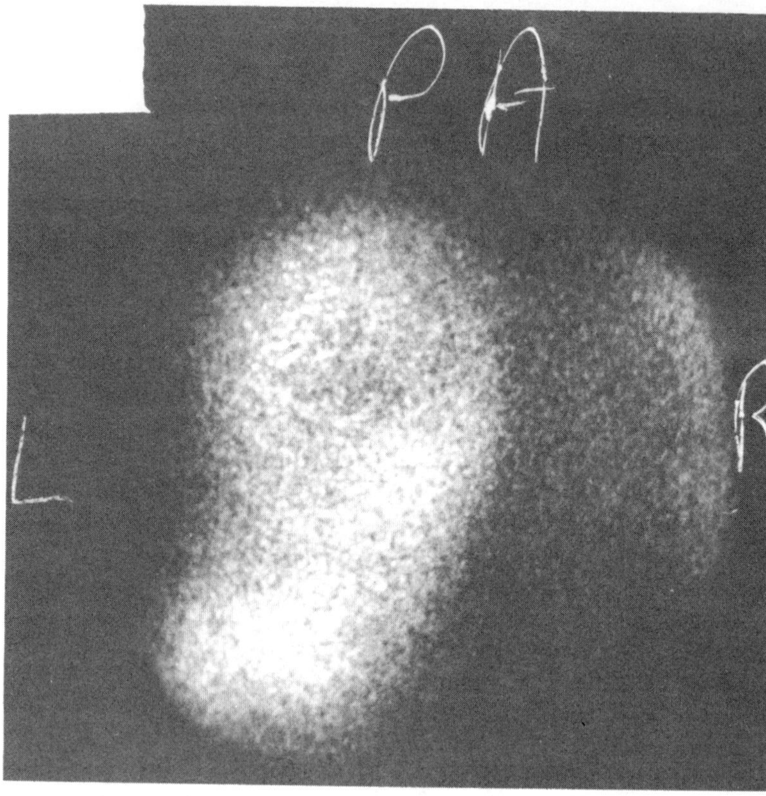

FIGURE 8. Posterior scintiphoto (^{99m}Tc-sulfur colloid) in a 77-year-old woman with lymphosarcoma. The spleen was 24 cm in length and contained multiple filling defects. Case 67-759.

appears to occur,[59] although newer techniques suggest that these so-called mixed types may in fact be monocytic. Proliferation of white cell masses accounts for most of the clinical signs and symptoms, although humoral effects of these cells or their precursors cannot be excluded. Leukemic cell infiltration accounts for hepatosplenomegaly, lymphadenopathy, and symptoms referable to specific organs. The growth of these cells in bone marrow produces a decrease in platelets and other hematologic formed elements, resulting in thrombocytopenic bleeding, anemia, and susceptibility to bacterial infection. Still other manifestations (Table 1) of the disease may be due to breakdown of the leukemic cells or alterations they produce in cellular metabolism (such as excess production of uric acid, weight loss, and fever).

Radioisotopic studies, primarily by use of ^{14}C or ^{3}H precursors of DNA, indicate an abnormally high rate of production of leukocytes in chronic myelocytic leukemia and the acute leukemias. This production is due to an expanded compartment of precursor cells. It also follows, when the counts are stable, that there is also an elevated destruction of leukocytes. ^{32}P-diisopropylfluorophosphate has also been used to label white cells in myelogenous leukemia in order to follow their disappearance curves.[60] Cyclic fluctuations in the white cell and platelet counts in chronic granulocytic leukemia have also been studied by means of ^{32}P-diisopropylfluorophosphate.[61] It has been hypothesized that there is negative feedback, controlled by a humoral substance. In addition to leukocyte turnover, survival of fibrinogen (tagged by use of ^{75}Se-selenomethionine) has been studied in leukemia.[62] The ability to culture leukemic cells in vitro[63,64] provides an opportunity to study their characteristics; it might also be possible to incorporate radionuclides into these cells for reintroduction into the host, but this has not as yet been performed.

There has been recent interest in the Epstein-Barr virus since some cases of acute lymphocytic leukemia have been reported to be preceded by infectious mononucleosis.[65] The widespread presence of antibodies to this virus[66,67] and the

TABLE 1

Commentary on the Major Types of Leukemia

Acute myeloctyic (blastic) leukemia	The leukocyte count may not be elevated in the peripheral blood in about one third of the cases when first seen. Blast cells in the blood may range as high as one million. Anemia and thrombocytopenia are present.
Chronic myelocytic leukemia	Usual leukocyte count is over 100,000/mm³ in blood. When the count is below 50,000, few immature forms may appear. Otherwise, multiple forms (blasts to segmented) occur. The fraction of immature cells in the marrow is still more elevated, suggesting some surviving block to their release. A blastic crisis may occur as a terminal event, resembling the acute leukemias. There can be a Philadelphia chromosome and a low leukocyte alkaline phosphatase. Serum vitamin B_{12} may be elevated.
Acute lymphocytic (blastic) leukemia	Most common type of leukemia in children. Lymph node and visceral involvement are usual, and central nervous system infiltration can occur.
Chronic lymphocytic leukemia	The most slowly progressing of these diseases; lymphadenopathy and splenomegaly are common. Many have white cell counts of under 100,000/mm³. Normal leukocytes appear on the smear interspersed between the abnormal cells. The population is usually older. A variant may be the Sezary syndrome in which the lymphocytes contain more PAS-staining material.
Rare forms of leukemia	Eosinophilic, plasmacytic, erythroleukemia.

ability of the virus to induce DNA synthesis in leukocytes deserve further study.

Splenomegaly can occur in each of the forms of leukemia. The organ is palpable in nearly all cases of chronic myelocytic leukemia and 60 to 80% of those with other types of leukemia.[68] Utilizing ^{198}Au as the scanning agent, Goswitz and Vodopick[69] noted that splenic infarcts can occur in chronic myelocytic leukemia. Both irradiation and ^{32}P therapy[70,71] have been used in treating leukemias. Additional discussion can be found in the section on the effects of radiation on the spleen.

Palmer and associates[72,73] carried out studies utilizing ^{131}I-microaggregated albumin in normal subjects and those with leukemia. Blood samples were drawn periodically and then fractionated to measure activity due to colloid (to quantify uptake by reticuloendothelial cells), as well as that due to inorganic ^{131}I, which was a measure of the catabolic function of the reticuloendothelial system (that is, the ^{131}I was cleaved from the radiocolloid). To correct for variations in the handling of radioiodide between patients, each was given Na ^{125}I to act as a separate tracer of iodide. A mathematical model was developed, from which rate constants for the events of colloid uptake and ^{131}I discharge from the reticuloendothelial system could be calculated. Leukemic patients had a rate of phagocytosis (of much of the colloid) which was indistinguishable from controls. However, the percent of particles undergoing slow clearance was slightly increased (that is, fewer were taken rapidly). Perhaps this is related to impaired bacterial clearance and the increased rate of infection in leukemia. In addition, leukemic subjects had an increased rate of catabolism of the particles.[73]

Badrawi and associates[74] studied the rate of blood clearance of ^{51}Cr-erythrocytes which had been heat denatured (50° for 60 min). The assumption was that these cells were quantitatively trapped in the spleen, and hence trapping was an index of splenic function. The normal clearance half-time of the cells was said to be 172 ± 69 min in control subjects. A half-time of 74 min or less was considered to indicate rapid clearance (and hence increased splenic activity). Four of 6 patients with acute leukemia and 4 of 15 with chronic myelocytic leukemia showed rapid clearance of the labeled cells. No abnormality of the disappearance rate was noted in patients with chronic lymphatic leukemia.

Bowie and associates[75] studied anemia in patients with leukemia, using both ^{51}Cr-tagged erythrocytes and ^{59}Fe. They concluded that in acute leukemia, anemia resulted from failure of bone marrow production to keep up with erythrocyte destruction. In two cases of chronic granulocytic leukemia, there was impaired erythropoiesis and a high plasma volume (possible hemodilution).

In our experience, spleen scans have had a small but finite role in the leukemias.

1. They can be used to determine whether a left upper quadrant mass is the spleen or another structure, such as a group of nodes or the liver (Figure 9).

2. The scans can be utilized to show the presence of intrahepatic defects (Figure 10), but recall that many diseases can cause such lesions.

3. Spleen scans can be utilized to document splenomegaly when the organ is not palpable (Figure 11), as well as rapid changes in liver and spleen size.

4. The scans can be used to indicate the presence of intrasplenic defects (Figure 12) or to follow the effect of medication (Figure 13). While extracorporeal irradiation has been used to reduce the white cell count in leukemia, we are not aware of the use of spleen scans to follow the size of the organ during such therapy.

Infiltration of the spleen, or deposition of materials, occurs in many other disorders. For example, fibrin deposits were mentioned in an earlier section. In this chapter we will also consider sarcoid infiltration of the spleen, splenic amyloidosis, and the presence of eosinophils in the organ.

SARCOIDOSIS

The granulomatous disease referred to as sarcoidosis is of uncertain etiology. Almost all organs can be involved, including the spleen.

1. A palpable spleen is noted in about one third of the cases of sarcoidosis (Figure 14). On rare occasions, the spleen may be massively enlarged.[76] The triad of leukopenia, anemia, and thrombocytopenia can occur, although splenomegaly in other cases may persist for many years without specific symptoms. Hepatosplenomegaly is said to indicate a less favorable prognosis.

2. When a suspension (heat sterilized) of human sarcoid-involved spleen or lymph nodes is injected intracutaneously, about two thirds of patients with sarcoidosis show a papulonodular response (Kveim test).

There are a number of observations that center around the reactivity of leukocytes from patients with sarcoidosis. For example, adding the Kveim antigen to such leukocytes produces increased transformation in tissue cultures.[77] The activity of circulating leukocytes in sarcoidosis can be studied in vitro and the response to medications noted.[78] Leukocyte migration was inhibited in vitro by sarcoid spleen suspensions in 4 out of 10 patients with celiac disease and 16 out of 17 patients with dermatitis herpetiformis.[79] This is consistent with the view that cross reaction occurs in disorders in which the epithelioid reaction is not obvious. It may also be recalled that celiac disease and dermatitis herpetiformis are among the diseases

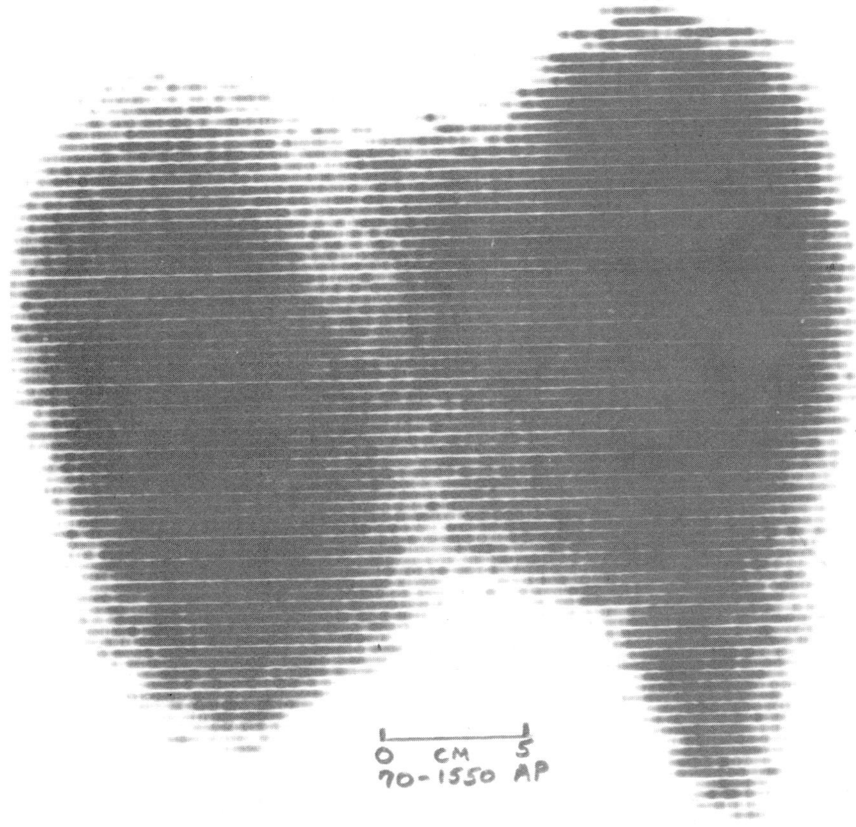

FIGURE 9. Anterior rectilinear scan (^{99m}Tc-sulfur colloid) in a 44-year-old man. This extraordinary picture resulted from the combination of Kartagener's syndrome and chronic lymphatic leukemia. Hepatosplenomegaly and reversal of the organs can be noted. Case 70-1550

occasionally associated with splenic atrophy. The Kveim antigen also inhibited leukocyte migration from 12 out of 18 patients with Crohn's disease.[80] There is, however, no effect in ulcerative colitis. Papamichail and associates[81] studied human lymphocytes (by fluorescence) for surface immunoglobulins and for rosette formation with sheep erythrocytes. In five cases of sarcoidosis, the fraction of immunofluorescent cells was increased and the fraction of rosette-forming cells was diminished. How this interrelates to other parameters of splenic function in sarcoidosis has still to be determined. Reports of sarcoidlike lesions in lymph nodes draining a malignant area [82] suggest that the tissue response is an important factor in development of sarcoid.

Splenic involvement in sarcoidosis appears to be independent of whether pulmonary problems are present (Figure 15). Dickerman and associates[83] have discussed the thrombocytopenia that occurs in sarcoidosis. They point out that in some of the patients, bleeding may be severe and can require corticosteroids or splenectomy. Steroids may have little effect on the pulmonary manifestations of sarcoidosis.[84] However, steroids can result in a decrease in the size of the spleen in patients with giant splenomegaly sarcoidosis. Burt and Kuhl[85] have documented such a case by scintillation scanning, and we have commented on quantifying the rate of change of splenic size.[86]

AMYLOIDOSIS

Among the reasons that amyloidosis is of interest is that animal models of the disease are well recognized.[87,88] Indeed, at least 30 mammalian species can have spontaneous amyloidosis (and induced amyloidosis is mentioned briefly below). Although the amorphous and eosinophilic substance was first termed amyloid because of

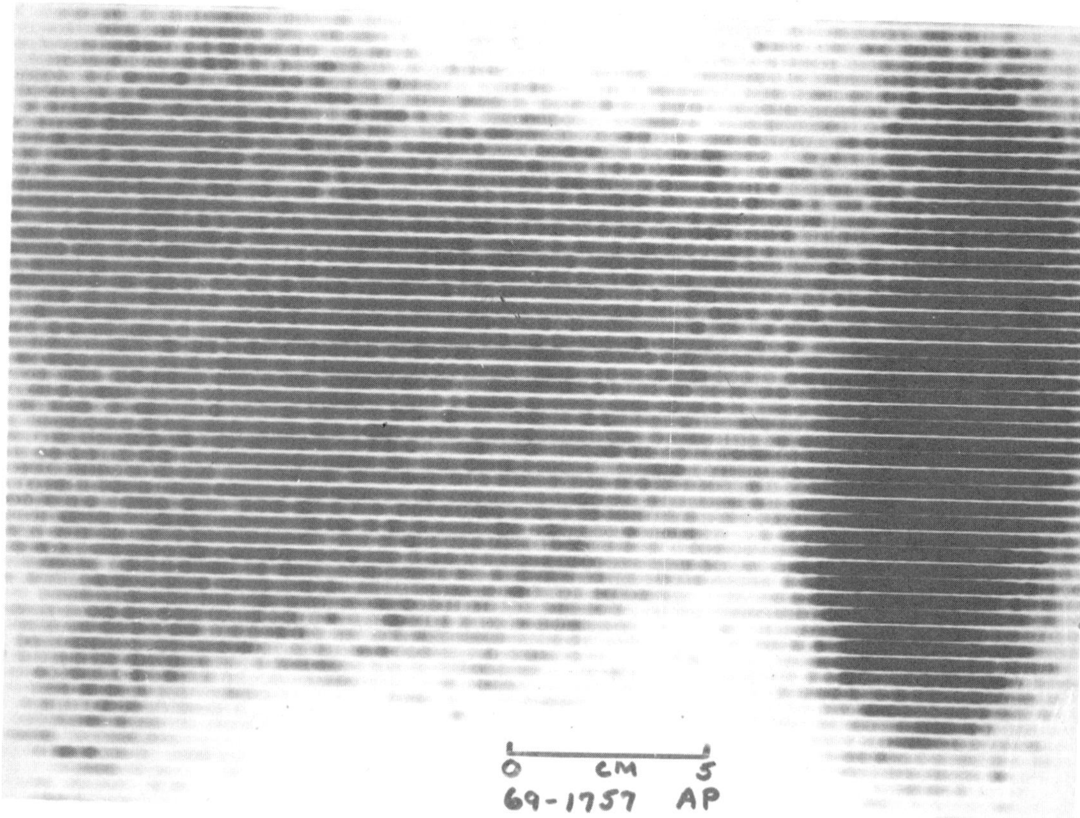

FIGURE 10. Anterior rectilinear scan (^{99m}Tc-sulfur colloid) in a 65-year-old man with chronic lymphocytic leukemia. Intrahepatic defects can be seen. Case 69-1757.

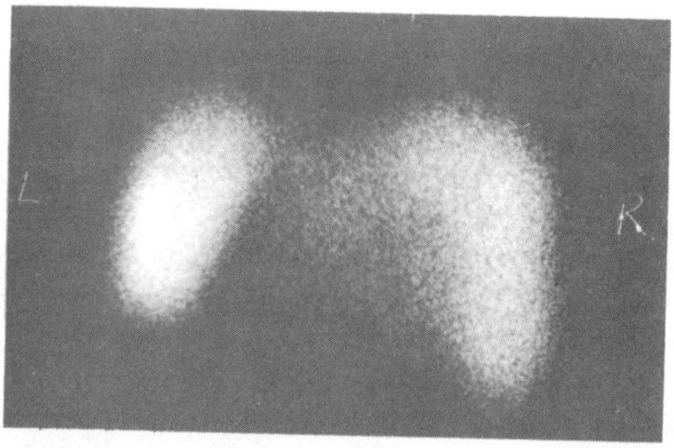

FIGURE 11. Posterior scintiphoto (^{99m}Tc-sulfur colloid) in a 28-month-old boy, who had been recently diagnosed as having acute lymphoblastic leukemia. The spleen was enlarged (9 cm), and there was a shift of the radioactive colloid. Case 72-1361.

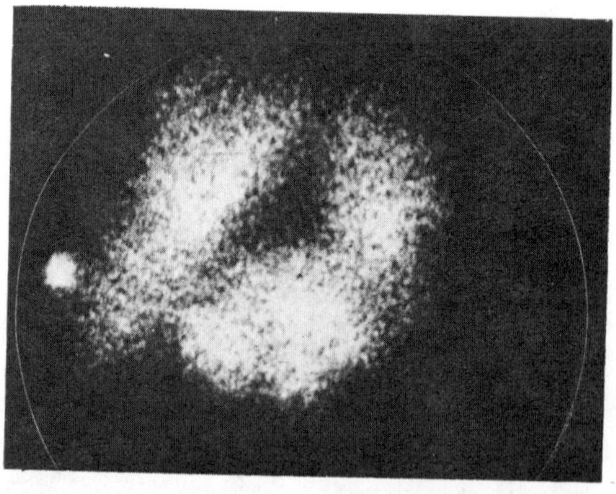

FIGURE 12. Left lateral, slightly obliqued scintiphoto (dot is anterior) obtained using ^{99m}Tc-sulfur colloid. The patient is a 71-year-old man with acute myelogenous leukemia in exacerbation (temperature of 102°). Whether the intrasplenic defects represent accumulation of leukemic cells, infarcts, or another process is unknown. Case 70-2061.

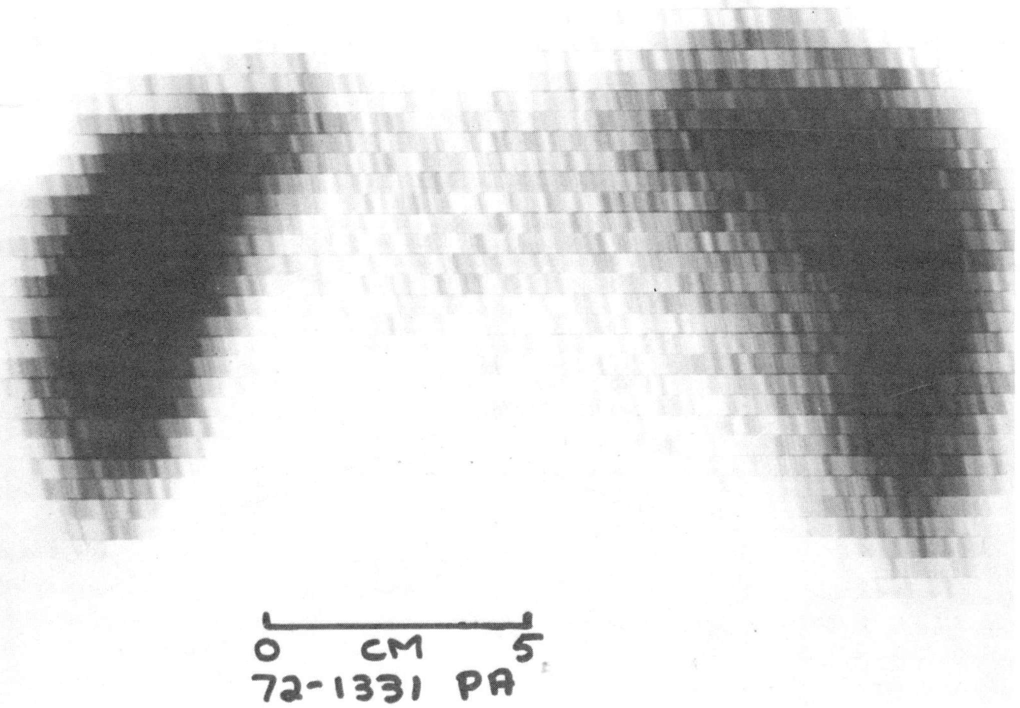

FIGURE 13. Posterior rectilinear scan (^{99m}Tc-sulfur colloid) in a 6-year-old girl. The patient had acute myelocytic leukemia and was on massive doses of methotrexate. The spleen was functional. Case 72-1331.

staining with iodine (and hence a similarity to starch), it is now clear that a protein is involved. Congo red staining, with green birefringence, and fibrillar appearance under the electron microscope mark this material[89] (and the properties of amyloid have been summarized).[90] From human tissues (particularly the spleen involved by amyloid), a protein can be obtained in high purity; however, some of the typical properties may be altered in the purified products.[89] For monkey amyloid protein, the amino acid composition has been determined.[91]

Secondary amyloidosis is the term applied to amyloid deposition found in association with chronic diseases involving infection or inflammation. Although the kidney is the organ principally affected, hepatosplenomegaly can occur. It is of interest that a significant number of patients with multiple myeloma also have amyloid deposits (Figure 16).

Even so-called "primary amyloidosis" may be comprised of a number of disorders. There appears to be a familial type as well as spontaneous appearance of the disorder. Intrahepatic obstruction due to amyloid deposition is quite rare, but the five reported cases (all males) had hepatomegaly and splenomegaly.[92]

Amyloidosis can be induced in animals by casein injections. In mice, splenectomy apparently enhances the development of amyloidosis following use of casein.[93] Amyloid formation can be fostered in guinea pigs by intraperitoneal introduction of spleen cells especially prepared by prior casein injection into the donors.[94] In pheasants, a "marble spleen disease" can occur with extensive amyloid deposition on the spleen.[95] Whether the disorder is caused by a virus is uncertain.

EOSINOPHILS

On the basis of studies involving injection of tritiated thymidine and then quantitation of radioactivity in eosinophils, Bro-Rasmussen[96] concluded that little splenic eosinopoiesis occurred in the rat but that the spleen stored some eosinophils. The relationship (if any) of the spleen to maintaining eosinophilic heomeostasis is unknown. A triad of eosinophilia, splenomegaly, and cardiac disease has been reported.[97] The relationship to an eosinophilic leukemic process is uncertain. Eosinophilic leukemia may be associated with a palpable spleen, [98] but splenic function in this

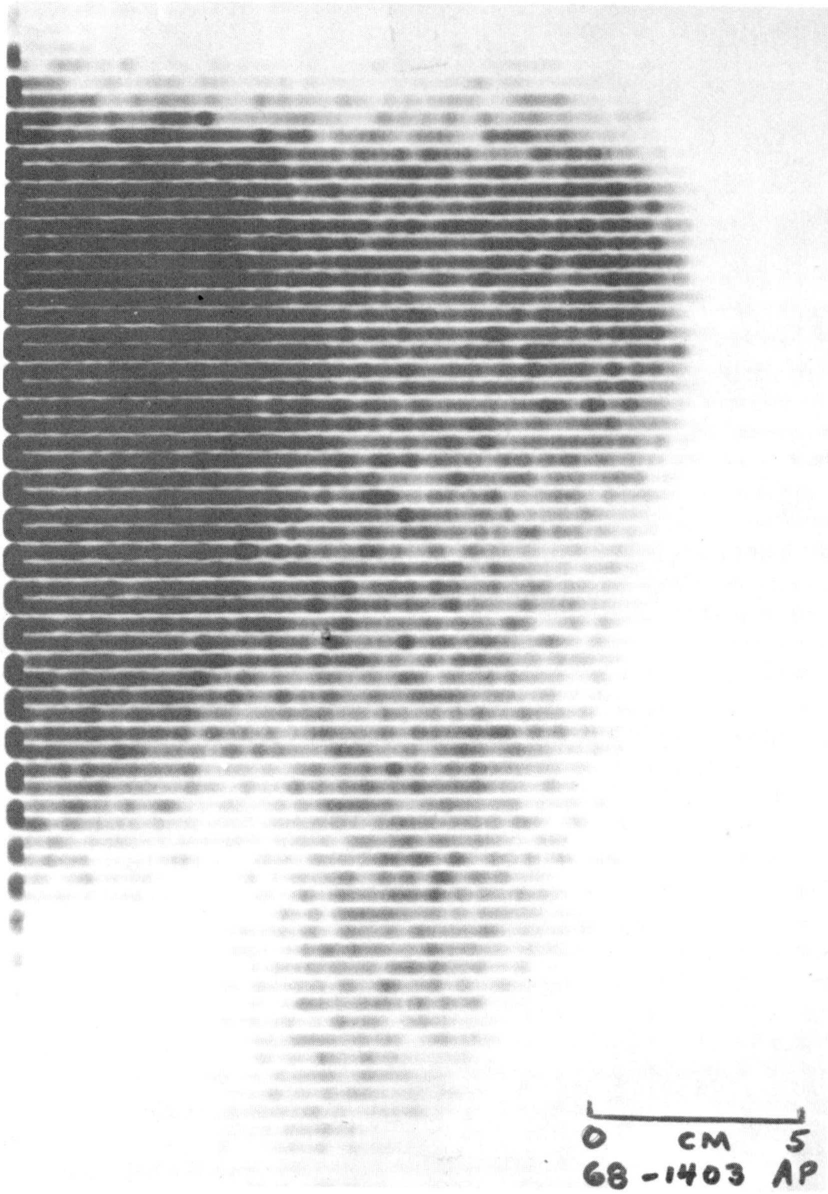

FIGURE 14. Anterior rectilinear scan (^{99m}Tc-sulfur colloid) in a 24-year-old woman with sarcoidosis. The patient had pancytopenia and probable hypersplenism. The spleen was massively enlarged, and there was pain over the organ. Case 68-1403.

disease has not been clearly defined by radioisotopic techniques.

Certain patients with severe rheumatoid arthritis have eosinophilia[99] (and splenic involvement in rheumatoid arthritis is discussed in another section). There has been speculation that Charcot-Leyden crystals in human tissues may arise from eosinophils, but the evidence is unclear.[100] It will be recalled that several syndromes characterized by histiocytosis, eosinophils, and giant cells are grouped under the heading of histiocytosis X. This grouping does not prove, however, that the disorders are of common pathogenesis. One of these conditions is designated eosinophilic granuloma. Localized eosinophil collections, as in eosinophilic granuloma in bone, are associated with apparently

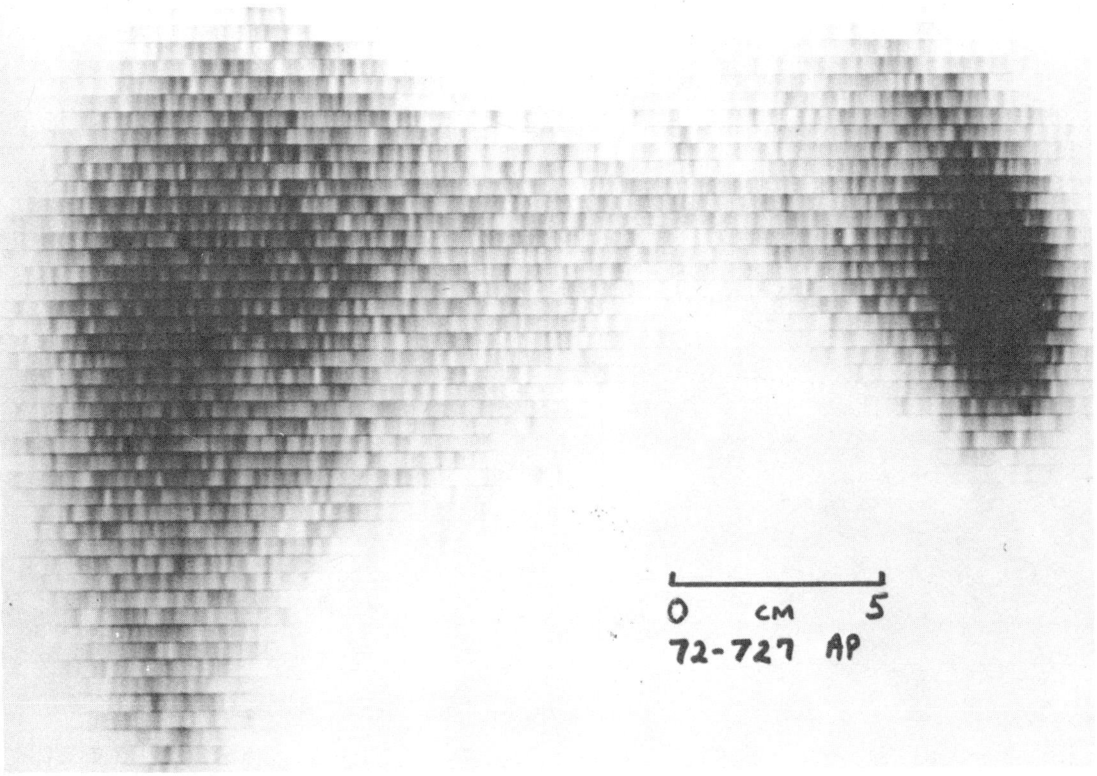

FIGURE 15. Anterior rectilinear scan (^{99m}Tc-sulfur colloid) in a 45-year-old woman. The patient, with severe pulmonary changes of sarcoidosis, does not have splenomegaly. Case 72-727.

normal splenic capacity to concentrate radiocolloid (Figure 17). Another of these disorders is Letterer-Siwe disease,[101] which often has associated splenomegaly (Figure 18). Letterer-Siwe disease with combined immunodeficiency has been described.[103,104] In Schuller-Christian disease, only 3 of 29 patients seen by Avery and her co-workers had splenomegaly.[101] We have also had the opportunity to study a 20-year-old woman with thrombocytosis and eosinophilia (case 72-2424). Both splenic size and function were apparently normal. The relationship of the eosinophilia of parasitic infestation to splenic function has not been studied. Eosinophilic fibrohistiocytic lesions of bone have been described,[102] but splenic function in the disorder has still to be elucidated.

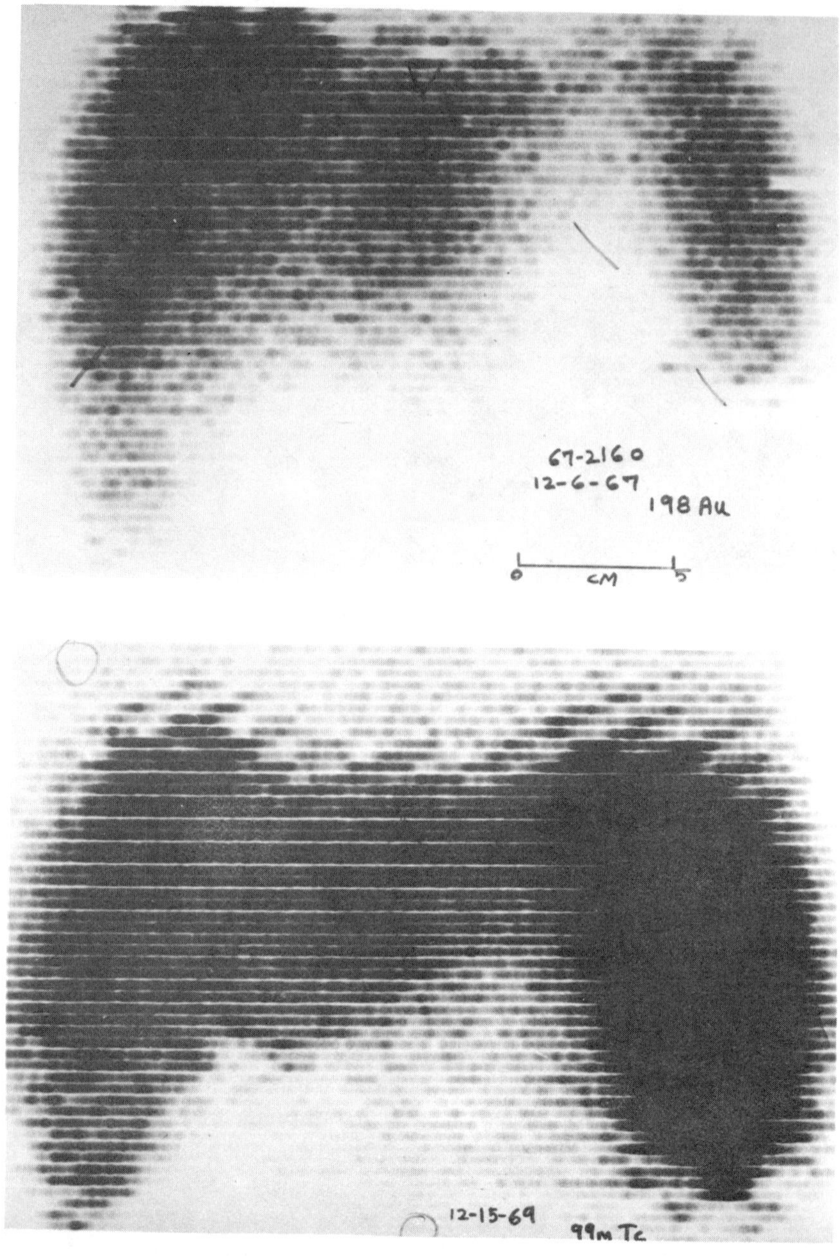

FIGURE 16. Anterior rectilinear scans (^{198}Au-colloid, top view; ^{99m}Tc-sulfur colloid, bottom view) taken 2 years apart. The patient is a 72-year-old man with probable multiple myeloma. There were plasma cells in the bone marrow and increased gamma globulins. Case 67-2160.

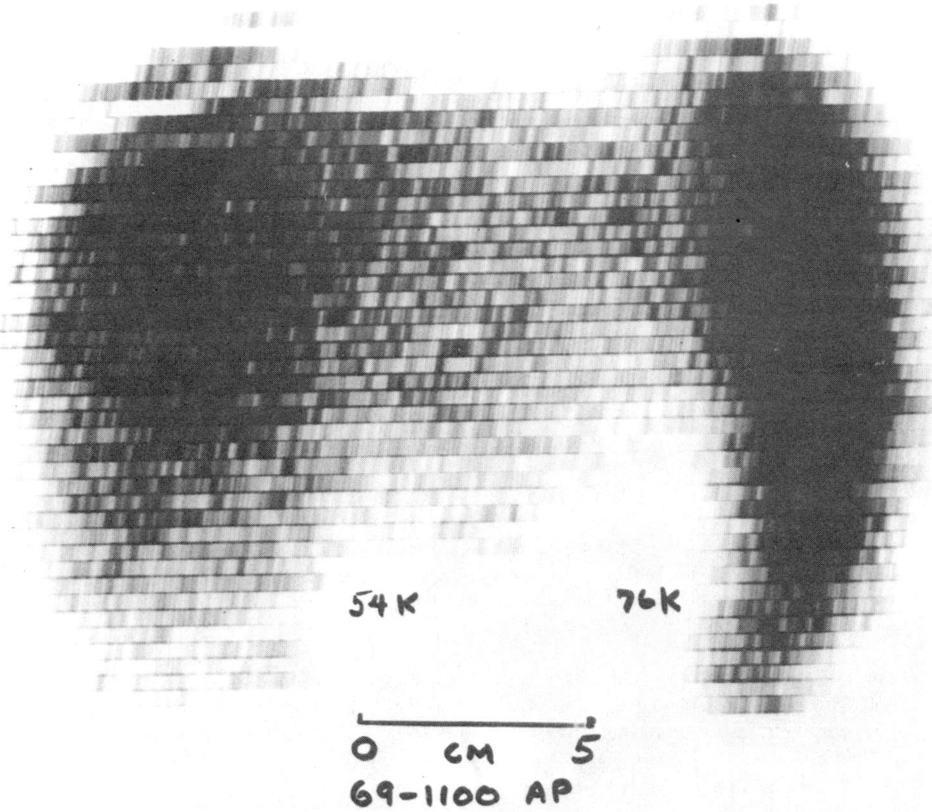

FIGURE 17. Anterior rectilinear scan (^{99m}Tc-sulfur colloid) in a 12-year-old girl with extensive bone damage in the region of the left ear due to eosinophilic granuloma. Splenomegaly and a slight shift of radiocolloid are apparent. Case 69-1100.

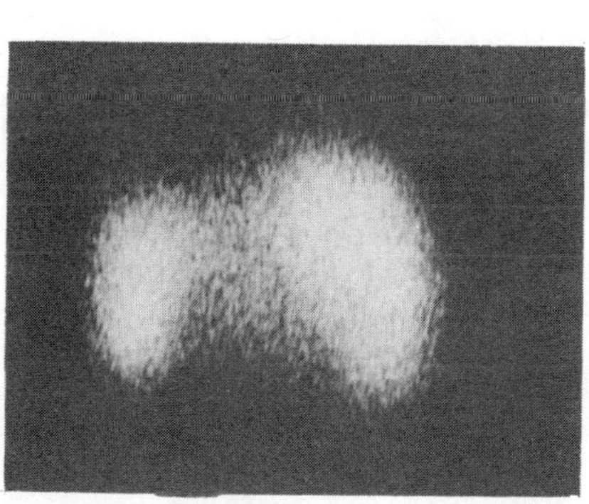

FIGURE 18. Posterior scintiphoto (^{99m}Tc-sulfur colloid) in an 8-month-old boy with Letterer-Siwe disease. The spleen is 6 cm in length, which is normal. Case 72-535.

REFERENCES

1. **Moss, W. T. and Brand, W. N.,** *Therapeutic Radiology,* 3rd ed., C. V. Mosby, St. Louis, 1969, 455.
2. **Strum, S. B. and Rappaport, H.,** Hodgkin's disease in the first decade of life, *Pediatrics,* 46, 748, 1970.
3. **Rosenthal, S. R.,** Significance of tissue lymphocytes in prognosis of lymphogranulomatosis, *Arch. Pathol.,* 21, 628, 1936.
4. **Jackson, H., Jr. and Parker, F., Jr.,** *Hodgkin's Disease and Allied Disorders,* Oxford University Press, New York, 1947, 117.
5. **Lukes, R. J.,** Relationship of histological features to clinical stages in Hodgkin's disease, *Am. J. Roentgenol.,* 90, 944, 1963.
6. **Kaplan, H. S.,** quoted by Rubin, P., Hodgkin's disease, *JAMA,* 190, 132, 1964.
7. **Ultmann, J. E.,** Clinical features and diagnosis of Hodgkin's disease, *Cancer,* 19, 297, 1966.
8. **Cohen, S. M., Weiner, M. J., Ratner, L. H., and Greenspan, E. M.,** Hodgkin's disease. Recent concepts in management, *N.Y. State J. Med.,* 72, 2189, 1972.
9. **Rappaport, H. and Strum, S. B.,** Vascular invasion in Hodgkin's disease: its incidence and relationship to the spread of disease, *Cancer,* 25, 1304, 1970.
10. **Carbone, P. E., Kaplan, H. S., Musshoff, K., Smithers, D. W., and Tubiana, M.,** Report of the committee on Hodgkin's disease staging classification, *Cancer Res.,* 31, 1860, 1971.
11. **Lipton, M. J., DeNardo, G. L., Silverman, S., and Glatstein, E.,** Evaluation of the liver and spleen in Hodgkin's disease. I. The value of hepatic scintigraphy, *Am. J. Med.,* 52, 356, 1972.
12. **Dibos, P. E., Judisch, J. M., Spaulding, M. B., Wagner, H. N., Jr., and McIntyre, P. A.,** Scanning the reticuloendothelial system (RES) in hematological diseases, *Johns Hopkins Med. J.,* 130, 68, 1972.
13. **Castellino, R. A., Silverman, J. F., Glatstein, E., Blank, N., and Wexler, L.,** Splenic arteriography in Hodgkin's disease. A roentgenologic-pathologic study of 33 consecutive untreated patients, *Am. J. Roentgenol.,* 114, 574, 1972.
14. **Silverman, S., DeNardo, G. D., Glatstein, E., and Lipton, M. J.,** Evaluation of the liver and spleen in Hodgkin's disease. II. The value of splenic scintigraphy, *Am. J. Med.,* 52, 362, 1972.
15. **Fischer, J. and Wolf, R.,** Resultats de l'application clinique de la scintigraphie de la rate dans 500 cas: possibilities et limites, *Medical Radioisotope Scanning. Vol. ii. Symposium Proceedings,* I.A.E.A., Vienna, 1964, 337.
16. **Wagner, S. C. and Verdon, T. A., Jr.,** Use of the liver-spleen scan in the clinical staging of patients with Hodgkin's disease, *J. Nucl. Med.,* 10, 450, 1969.
17. **Delarue, J. and Diebold, J.,** La rate dans la maladie de Hodgkin, *Virchows Arch. A,* 353, 27, 1971.
18. **Parmentier, C., Askienazy, S., Gerard-Marchant, R., Lacour, J., Amiel, J. L., Lemerle, J., and Tubiana, M.,** Confrontations entre les donnees de la scintigraphie splenique et les constatations anatomiques dans la maladie de Hodgkin, *Ann. Radiol.,* 12, 43, 1969.
19. **Juillard, G., Pierotti, T., Abbes, M., and Kermarec, J.,** Interet de la scintigraphie splenique dans la maladie de Hodgkin, *Presse Med.,* 77, 1241, 1969.
20. **Pettit, J. E., Wiliams, E. D., Glass, H. I., Lewis, S. M., Szur, L., and Wicks, C. J.,** Studies of splenic function in the myeloproliferative disorders and generalized malignant lymphomas, *Br. J. Hematol.,* 20, 575, 1971.
21. **Sharma, S. M., Ramanathan, P., and Canatra, R. D.,** Role of spleen scanning in planning the treatment and assessment of splenic response in blood dyscrasias, *Am. J. Roentgenol.,* 101, 656, 1967.
22. **Glatstein, E., Guernsey, J. M., Rosenberg, S. A., and Kaplan, H. S.,** The value of laparatomy and splenectomy in the staging of Hodgkin's disease, *Cancer,* 24, 709, 1969.
23. **Smithers, D. W.,** Spread of Hodgkin's disease, *Lancet,* 1, 1262, 1970.
24. **Nuland, S. B., Cornelius, E. A., and Spencer, R. P.,** Scan evidence of organ involution and improvement of hypersplenism in Hodgkin's disease following splenic artery ligation, *J. Nucl. Med.,* 11, 693, 1970.
25. **Kadin, M. E., Donaldson, S. S., and Dorfman, R. F.,** Isolated granulomas in Hodgkin's disease, *N. Engl. J. Med.,* 283, 859, 1970.
26. **Wilson, F. E., Preston, D. F., and Overholt, E. L.,** Detection of hepatic neoplasms, hepatic scanning combined with liver-function studies, *JAMA,* 209, 676, 1969.
27. **Sheagren, J. N., Black, J. B., and Wolff, S. M.,** Reticuloendothelial system phagocytic function in patients with Hodgkin's disease, *J. Clin. Invest.,* 46, 855, 1967.
28. **Abrahamsen, A. F.,** Effects of an enlarged splenic platelet pool in Hodgkin's disease, *Scand. J. Haematol.,* 9, 153, 1972.
29. **Ravry, M., Maldonado, N., Velez-Garcia, E., Montalvo, J., and Santiago, P. J.,** Serious infection after splenectomy for the staging of Hodgkin's disease, *Ann. Intern. Med.,* 77, 11, 1972.
30. **Kinns, A. M.,** Growth in the rat's brown fat of a Hodgkin's-like transplantable reticuloendothelial tumour, *Br. J. Exp. Pathol.,* 51, 411, 1970.
31. **Order, S. E., Porter, M., and Hellman, S.,** Hodgkin's disease: evidence for a tumor-associated antigen, *N. Engl. J. Med.,* 285, 471, 1971.
32. **Forbes, J. F. and Morris, P. J.,** Leucocyte antigens in Hodgkin's disease, *Lancet,* II, 849, 1970.
33. **Falk, J. and Osoba, D.,** HL-A antigens and survival in Hodgkin's disease, *Lancet,* II, 1118, 1971.

34. **Zervas, J. D., Delamore, I. W., and Israels, M. C. G.,** Leucocyte phenotypes in Hodgkin's disease, *Lancet,* II, 634, 1970.
35. **Vianna, N. J., Greenwald, P., and Davies, J. N. P.,** Nature of Hodgkin's disease agent, *Lancet,* I, 733, 1971.
36. **DeVita, V. T., Chabner, B. A., Livingston, D. M., and Oliverio, V. T.,** Anergy and tryptophan metabolism in Hodgkin's disease, *Am. J. Clin. Nutr.,* 24, 835, 1971.
37. **Young, R. C., Corder, M. P., Haynes, H. A., and DeVita, V. T.,** Delayed hypersensitivity in Hodgkin's disease: a study of 103 untreated patients, *Am. J. Med.,* 52, 63, 1972.
38. **Edwards, C. L. and Hayes, R. L.,** Tumor scanning with ^{67}Ga citrate, *J. Nucl. Med.,* 10, 103, 1969.
39. **Langhammer, H., Glaubitt, G., Grebe, S. F., Hampe, J. F., Haubold, U., Hor, G., Kaul, A., Koeppe, P., Koppenhagen, J., Roedler, H. D., and van der Schoot, J. B.,** ^{67}Ga for tumor scanning, *J. Nucl. Med.,* 13, 25, 1972.
40. **Edwards, C. L., Hayes, R. L., and Nelson, B.,** The "normal" ^{67}Ga scan, *J. Nucl. Med.,* 13, 428, 1972.
41. **Larson, S. M., Milder, M. S., Tretner, I. H., and Johnston, G. S.,** Interpretation of ^{67}Ga in lymphoma and leukemia, *J. Nucl. Med.,* 13, 448, 1972.
42. **Nelson, B., Hayes, R. L., Edwards, C. L., Kniseley, R. M., and Andrews, G. A.,** Distribution of ^{67}Ga in human tissues at autopsy, *J. Nucl. Med.,* 12, 452, 1971.
43. **Pinsky, S. M., Hoffer, P. B., Turner, D. A., Harper, P. V., and Gottschalk, A.,** Place of ^{67}Ga in the staging of Hodgkin's disease, *J. Nucl. Med.,* 12, 385, 1971.
44. **Milder, M. S., Larson, S. M., Bagley, C. M., deVita, V. T., and Johnston, G. S.,** The liver-spleen scan in Hodgkin's disease, *J. Nucl. Med.,* 13, 453, 1972.
45. **Skarin, A. T., Davey, F. R., and Moloney, W. C.,** Lymphosarcoma of the spleen, *Arch. Intern. Med.,* 127, 259, 1971.
46. **Gutterman, J. U., Rodriguez, V., and McClure, J. B.,** Staging of malignant lymphoma by laparotomy and splenectomy: review of the literature, *Milit. Med.,* 137, 251, 1972.
47. **Peters, M. V.,** The contribution of radiation therapy in the control of early lymphomas, *Am. J. Roentgenol.,* 90, 956, 1963.
48. **Desai, D. V., Ezdinli, E. Z., and Stutzman, L.,** Vincristine therapy of lymphomas and chronic lymphocytic leukemia, *Cancer,* 26, 352, 1970.
49. **Newall, J. and Friedman, M.,** Reticulum cell sarcoma. III. Prognosis, *Radiology,* 97, 99, 1970.
50. **Fuzy, M., Karika, S., and Tarjan, G.,** The importance of spleen scintigraphy in malignant lymphomas, *Neoplasma,* 16, 447, 1969.
51. **Nishimura, E. T., Ross, E., Leslie, G., Yang, H. Y., and Hokama, Y.,** Epizootic reticulum cell sarcoma in a sequestered colony of Japanese quails, *Cancer Res.,* 30, 2119, 1970.
52. Editorial, Lymphoid stimulation and lymphoid neoplasia, *Lancet,* II, 596, 1970.
53. **Herrera, N. E., Gonzalez, R., Schwartz, R. D., Diggs, A. M., and Belsky, J.,** ^{75}Se methionine as a diagnostic agent in malignant lymphoma, *J. Nucl. Med.,* 6, 792, 1965.
54. **Spencer, R. P., Montana, G., Scanlon, G. T., and Evans, O. R.,** Uptake of selenomethionine by mouse and human lymphomas with observations on selenite and selenate, *J. Nucl. Med.,* 8, 197, 1967.
55. **Chaudhuri, Ta.K., Chaudhuri, Tu.K., Suzuki, Y., Go, R. T., and Christie, J. H.,** Splenic accumulation of ^{87m}Sr in a patient with Hodgkin's disease, *Radiology,* 105, 617, 1972.
56. **Ashburn, W. L. and McDonald, D. G.,** Malignant lymphoma demonstrated with ^{75}Se-selenomethionine and selective intra-arterial injection of ^{131}I-macroaggregated human serum albumin, *J. Nucl. Med.,* 11, 92, 1970.
57. **Anezyris, N., Sawas-Dimopoulou, C., Dontas, N., and Samaras, V.,** Thoracic lymph node scintiscan as a diagnostic test in mediastinal malignant enlargement, *Chest,* 59, 372, 1971.
58. **Kay, D. N. and McCready, V. R.,** Clinical isotope scanning using ^{67}Ga citrate in the management of Hodgkin's disease, *Br. J. Radiol.,* 45, 437, 1972.
59. **Saarni, M. I. and Linman, J. W.,** Myelomonocytic leukemia: disorderly proliferation of all marrow lines, *Cancer,* 27, 1221, 1971.
60. **Galbraith, P. R., Chikkappa, G., and Abu-Zahra, H. T.,** Patterns of granulocyte kinetics in acute myelogenous and myelomonocytic leukemia, *Blood,* 36, 371, 1970.
61. **Vodopick, H., Rupp, E. M., Edwards, C. L., Goswitz, F. A., and Beauchamp, J. J.,** Spontaneous cyclic leukocytosis and thrombocytosis in chronic granuloyctic leukemia, *N. Engl. J. Med.,* 286, 284, 1972.
62. **Brodsky, J., Kahn, S. B., Vash, G., Ross, E. M., and Petkov, G.,** Fibrinogen survival with ^{75}Se selenomethionine during L-asparaginase therapy, *Br. J. Haematol.,* 20, 477, 1971.
63. **Chervenick, P. A., Ellis, L. D., Pan, S. F., and Lawson, A. L.,** Human leukemic cells: in vitro growth of colonies containing the Philadelphia (Ph) chromosome, *Science,* 174, 1134, 1971.
64. **Greenberg, P. L., Nichols, W. C., and Schrier, S. L.,** Granulopoiesis in acute myeloid leukemia and preleukemia, *N. Engl. J. Med.,* 284, 1225, 1971.
65. **Levine, P. H., Stevens, D. A., Coccia, P. F., Dabich, L., and Roland, A.,** Infectious mononucleosis prior to acute leukemia: a possible role for the Epstein-Barr virus, *Cancer,* 30, 875, 1972.
66. **Gerber, P. and Hoyer, B. H.,** Induction of cellular DNA synthesis in human leucocytes by Epstein-Barr virus, *Nature,* 231, 46, 1971.
67. **Lehane, D. E.,** A seroepidemiologic study of infectious mononucleosis – the development of EB virus antibody in a military population, *JAMA,* 212, 2240, 1970.

68. **Coeur, P., Revol, L., Viala, J. J., and Croizat, P.,** Consideration statistiques sur l'atteinte ou l'integrite des organes hematopoietieuqes (moelle, ganglions, rate et foie) au cours de la leucemie lymphoide chronique, *Sem. Hop. Paris,* 47, 2171, 1971.
69. **Goswitz, F. A. and Vodopick, H.,** Radiocolloid scans in chronic granulocytic leukemia, *J. Nucl. Med.,* 11, 630, 1970.
70. **Osgood, E. E.,** Treatment of chronic leukemias, *J. Nucl. Med.,* 5, 139, 1964.
71. **Osgood, E. E.,** The relative dosage required of total body X-ray vs. intravenous ^{32}P for equal effectiveness against leukemic cells of the lymphocytic series or granulocytic series in chronic leukemia, *J. Nucl. Med.,* 6, 421, 1965.
72. **Palmer, D. L., Rifkind, D., and Brown, D. W.,** ^{131}I-labeled colloidal human serum albumin in the study of reticuloendothelial system function. II. Phagocytosis and catabolism of a test colloid in normal subjects, *J. Infect. Dis.,* 123, 457, 1971.
73. **Palmer, D. L., Rifkind, D., and Brown, D. W.,** ^{131}I-labeled colloidal human serum albumin in the study of reticuloendothelial system function. III. Phagocytosis and catabolism compared in normal, leukemic and immunosuppressed human subjects, *J. Infect. Dis.,* 123, 465, 1971.
74. **Badrawi, H. S., Razzak, M. A., and Guirgis, B.,** Splenic trapping of heated-erythrocytes in leukemia and allied conditions, *J. Nucl. Med.,* 8, 379, 1967.
75. **Bowie, E. J. W., Kiely, J. M., Tauxe, W. N., and Stickney, J. M.,** The anemia of leukemia, *J. Nucl. Med.,* 3, 423, 1962.
76. **Young, H. B. and Mooney, R. A. H.,** Giant splenomegaly in sarcoidosis, *Br. J. Surg.,* 55, 554, 1968.
77. **Hirschorn, K., Schreibmann, R. R., Bach, F., and Siltzbach, L. E.,** In-vitro studies of lymphocytes from patients with sarcoidosis and lymphoproliferative diseases, *Lancet,* 2, 842, 1964.
78. **Schweiger, O.,** Biologic activity of circulating leukocytes in sarcoidosis. I. Influence of spleen extract of guinea pigs inoculated with leukocytes of patients with sarcoidosis on the respiration of leucocytes of patients with pulmonary sarcoidosis and other pulmonary diseases, *Am. Rev. Resp. Dis.,* 101, 600, 1970.
79. **Pagaltsos, A. S., Kumar, P. J., Willoughby, J. M. T., and Dawson, A. M.,** In-vitro inhibition of leucocyte migration by sarcoid spleen suspension in coeliac disease and dermatitis herpetiformis, *Lancet,* 2, 1179, 1971.
80. **Willoughby, J. M. T. and Mitchell, D. N.,** In-vitro inhibition of leukocyte migration in Crohn's disease by a sarcoid spleen suspension, *Br. Med. J.,* 3, 155, 1971.
81. **Papamichail, M., Holborow, E. J., Keith, H. I., and Currey, H. L. F.,** Subpopulations of human peripheral blood lymphocytes distinguished by combined rosette formation and membrane immunofluorescence, *Lancet,* 2, 64, 1972.
82. **Sumiyoshi, A., Sannoe, Y., and Tanaka, K.,** Rhabdomyo sarcoma of the esophagus – a case report with sarcoid-like lesions in its draining lymph nodes and the spleen, *Acta Pathol. Jap.,* 22, 581, 1972.
83. **Dickerman, J. D., Holbrook, P. R., and Zinkham, W. H.,** Etiology and therapy of thrombocytopenia associated with sarcoidosis, *J. Pediatr.,* 81, 758, 1972.
84. **Young, R. L., Harleroad, L. E., Lordon, R. E., and Weg, J. G.,** Pulmonary sarcoidosis: a prospective evaluation of glucocorticoid therapy, *Ann. Intern. Med.,* 73, 207, 1970.
85. **Burt, R. W. and Kuhl, D. E.,** Giant splenomegaly in sarcoidosis demonstrated by radionuclide scintiphotography, *JAMA,* 215, 2110, 1971.
86. **Spencer, R. P., Pearson, H. A., and Binder, H. A.,** Identification of cases of "acquired" functional asplenia, *J. Nucl. Med.,* 11, 763, 1970.
87. **Jakob, W.,** Spontaneous amyloidosis of mammals, *Vet. Pathol.,* 8, 292, 1971.
88. **Cohen, A. S. and Shirahama, T.,** Animal model for human disease: spontaneous and induced amyloidosis, *Am. J. Pathol.,* 68, 441, 1972.
89. **Zuckerberg, A., Gazith, J., Rimon, A., Reshef, T., and Gafni, J.,** The structural subunit of amyloid; isolation and characterization of polypeptide capable of fibril formation, *Eur. J. Biochem.,* 28, 161, 1972.
90. **Black, M. M.,** The nature, pathogenesis and staining properties of amyloid, *Br. J. Dermatol.,* 87, 280, 1972.
91. **Hermodson, M. A., Kuhn, R. W., Walsh, K. A., Neurath, H., Eriksen, N., and Benditt, E. P.,** Amino acid sequence of monkey amyloid protein A, *Biochemistry,* 11, 2934, 1972.
92. **Levy, M., Fryd, C. H., and Eliakim, M.,** Intrahepatic obstructive jaundice due to amyloidosis of the liver, *Gastroenterology,* 61, 234, 1971.
93. **Dreher, R.,** Experimentelle Amyloidose bei splenktomierten Mausen, *Z. Immunitaetsforsch. Allerg. Klin. Immunol.,* 140, 1, 1970.
94. **Cathcart, E. S., Rodgers, O. G., and Cohen, A. S.,** Amyloid-inducing factor and immunological unresponsiveness, *Ann. Rheum, Dis.,* 31, 303, 1972.
95. **Wyand, D. S., Jakowski, R. M., and Burke, C. N.,** Marble spleen disease in ring necked pheasants: histology and ultrastructure, *Avian Dis.,* 16, 319, 1972.
96. **Bro-Rasmussen, F.,** Eosinopoiesis in the spleen of normal rats, *Scand. J. Haematol.,* 9, 8, 1972.
97. **Shepherd, A. J. N., Walsh, C. H., Archer, R. K., and Wetherly-Mein, G.,** Eosinophilia, aplenomegaly and cardiac disease, *Br. J. Haematol.,* 20, 233, 1971.
98. **Flannery, E. P., Dillan, D. E., Freeman, M. V. R., Levy, J. D., D'Ambrosio, V., and Bedynek, J. L.,** Eosinophilic leukemia with fibrosing endocarditis and short Y chromosome, *Ann. Intern. Med.,* 77, 223, 1972.

99. **Winchester, R. J., Litwin, S. D., Koffler, D., and Kunkel, H. G.,** Observations on the eosinophilia of certain patients with rheumatoid arthritis, *Arch. Rheum.*, 14, 650, 1971.

100. **Smith, H. and Forbes, I. M.,** Charcot-Leyden crystals in human bone marrow, *Pathology,* 4, 279, 1972.

101. **Avery, M. E., McAfee, J. G., and Guild, H. G.,** The course and prognosis of reticuloendotheliosis (eosinophilic granuloma, Schuller-Christian disease and Letterer-Siwe disease), *Am. J. Med.*, 22, 636, 1957.

102. **Rywlin, A. M., Hoffman, E. P., and Orteya, R. S.,** Eosinophilic fibrohistiocytic lesion of bone marrow: a distincitve new morphologic finding, probably related to drug hypersensitivity, *Blood*, 40, 464, 1972.

103. **Cederbaum, S. D., Niwayama, G., Stiehm, E. R., Neehout, R. C., Ammann, A. J., and Berman, W., Jr.,** Combined immunodeficiency presenting as the Letterer-Siwe syndrome, *J. Pediatr.*, 85, 466, 1974.

104. **Ochs, H. D., Davis, S. D., Mickelson, E., Lerner, K. G., and Wedgwood, R. J.,** Combined immunodeficiency and reticuloendotheliosis with eosinophilia, *J. Pediatr.*, 85, 463, 1974.

Chapter 12

CYSTS, ABSCESSES, METASTATIC DISEASE, INFARCTS, AND TRAUMA

SPACE-OCCUPYING LESIONS

There are multiple causes of splenic filling defects on radiocolloid scans. The commonest of these can be briefly outlined as follows.

Extrinsic Causes

1. Pancreatic cysts.
2. Space-occupying lesions extending from other neighboring organs or tumors.

Intrinsic Causes

1. Vascular occlusion (infarct).
2. Trauma (hematoma, rupture).
3. Tumors.
4. Abscesses or inflammation, granulomas.
5. Cysts (true, other, parasitic).

It must be pointed out that any process that displaces reticuloendothelial cells will create a "void" on a radiocolloid scan. The findings are thus not pathognomonic. It is crucial to obtain as much ancillary information as possible in order to arrive at a correct diagnosis. Thus, careful history taking and a physical examination are in order. The finding of hemoglobinopathy, specifically one involving hemoglobin S, may suggest vascular occlusion and splenic infarction.

CYSTS

Extrinsic lesions can involve the spleen. Warshaw and associates[1] described four patients with pancreatic pseudocysts which ruptured into the substance of the spleen. In these cases, ^{99m}Tc-sulfur colloid scans revealed compression of the splenic pulp and some displacement of the organ.

Some years ago we had the opportunity to perform a spleen scan (with ^{197}Hg-mercurihydroxypropane) on a 59-year-old woman with a left upper quadrant mass. The scan revealed a small region below the costal margin to be functional in terms of ability to accumulate erythrocytes tagged with the mercury-labeled compound. The area above the costal margin was nonfunctional (case 66-481). At operation, the major portion of the left upper quadrant mass was found to be a cystic metastasis, which had indented the upper portion of the spleen and displaced the spleen downward. Such extrinsic causes of splenic derangement are unusual and rarely diagnosed preoperatively.

Splenic cysts are uncommon. Davis and coworkers[2] have reviewed the literature and referred to the classification first put forth by Martin.[3] This classification lists cysts as primary if they have a cellular lining (parasitic and two types of nonparasitic: congenital and neoplastic). Secondary or false cysts are considered to be those without cellular lining (and these are the most frequent). Angiography appears to be a useful tool for delineating splenic cysts, and two recent discussions have appeared.[4,5] The other contribution that may be made by the radiograph is the demonstration of calcification around the wall of the cyst (particularly common in parasitic cysts and in those that appear to follow resolution of a hematoma within the spleen). Although there is at least one report of the puncture of a splenic cyst and introduction of contrast media,[6] such a procedure (either by the percutaneous route or under operative control) appears too hazardous for routine use.

The combination of radionuclide scanning and radiographic contrast tomography has been reported of value in evaluating splenic masses.[12] Wright and Williams[76] have noted the value of radiographs (displaced organs), scans, and ultrasound in establishing the diagnosis of a post-traumatic splenic cyst. Spleen scanning has been used in establishing the diagnosis of intrasplenic defects (and cysts, of course, fit into this class).[7] On the basis of the scan alone, it may be impossible to determine the nature of the intrasplenic defect. Two reports on scintiscanning of splenic cysts[7,8] noted a small functional mass with a large nonfunctional area representing the cyst (which is devoid of reticuloendothelial cells). We have seen two cases showing related findings (Figures 1 and 2).

We have also seen two children with a finding

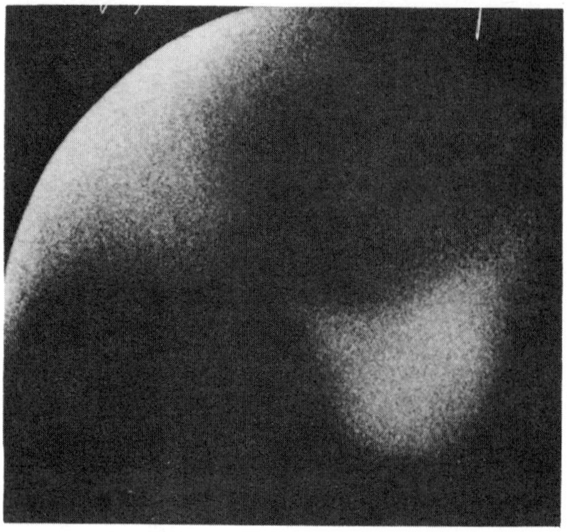

FIGURE 1. Anterior scintiphoto of the spleen and portion of the liver (^{99m}Tc-sulfur colloid). The patient, a 14-year-old girl, was studied because of left upper quadrant pain. At operation, the large, rounded defect was noted to correspond to a splenic cyst. Splenectomy was performed. On microscopic examination, the cyst had an epithelial lining. Case 73-1557.

that now suggests to us an expanding intrasplenic mass (and hence possibly a cyst).[9] The finding is what we have referred to as "the binary spleen." Figure 3 depicts possible stages in the development of this situation. As the intrasplenic mass enlarges, remaining functional splenic tissue is separated, creating the scan appearance of two distinct splenic masses removed from each other. In both of these cases, the cysts were secondary, ("false" or "pseudo") since they did not contain an epithelial lining. It is clear that we have no solid information as to the etiology or temporal development of nonparasitic or nontraumatic splenic cysts. In some cases they may contain large trabeculae,[72] which resemble chorda tendinae, and are probably below the limits of resolution of scanning techniques. We have no personal experience with hydatid cysts of the spleen; these have been reported to reach enormous size.[10,11]

ABSCESS

Splenic abscess is an unusual occurrence. In a series of (general) autopsies quoted by Reid and Lang,[13] the incidence was 0.4%. Pickleman and co-workers[14] reviewed much of the pertinent literature. They stated that infection in the spleen resulted from:

1. Hematogenous spread from a focus of infection (one case has been reported to follow prostatic biopsy).[15]
2. Direct spread (intraabdominal process).
3. Trauma, with a hematoma of the spleen that becomes infected.

Pickleman and co-workers[14] further state that if untreated, the disorder is uniformly fatal and that wide use of antibiotics has masked symptoms, in some cases, until rupture of the spleen occurs. Splenectomy is essential if there is not widespread sepsis. Useful diagnostic tools are chest x-rays (left hemidiaphragm elevated, pneumonitis of the left base), abdominal x-rays (displacement of gastric or colonic shadows), and radionuclide spleen scans. Drainage of splenic abscesses has not been very successful,[16] and total splenectomy may offer better hope of cure. Sometimes the focus of the infection that led to splenic abscess formation is not apparent. Splenic and hepatic abscesses can occur simultaneously.[17]

Splenic abscesses displace functional reticuloendothelial cells in the spleen and therefore appear as nonfunctional defects on radiocolloid scans. In addition to the scan of a splenic abscess reported by Pickleman and co-workers[14] (using ^{99m}Tc-sulfur colloid), an earlier report (employing heat-denatured ^{51}Cr-erythrocytes) also pictured such an abscess.[8] LePage and associates noted a splenic abscess on a scan[18] and correlated this with the splenic arteriogram. Zook and co-workers[15] also documented two cases with scans. In one case we have studied, the splenic abscesses were well seen on scan.

A number of workers have studied the experimental basis for localizing abscesses by means of radiolabeled antibodies[19] (against bacteria) or leukocytes.[20] What role these techniques will have in outlining splenic abscesses is uncertain. Although ^{67}Ga has some affinity for abscesses, its role in outlining splenic lesions has still to be defined.

The relationship of splenic infarcts to infection in the organ is likely a complex one.

1. Certain splenic infarcts may be caused by infected emboli. Buchbinder and Roberts[21] reported that 33% of 45 necropsies of patients with left-sided infective endocarditis revealed splenomegaly. We have had the opportunity to perform a spleen scan on a 35-year-old man who

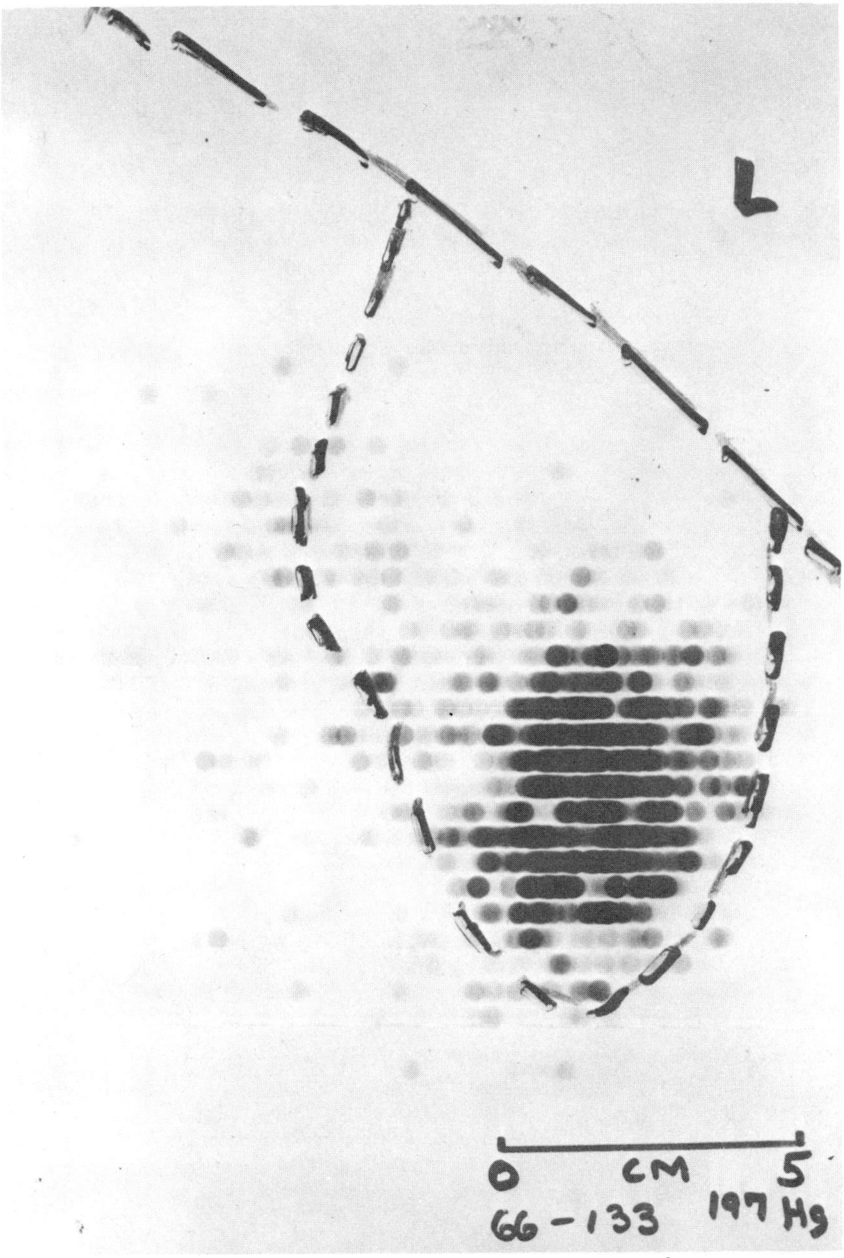

FIGURE 2. Anterior rectilinear scan (performed with ^{197}Hg-mercurihydroxypropane) in a 23-year-old woman. The patient presented with a left upper quadrant mass. An arteriogram revealed a large avascular area of the spleen. The scan shows that only the lower pole of the spleen has functional reticuloendothelial cells. At splenectomy, a 1,400-g organ was removed. It contained a serous fluid-filled cyst. The cyst was lined by a single layer of endothelium. It might have represented a malformation of an intravascular channel (perhaps lymphatic). Case 66-133.

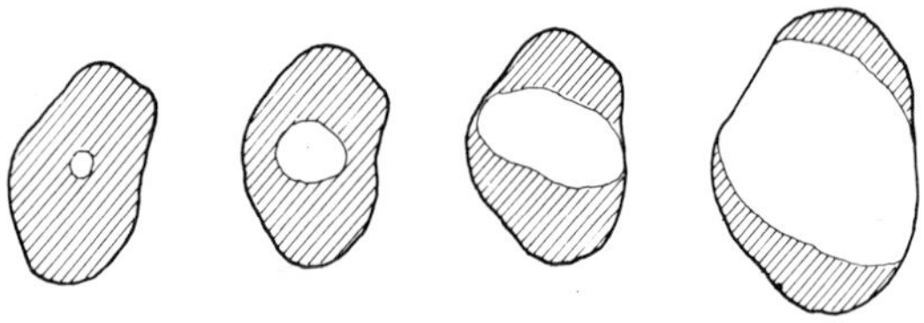

FIGURE 3. Possible stages in the development of the "binary spleen." In essence, an expanding intrasplenic mass forces functional tissue toward the poles (or destroys all function not at the extreme poles of the spleen). The increased intrasplenic tension may also contribute to compromising the remaining function.

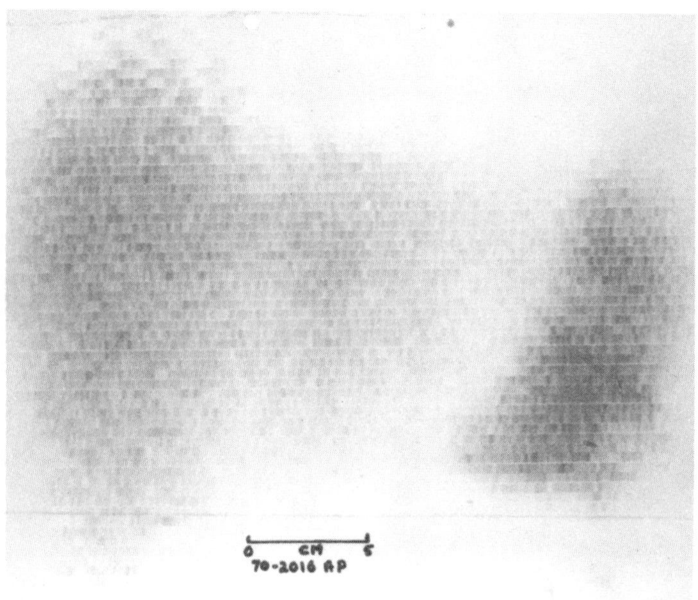

FIGURE 4. Anterior rectilinear scan (^{99m}Tc-sulfur colloid) in a 35-year-old man who had replacement of the aortic and mitral valves and bacterial endocarditis. Although the scan is technically suboptimal, splenomegaly, shift of radiocolloid to the spleen, and multiple splenic defects can be seen. This was confirmed on several views obtained under a gamma ray camera. Case 70-2016.

had aortic and mitral valve replacements and bacterial endocarditis (Figure 4). Multiple splenic defects were seen on the scan. A 59-year-old woman with massive necrotizing pneumonia, splenic infarcts, and pneumococcal foci in the spleen has also been seen in this hospital. The literature also contains reports of splenic arterio-venous fistulae (bruit) and endocarditis.[22]

2. Some diseases, associated with splenic infarction, also have a high incidence of infections. The classical example is sickle cell disease, where the likelihood of pneumococcal meningitis may be increased 600 times above normal. The reasons for the propensity to these types of infection are likely multiple and may result from functional asplenia, diminished splenic production of tuftsin and other opsonins, reduced properdin, and decreased ability to react to foreign antibodies.

3. Cockshott and Weaver[23] have discussed an interesting variant termed "primary tropical splenic abscess." They have related this to splenic infarction, liberation of oxygen by erythrocytes, and production of carbon dioxide within the spleen.

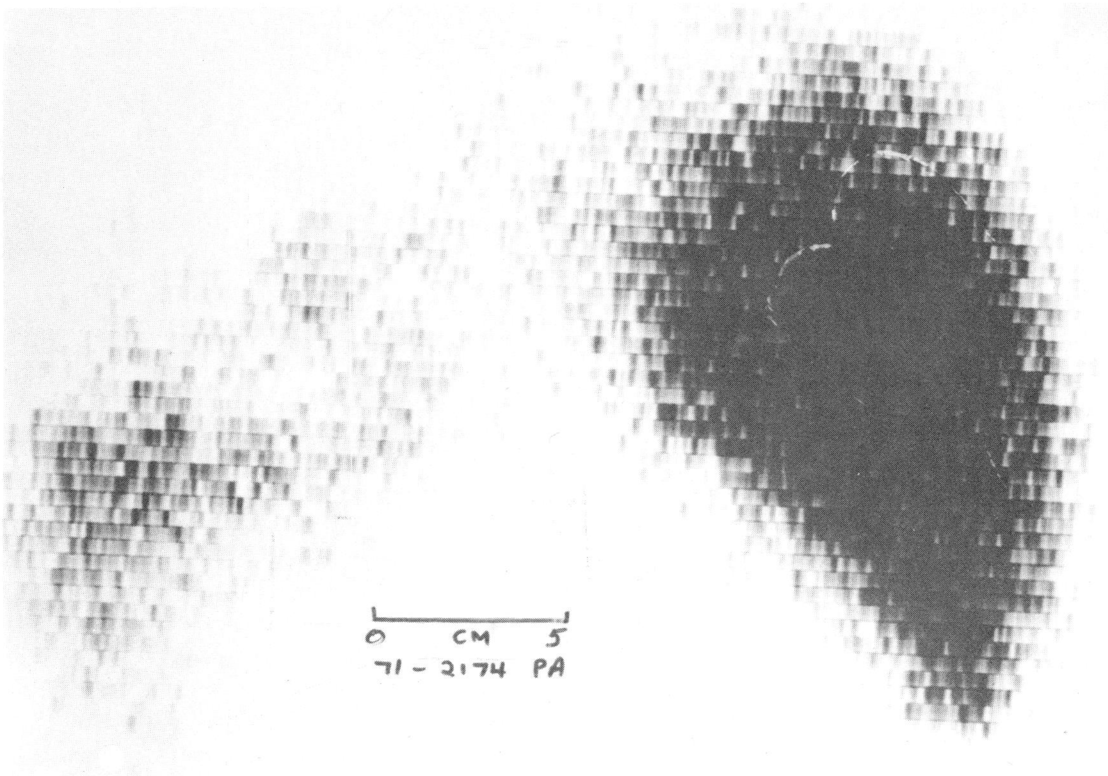

FIGURE 5. ^{99m}Tc-sulfur colloid scan of the spleen. This posterior view was obtained on a 21-year-old man with left upper quadrant pain. At laparotomy, an anaplastic tumor was observed to be infiltrating the spleen and surrounding tissues. Case 71-2174.

The spleen is frequently enlarged in the course of infectious diseases. In some cases this might represent direct invasion of the organ. In others, however, the spleen may be acting as a filter or as an organ for producing immunoreactive substances, with reticuloendothelial hyperplasia. Injecting killed *Bordetella pertussis* into mice, for example, results in an increase in splenic weight, casued by an increased number of cells. The response, however, is lost in aged mice.[24] Katsura and associates[25] noted that certain splenic reticulum cells were increased in the course of bacterial diseases.

Whether the spleen plays a role in processing leukocyte inclusions (by analogy to the removal of erythrocytic inclusions) is unknown. Circulating white blood cells can show "toxic granulations" or Dohle bodies in the course of bacterial disorders.[26] However, this finding also apparently occurs in the course of therapy with cyclophosphamide[27] and in pregnancy.[28] Whether or not it is related to splenic dysfunction is presently unknown.

METASTATIC DISEASE IN THE SPLEEN

While perhaps half of all patients with malignant disease eventually show metastases to the liver, involvement of the spleen has been noted to occur in only 2 to 4% of cases in compilations on the location of tumor metastases (Gould and co-workers[29] have summarized much of the literature). Although an isolated splenic metastasis can occur without metastases elsewhere, it is quite rare. Also unusual is the finding of a splenic metastasis as the first indication of a malignancy (Figure 5). Statistically, metastases in the spleen are most frequently related to the malignant lymphomas, especially Hogkin's disease and reticulum cell sarcoma; perhaps these can be considered as independent foci of the disease. The lymphomas are discussed in Chapter 11. In the staging of the lymphomas, the spleen is considered equivalent to a subdiaphragmatic lymph node. When grossly positive, a spleen scan may be of value in staging Hodgkin's disease. However, the overall value of the spleen scan in this disease is still open to question[30] since a number of centers perform splenectomy for diagnostic purposes.

There is one metastatic tumor which frequently involves the spleen. This is the malignant melanoma. In perhaps one half of the cases of disseminated melanoma, splenic metastases can be found.[29] A splenotropic tumor (reticulum cell sarcoma) has been reported in mice,[31] but the only other known tumor (aside from melanoma) with a tendency to frequently spread to the spleen in humans is the chorionepithelioma.[32] Splenomegaly, in the course of tumor spread, does not necessarily mean that the spleen is involved by metastases. In man, blockade of the liver by tumor may cause portal hypertension and resultant splenomegaly. In animals, splenomegaly can occur where transplanted tumors are present elesewhere. Kerr has commented as to possible mechanisms.[33,34]

An intrasplenic defect, on a radiocolloid scan, is certainly not pathognomonic of metastasis. However, an irregular ("nodular") appearance to the lesion, the presence of splenomegaly, the occurence of hepatic defects, and the past history are all suggestive clues. Gould and co-workers[29] have discussed the use of angiography and spleen scans in establishing the diagnosis. In some instances, the distinction between primary and metastatic tumor in the spleen is difficult if not impossible to make preoperatively. For example, hemangioma of the spleen can occur (perhaps the most frequent benign tumor of the organ). Coincident hemangiomas may be present in the liver, bone, or elsewhere.[35]

Tumor spread to the spleen was stated by Strauli[36] to occur through the bloodstream. He stated that afferent lymphatic spread of tumor to the spleen could not be confirmed by demonstration of corresponding lymphatic pathways. Bengmark and associates[37] have noted that in abdominal cancers, lymph nodes may be involved up to, and including, the hilus of the spleen. Whether to perform splenectomy in such cases (when removing the primary tumor) is still uncertain.

Watanabe and Tanaka[32] reported an interesting study of the incidence of splenic metastases. In 595 autopsies of patients with carcinoma, but without treatment with carcinostatic agents, splenic metastases were found in 4.9%. However, in 247 cases in which carcinostatic therapy had been used, splenic metastases were present in 9.3%. It is known that "resistance" is lowered by carcinostatics, but how this is related to the higher involvement of the spleen is unknown. The types of splenic metastasis were summarized as follows:

Microscopic	42.3%
Solitary or multiple nodular	55.8%
Almost complete replacement of spleen	1.9%

Another interesting figure to come out of this study was that when the spleen was involved by metastases, the number of other organs affected was twice as great as in cases without splenic metastases.

Plain films of the abdomen and splenic scans likely will not establish the etiology of a splenic defect. Pellerin and Bertin[38] believe that (in children) arteriography is capable of determining the benign or malignant nature of a splenic tumor. Morgan and Johnson[12] have described contrast infusion tomography for obtaining additional information on splenic masses.

Information on the growth of intrasplenic tumors is quite sparse. Fidler[39] labeled B 16 melanoma cells, grown in tissue culture, with ^{125}I-5-iodo-2′-deoxyuridine. After injection into C57BL/6 mice, animals were sacrificed at various time intervals; the assumption was that radiolabel was released from the cells only at the time of their death. Following injection of 200,000 labeled cells, the spleen contained a maximum of only 0.44 of 1% of the cells. The peak occurred at 4 hr, and the number of cells then declined (none were left at 14 days).

SPLENIC INFARCTS

The incidence of splenic infarction is unknown since the disorder appears to be rarely substantiated during life by objective criteria. It is here that spleen scanning may have a real contribution to make. Despite isolated case reports, there have been no systematic studies of the production and repair of splenic infarcts.

The reason for the occurrence of splenic infarcts is likely related to the peculiarities of the circulation with the organ. In sickle cell disease, during reduced oxygen tension, any organ may be subjected to vascular occlusion and infarction. However, the spleen appears to be particularly involved in many cases. This is probably the result

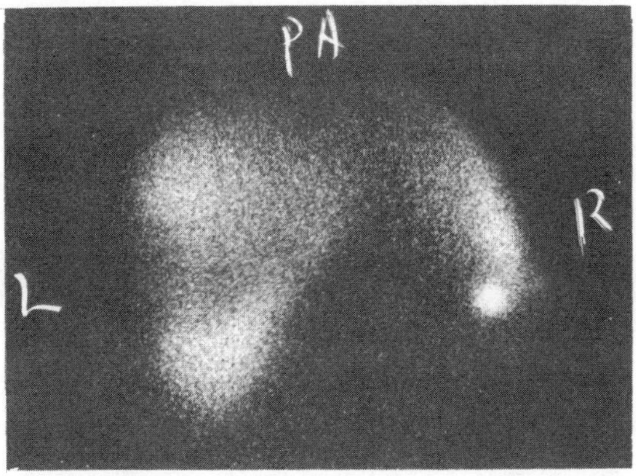

FIGURE 6. Posterior scintiphoto (^{99m}Tc-sulfur colloid) of a 26-year-old man who had the sudden onset of left upper quadrant pain while climbing at an altitude of 2,500 ft. The patient was shown to have sickle cell trait. The scan revealed a large intrasplenic defect, most likely an infarct. This was unchanged 9 days later but completely healed within 4 months. Additional data on this case have been published. Case 71-1678.

of vascular blockade by sickled cells, border line anoxia, and then tissue destruction when the oxygen tension falls further. At sea level, the pressure of air is 760 mm Hg. The oxygen tension is 94 mm Hg. At 10,000 feet above sea level, the pressure of air is 523 mm Hg, and the oxygen tension has fallen to 53 mm Hg. Because of the dangers of reduced oxygen tension, it has been recommended that individuals with sickle cell anemia and sickle cell hemoglobin C should not fly.[40] While usually true that sickle cell trait is benign, as compared with homozygous sickle cell disease, we have, however, seen a young man with sickle cell trait who suffered splenic infarction after climbing at an altitude of 2,500 ft[41] (another view of this is shown in Figure 6).

In dogs and man, massive infarction does not occur following splenic artery occlusion. We have reported a case in which ligation of the splenic artery, necessitated by inability to remove the spleen in case of Hodgkin's disease with hypersplenism, resulted in a decrease in the size of the spleen and temporary cure of hypersplenism.[42] Our experience has been extended to three patients. In each case, ligation of the splenic artery resulted in a decrease in the size of the spleen, with only small infarction. Perhaps this is related to the rich collateral blood supply of the spleen via the gastric vessels and occasionally the mesenteric artery.

There can be multiple factors contributing to splenic infarction.

I. Septic causes. Endocarditis and endarteritis can produce septic emboli (these were also discussed in the section on splenic abscess). Splenic infarcts may be followed by abscesses in some cases.[23]

II. Nonseptic causes:

a. Associated with increased coagulability or thrombus formation (such as polycythemia vera).

b. Emboli, such as those coming from atrial fibrillation and mural thrombi.

c. Vascular blockade, such as sickle cell disease (exaggerated by hypoxia).

d. Uncertain mechanisms, possibly due to vasculitis, as in leukemias, myeloproliferative diseases.

It is of note that use of scans in diagnosing splenic infarcts has received relatively little attention in the literature. We have summarized some of the pertinent reports in Table 1. Perhaps in no other disorder does spleen scanning have more to offer as an initial procedure. That is, the patient with a splenic infarct, perhaps troubled by a bacterial infection or hypoxia, may not be able to stand involved diagnostic studies. Despite occasional limitations of scanning for infarcts,[43] a spleen scan should be one of the initial procedures carried out when an infarct is suspected. There are a number of notes of caution.

1. Small infarcts (or perhaps vascular occlusions) may not show on the scan, and hence a negative scan does not rule out the disorder.

2. Care must be observed that anatomic variants are not mistaken for splenic filling defects (Figure 7).

3. A filling defect on a spleen scan does not carry with it absolute assurance as to the nature of its cause. That is, intrasplenic bleeds and other processes will resemble infarcts on the scan. Relevant additional data, such as the presence of hemoglobinopathies, are essential.

The time course of splenic infarcts has not been well defined. In the case reported by Vagenakis and co-workers,[44] a large infarct was undetectable by scan about 6 months later. We can contribute brief information on two cases. In the first, a

TABLE 1

A Summary of Some Literature Data on Spleen Scans in Splenic Infarction

Scanning agent used	Comment	Ref.
^{51}Cr-denatured erythrocytes	Fever, tenderness, and probable septic splenic embolus in a male with aortic valvular disease and Klebsiella-Aerobacter infection. A second case involved a man with an aortic prosthesis and infection. Scans showed a splenic defect in each case.	45
^{203}Hg bromomercuri hydroxypropane	A 39-year-old man had tachycardia, fever, a cardiac murmur, anemia, and decreased breath sounds on the left. The scan revealed a band of nearly absent activity across the lower third of the spleen. At autopsy, the patient was noted to have left-sided bacterial endocarditis. The second case was an 18-year-old male with splenomegaly and probable sickle cell thalassemia (hemoglobin S present, with 8.8% hemoglobin F). The ^{51}Cr-erythrocyte survival T1/2 was 14 days (shortened). Splenomegaly, fever, and left upper quadrant pain resulted in splenectomy. Defects on the scan were shown to correspond to infarcts of the spleen.	46
^{99m}Tc-sulfur colloid	A 47-year-old woman with a positive blood culture (Gram-negative rod) developed left upper quadrant pain. The spleen was enlarged with a defect on scan. The scan had returned to normal 6 months later.	44
^{198}Au-colloid	Two cases of splenic infarction, in chronic granulocytic leukemia, were diagnosed by decreased uptake in localized areas on the spleen scan (we must be concerned, however, that leukemic infiltrates and hemorrhage may also occur in the spleen in this disorder).	47

26-year-old man with sickle cell trait (Figure 6), the large splenic infarct was essentially unchanged 9 days later but had cleared by 4 months. The second case involved a 52-year-old woman with mitral valve prosthesis who developed left upper quadrant pain. A clearly demonstrable splenic infarct was reduced in size on the 5th subsequent day and undetectable on the 17th day. A third case was also rather interesting since it raised questions as to possible volume changes occurring in the spleen after part of the organ has been infarcted. A 37-year-old woman with chronic myelogenous leukemia had massive splenomegaly. Radiation therapy was begun. The patient experienced an episode of severe left upper quadrant pain. The spleen scan was repeated. Superimposition of the two scans (Figure 8) revealed a large loss of volume.

In sickle cell disease, after multiple infarcts, the spleen tends to be small and may completely lose the ability to accumulate ^{99m}Tc-sulfur colloid. In sickle thalassemia the spleen may suffer multiple infarcts and yet still retain considerable size and reticuloendothelial function (Figure 9).

It should be apparent that, despite its potential value, radioisotopic scanning has not been widely used in the diagnosis of splenic infarction. If the diagnosis is considered, then spleen scans should be called upon as an important diagnostic aid.

SPLENIC INJURY AND RUPTURE

Trauma to the spleen can occur in a number of ways. Shirkey and co-workers,[48] in a study of 189 cases of injury to the spleen, noted that 125 of the patients (66%) had penetrating injuries (stab,

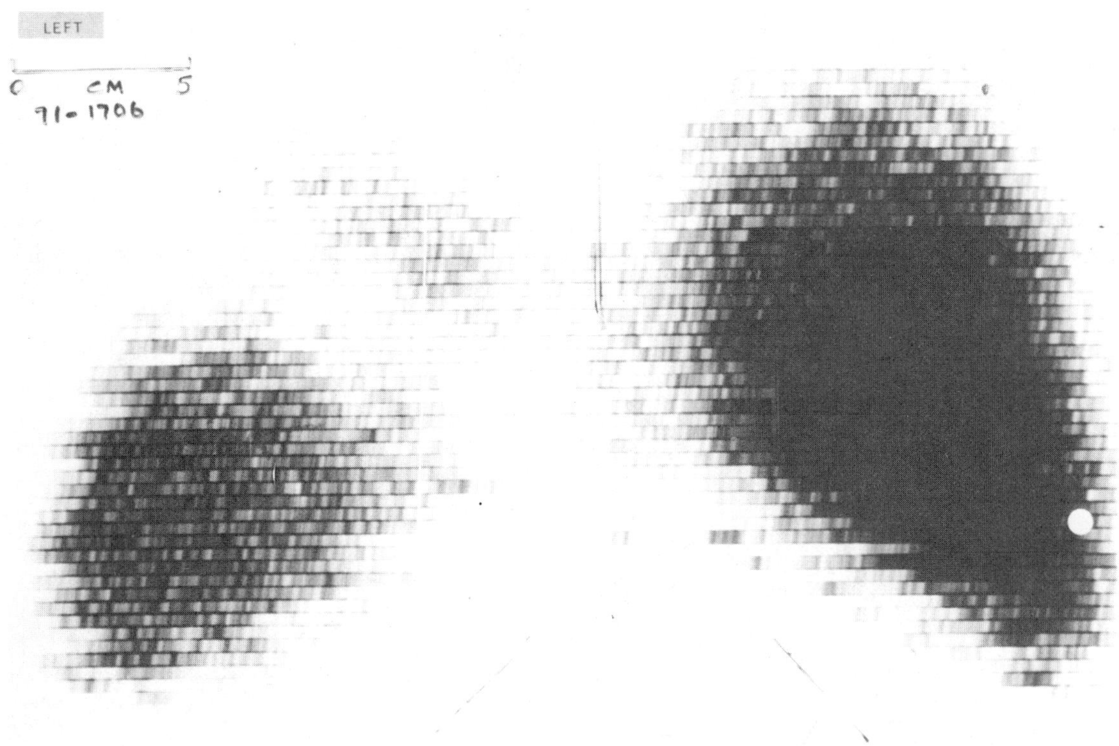

FIGURE 7. Posterior rectilinear scan (^{99m}Tc-sulfur colloid) in a 34-year-old man with thrombotic thrombocytopenic purpura. At first glance, it appears that there is a large filling defect in the superior portion of the spleen. On closer inspection, it can be noted that the uppermost activity on the left is contiguous with the liver. This was confirmed on multiple angulated views. Hepatic tissue in the left upper quadrant can readily be confused with the spleen. Case 71-1706.

bullet wound, shotgun wound), while 64 (34%) had sustained blunt injuries (auto accidents, falls, blows, or injury of uncertain etiology). In some cases, association with trauma may be less specific. For example, neonatal rupture of the spleen can occur.[49] Of the 19 reported cases, 6 were associated with a difficult or breech delivery or with prolonged labor. When a known cause of neonatal splenomegaly, such as erythroblastosis fetalis is present, rupture of the spleen should be suspected if the child develops a distended abdomen and shock.

Whether the "normal" spleen can rupture spontaneously is open to considerable debate. Some disease states, however, have been associated with apparent spontaneous rupture of the spleen. Amir and co-workers[50] have listed some of these conditions as infectious mononucleosis, viral hepatitis, pancreatitis, typhoid fever, malaria, sarcoidosis, actinomycosis, Gaucher's disease, leukemia, erythroblastosis fetalis, splenic hemangioma, and labor (and they described a case associated with myeloid metaplasia). It would appear reasonable to assume that if the spleen or its capsule were diseased, then minor insults might initiate bleeding or other events that would lead to rupture. An interesting aspect, which we have not seen discussed in the literature, is that the changing indentation of the spleen (by the stomach) might be a potential "cushion," protecting the medial surface of the spleen from injury.

Terry and co-workers[51] described the anatomic types of splenic injury as capsular tear, single laceration or perforation, multiple or stellate tears, fragmentation of the spleen, tears of the splenic pedicle, and multiple or diffuse hemorrhages. The diagnosis of such splenic injuries is readily made in some cases, but in others is fraught with difficulty. The most pertinent points are as follows:

History – Trauma, or the existence of a "predisposing" disease, should be an alerting signal. The number of cases of splenic rupture seen

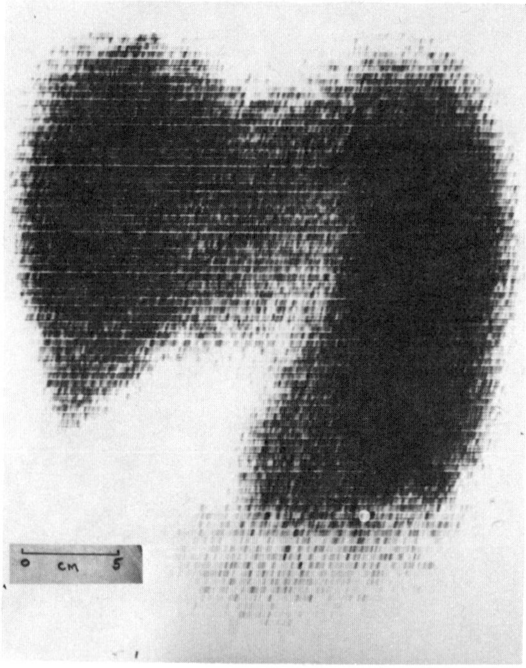

FIGURE 8. Superimposed anterior rectilinear scans (^{99m}Tc-sulfur colloid) in a 37-year-old woman with chronic myelogenous leukemia. The patient had begun a course of radiation to the spleen and suddenly experienced left upper quadrant pain. At the bottom of the figure, the massive loss of splenic volume can be appreciated. We can only speculate as to how much loss was due to the radiation and how much to splenic infarction. Case 70-2530.

in Egypt[68] may be related to underlying parasitic disorders.

Physical – Left upper quadrant guarding or tenderness, as well as referred pain to the left shoulder, are classical (phrenic distribution). Foster[61] has given particular diagnostic importance to the presence of shoulder pain ("Kehr's sign"). In the extreme, shortness of breath and shock can occur.

Laboratory – A falling hematocrit, of course, indicates continued bleeding. Recovery of blood from peritoneal aspiration is an indication of bleeding outside of an organ, but the technique is sometimes not rewarding. The significance of ahaptoglobinemia is discussed later.

Radiographically, the only sign occurring with any degree of frequency (7/12 cases, or 58% in the series of Schwartz and co-workers[52]) was an exaggeration of the mucosal folds on the greater curvature at the stomach. However, this finding was not specific and occurred in 6% of controls. These investigators summarized previous work showing that two thirds of 33 children with rupture of the spleen failed to show symptoms, signs, or laboratory indications of blood loss.

Abrams[53] states that splenic arteriography should be performed when the diagnosis is uncertain but suspected. He notes that the spleen is ruptured more frequently than other intra-abdominal organs after nonpenetrating trauma. A frequently associated injury is fracture of a rib. Sadler and Chinn[54] note that aortography may give normal findings in splenic hemorrhage, while studies of the splenic artery in particular may then show functional arteriovenous shunts secondary to hemorrhage. An extensive literature has developed on angiography in cases of splenic trauma.[55-57]

Ultrasonic scanning for splenic hematoma[58] might play an increasingly important role but has to be evaluated in additional centers.

Radionuclide imaging of the spleen, such as by use of ^{99m}Tc-sulfur colloid, provides an additional, relatively nontraumatic approach to the evaluation of splenic injury.[59] As to the disadvantages of the procedure, O'Mara and co-workers[73] list the limited spatial resolution (1.5 to 2 cm) and the nonspecific nature of a filling defect on the spleen scan. While ^{51}Cr-heat-denatured erythrocytes have been used in spleen scanning when searching for rupture,[58,59] it is likely that ^{99m}Tc-sulfur colloid is the present agent of choice.

We believe the following points should be made when scanning the spleen for suspected injury.

1. Since use of a radiocolloid allows visualization of the liver, the appearance of that organ should also be reported.
2. Multiple, angulated views are necessary (and hence the gamma camera may be easier to use than a rectilinear scanner). We have seen a case of splenic rupture in which the defect was only suggested on the posterior view but was elegantly demonstrated with the patient in the left posterior oblique position (Figure 10).
3. The ribs, midline, and body wall should be carefully delineated on the scan. A continuing outward slow leak of blood may be marked only by a progressive displacement of the spleen from the lateral body wall.
4. Aside from gross defects in the spleen and displacement of the organ, O'Mara and co-workers[73] point out that splenomegaly and non-

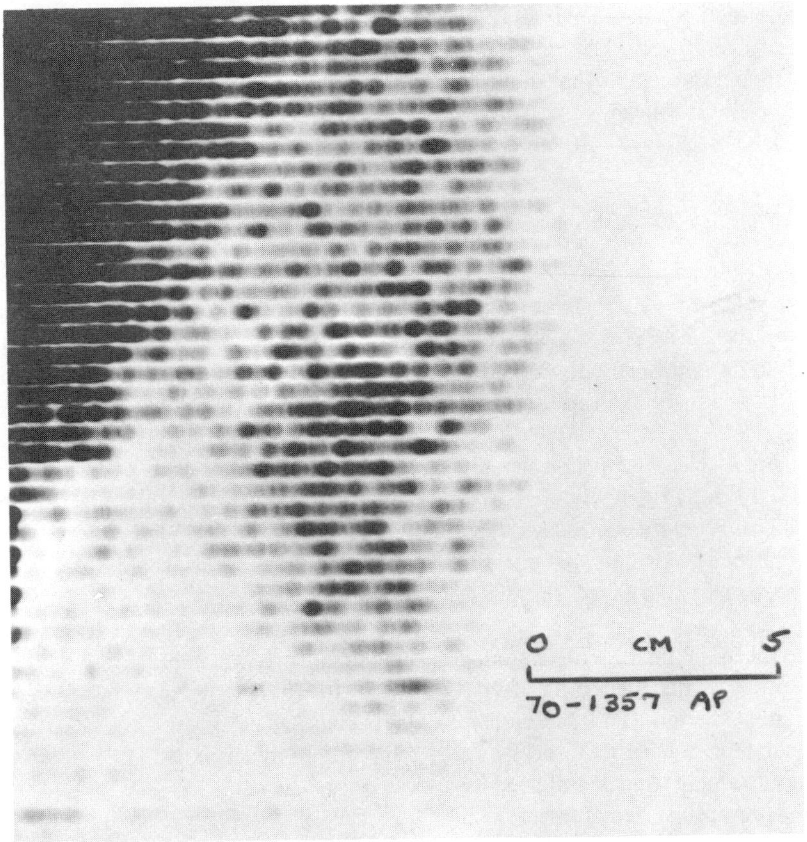

FIGURE 9. Anterior rectilinear scan (^{99m}Tc-sulfur colloid) of the spleen in a 14-year-old boy. The child had sickle thalassemia disease. Although there was uneven and poor uptake of the radiocolloid, the spleen was functional. The spleen was removed surgically and revealed multiple infarcts. Case 70-1357.

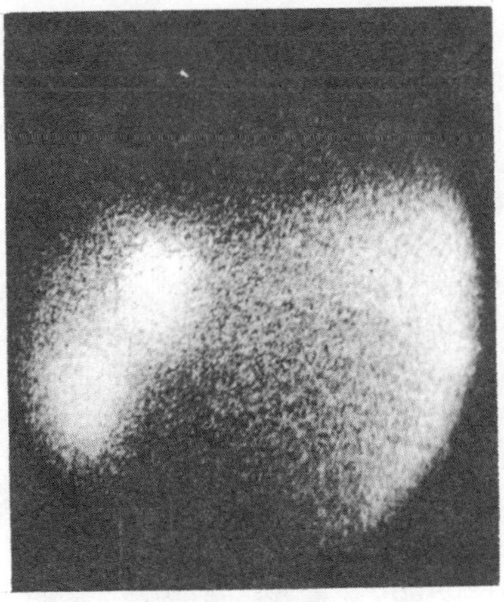

Posterior

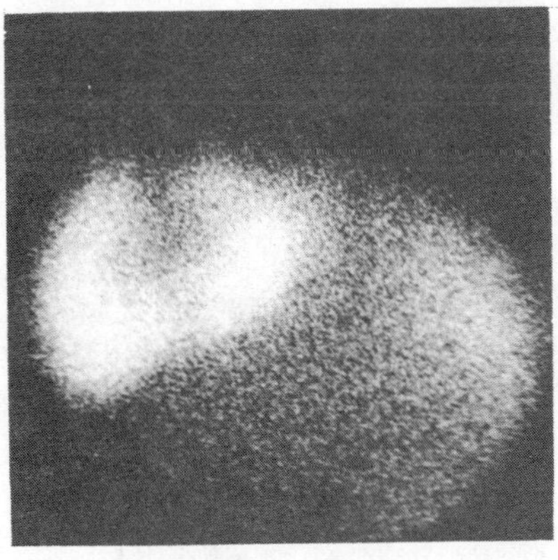

Left posterior oblique

FIGURE 10. A 12½-year-old girl fell while climbing and landed on her left side. She was described as having signs of diaphragmatic irritation on admission. After seeming to stabilize, her hematocrit dropped. The ^{99m}Tc-sulfur colloid spleen scan revealed a minimal defect on the posterior view. However, the left posterior oblique view clearly demonstrated a massive filling defect. At operation, a splenic rupture, with a "leaking" hematoma, was found. Case 71-2312.

homogeneous uptake of the radionuclide may be helpful in arriving at a diagnosis. They also state that angiography should be employed in those patients in whom a definitive diagnosis cannot be obtained by radionuclide scanning.

Our own experience with spleen scans in rupture of the organ has been rather good, and we recommend the procedure as an initial step. Of scans in 21 patients studied for suspected rupture, 12 were read as negative, 8 as positive, and 1 as equivocal (a repeat study in this patient was called negative). All eight of the suspected ruptures were confirmed surgically.[74] We have recently seen one case in which the initial spleen scan showed only an inferior decrease in activity, likely due to a renal hematoma. A repeat study 2 days later revealed a frank defect.[75] This points out the importance on repeat scans if delayed rupture is suspected.

McIndoe[63] has been credited with defining delayed splenic rupture as that occurring after a 48-hr or longer latent period. The mechanism might be postulated as a sequential process. In some cases, tearing of splenic tissue is followed by the formation of a subcapsular hematoma, which may cause cessation of further immediate bleeding. If the hematoma ruptures or lyses, vigorous bleeding might then start. Hence, there can be a delay between the time of trauma and the apparent splenic rupture. In the series of Shirkey and co-workers,[48] immediate rupture of the spleen occurred in 81% of the cases with blunt trauma. Delayed rupture represented 19% of the cases. An identical value of 19% for delayed splenic rupture occurs in the series of cases reported by Terry and co-workers.[51] Drapanas and associates[60] reported 14% of the cases of splenic rupture had delayed hemorrhage.

The time between injury and delayed rupture was reported by Terry and co-workers,[51] as 1 week in four cases, 2 weeks in four cases, and 4 or more weeks (up to 10 months) in three cases. They quote a figure of Boggs of a latent period of less than 1 week in half of the cases of splenic rupture and of under 2 weeks of 75% of cases. Although Terry and co-workers[51] had a higher mortality in patients with immediate rupture of the spleen (perhaps due in part to the other trauma) than in delayed rupture, this has not been the experience of more recent studies. The topic is summarized by Foster,[61] who states that in recent series the mortality in delayed hemorrhage of the spleen is 10% versus only 1% associated with "simple uncomplicated splenic rupture." This author stressed that delay in establishing a diagnosis was likely a major factor in the high mortality. A dissenting view has been expressed by Miller and Kelley,[62] who state that delay in the diagnosis of splenic rupture in children is not necessarily harmful.

Prager and associates,[64] in discussing "chronic, occult rupture of the spleen," stated that the ^{99m}Tc-spleen scan was abnormal in all four of their cases. These workers pointed out the common findings in each of their cases.

1. X-rays revealed a mass in the left upper quadrant.
2. The radioisotopic spleen scan showed a filling defect in each case.
3. Each of the patients had ahaptoglobinemia (blood haptoglobin = 0 mg/100 ml).
4. The bone marrow in each case was reported as showing absent iron stores and erythyroid hyperplasia.

The proposed explanation of the last two findings was that hemoglobin released from the splenic hematoma completely saturated the capacity of haptoglobin for carrying hemoglobin (little free hemoglobin is required in order to load haptoglobin). The specificity of this has not been measured in patients with retroperitoneal or intramuscular hematomas. The bone marrow findings were perhaps related to the massive blood (and iron) loss by pooling in the splenic hematoma. How available this iron is for reuse by the bone marrow is uncertain.

The true natural history of splenic rupture will perhaps never be known. Once the diagnosis is established, or even strongly suspected, operative intervention is the rule. Whether cases of minor trauma to the spleen go on to resolution is uncertain. Fontaine[65] reported a case of post-traumatic cystic hematoma of the spleen which was diagnosed angiographically. Kloth and Spagnuolo[66] have described a case of splenic rupture following degeneration of an aortic ball valve.

The treatment of splenic rupture is splenectomy. The risk of overwhelming infection following splenectomy is lower when the spleen is removed because of traumatic rupture than when it is removed because of certain systemic diseases. The late occurrence of a subphrenic hematoma following traumatic rupture of the spleen has been recorded.[67] Rupture of accessory splenic tissue has also been reported[69] and the use of spleen scanning noted in such a case.[70]

REFERENCES

1. **Warshaw, A. L., Chesney, T. M., Evans, G. W., and McCarthy, H. F.,** Intrasplenic dissection by pancreatic pseudocysts, *N. Engl. J. Med.*, 287, 72, 1972.
2. **Davis, C. E., Jr., Montero, J. M., and Van Horn, C. N.,** Large splenic cysts, *Ann. Surg.*, 173, 686, 1971.
3. **Martin, J. W.,** Congenital splenic cysts, *Am. J. Surg.*, 96, 302, 1958.
4. **Bron, K. M. and Hoffman, W. J.,** Preoperative diagnosis of splenic cysts, *Arch. Surg.*, 102, 459, 1971.
5. **Baltaxe, H. A., Watson, R. C., and Levin, D. C.,** The angiographic appearance of splenic masses, *Angiology*, 23, 316, 1972.
6. **Talerman, A. and Hart, S.,** Epithelial cysts of the spleen, *Br. J. Surg.*, 57, 201, 1970.
7. **Volpe, J. A. and Denardo, G. I.,** The preoperative diagnosis of spleen cysts by scintiscanning: report of a case, *Am. J. Roentgenol.*, 94, 839, 1965.
8. **Wagner, H. N., Jr., McAfee, J. G., and Winkelman, J. M.,** Splenic disease diagnosis by radioisotope scanning, *Arch. Intern. Med.*, 109, 673, 1962.
9. **Pearson, H. A., Touloukian, R. J., and Spencer, R. P.,** The binary spleen: a radioisotopic scan sign of splenic pseudocyst, *J. Pediatr.*, 77, 216, 1970.
10. **Rizk, G. K., Tayyarah, K. A., and Ghandur-Mnaymneh, L.,** The angiographic changes in hydatid cysts of the liver and spleen, *Radiology*, 99, 303, 1971.
11. **Sapkas, A. and Tierris, E.,** Complication spectaculaire d'un Kyste hydatique geant de la rate; la rupture dans le colon, *J. Chir.*, 103, 283, 1972.
12. **Morgan, H. and Johnson, P. M.,** Splenic masses detected by scintillation imaging and contrast tomography, *Radiology*, 97, 301, 1970.
13. **Reid, S. E. and Lang, S. J.,** Abscess of the spleen, *Am. J. Surg.*, 88, 912, 1954.
14. **Pickleman, J. R., Paloyan, E., and Block, G. E.,** The surgical significance of splenic abscess, *Surgery*, 68, 287, 1970.
15. **Zook, E. G., Bolivar, J. C., and Esptein, L. I.,** The value of scintiscans in the diagnosis of splenic abscess, *Surg. Gynecol. Obstet.*, 131, 1125, 1970.
16. **Sharr, M. M.,** Splenic abscess due to Salmonella agona, *Br. Med. J.*, 1, 546, 1972.
17. **Rabson, A. R., Koornhof, H. J., Notman, J., and Maxwell, W. G.,** Hepatosplenic abscess due to Yersinia enterocolitica, *Br. Med. J.*, 4, 341, 1972.
18. **LePage, J. R., Pratt, A. D., Jr., Miale, A., and Calvert, W. P.,** Diagnosis of splenic abscess by radionuclide scanning and selective arteriography, *J. Nucl. Med.*, 13, 331, 1972.
19. **Baker, G. H. and Powell, M. R.,** External localization of experimental abscesses: scanning staphylococcal abscesses with antibody to staphylococcus, *Invest. Radiol.*, 6, 266, 1971.
20. **Deysine, M., Robinson, R. G., and Wilder, J. R.,** Abscess detection by radioactive chromium labeled autologous white blood cells, *Surg. Gynecol. Obstet.*, 131, 216, 1970.
21. **Buchbinder, N. A. and Roberts, W. C.,** Left-sided valvular active infective endocarditis, *Am. J. Med.*, 53, 20, 1972.
22. **Quintiliani, R. and Ganguli, P.,** Splenic arteriovenous fistula with bacterial endarteritis and endocarditis, *JAMA*, 214, 727, 1970.
23. **Cockshott, W. P. and Weaver, E. J. M.,** Primary tropical splenic abscess: a misnomer, *Br. J. Surg.*, 49, 665, 1961.
24. **Emmerling, P., Finger, H., and Bertz, R.,** Non-appearance of splenomegaly after injection of filled Bordetella pertussis cells into aged mice, *Experientia*, 27, 1216, 1971.
25. **Katsura, S., Satodate, R., and Makita, Y.,** Demonstration of splenic metallophilic cells in bacterial infectious disease, *Acta Pathol. Jap.*, 20, 127, 1970.
26. **Easton, J. A., and Fessas, C.,** Incidence of Dohle bodies in various diseases and their association with thrombocytopenia, *Br. J. Haematol.*, 12, 54, 1966.
27. **Itoga, T. and Laszio, J.,** Dohle bodies and other granulocytic alterations during chemotherapy with cyclophosphamide, *Blood*, 20, 668, 1962.
28. **Abernathy, M. R.,** Dohle bodies associated with uncomplicated pregnancy, *Blood*, 27, 380, 1966.
29. **Gould, H. R., Clemett, A. R., and Ross, P.,** Radiologic diagnosis of splenic metastasis, *Am. J. Roentgenol.*, 109, 755, 1970.

30. **Silverman, S., de Nardo, G. L., Glatstein, E., and Lipton, M. J.**, Evaluation of the liver and spleen in Hodgkin's disease. II. The value of splenic scintigraphy, *Am. J. Med.*, 52, 362, 1972.
31. **Pilgrim, H. I.**, The metastatic behavior of a spleen-tropic reticulum cell sarcoma in splenectomized mice, *Proc. Soc. Exp. Biol. Med.*, 138, 178, 1971.
32. **Watanabe, T. and Tanaka, K.**, Effect of carcinostatic agents on carcinomatous metastasis in the spleen, *Gann*, 60, 611, 1969.
33. **Kerr, I. B.**,Spleen reaction following tumor growth, *Arch. Geschwulstforsch.*, 35, 13, 1970.
34. **Kerr, I. B.**, Experimental study on relationships between tumor growth and splenomegaly, *Arch. Geschwulstforsch.*, 38, 125, 1971.
35. **Sammis, A. F., Jr., Weitzman, S. and Arcomano, J. P.**, Hemangiolymphangioma of spleen and bone, *N. Y. State J. Med.*, 71, 1762, 1971.
36. **Strauli, P.**, Incidence and morphology of tumor metastases in the spleen, in *The Spleen*, Lennert, K. and Harms, D., Eds., Springer-Verlag, New York, 1970, 406.
37. **Bengmark, S., Domellof, L., and Olsson, A. M.**, The role of splenectomy in stomach cancer operations, *Digestion*, 4, 314, 1971.
38. **Pellerin, D. and Bertin, P.**, Les tumeurs de la loge splenique chez l'enfant (A propos de 11 observations), *Ann. Chir.*, 24, 1351, 1970.
39. **Fidler, I. J.**, Metastasis: quantitative analysis of distribution and fate of tumor emboli labeled with ^{125}I-5-iodo-2'-deoxyuridine, *J. Natl. Cancer Inst.*, 45, 773, 1970.
40. **Green, R. L., Huntsman, R. G., and Serjeant, G. R.**, The sickle-cell and altitude, *Br. Med. J.*, 4, 593, 1971.
41. **O'Brien, R. T., Pearson, H. A., Godley, J. A., and Spencer, R. P.**, Splenic infarct and sickel (cell) trait, *N. Engl. J. Med.*, 287, 720, 1972.
42. **Nuland, S. B., Cornelius, E. A., and Spencer, R. P.**, Scan evidence of organ involution and improvement of hypersplenism in Hodgkin's disease following splenic artery ligation, *J. Nucl. Med.*, 11, 693, 1970.
43. **Quinn, J. L., III**, Editorial comment, *Yearbook of Nuclear Medicine*, Year Book Med. Publ., Chicago, 1971, 161.
44. **Vagenakis, A. G., Abreau, C. M., and Braverman, L. E.**, Splenic infarction diagnosed by photoscanning, *J. Nucl. Med.*, 13, 563, 1972.
45. **Nelp, W. B. and Kuhn, I. N.**, Splenic infarction diagnosed by photoscanning, *JAMA*, 197, 368, 1966.
46. **Alarcon-Segovia, D., Mayorga-Cortes, A., Gonzalez-Jimenez, Y., and Maisterrena, J.**, Diagnosis of splenic infarction by scintillation scanning with Hg^{203}-bromomercurihydroxypropane (Hg^{203}-BMHP), *Am. J. Roentgenol.*, 109, 761, 1970.
47. **Goswitz, F. A. and Vodopick, H.**, Radiocolloid scans in chronic granulocytic leukemia, *J. Nucl. Med.*, 11, 630, 1970.
48. **Shirkey, A. L., Wukasch, D. C., Beall, A. C., Jr., Gordon, W. B., Jr., and DeBakey, M. E.**, Surgical management of splenic injuries, *Am. J. Surg.*, 108, 630, 1964.
49. **Leape, L. L. and Bordy, M. D.**, Neonatal rupture of the spleen, *Pediatrics*, 47, 101, 1971.
50. **Amir, J., Chaimov, C., Pinkhas, J., and DeVries, A.**, Spontaneous splenic rupture in myeloid metaplasia, *Isr. J. Med. Sci.*, 6, 658, 1970.
51. **Terry, J. H., Self, M. M., and Howard, J. M.**, Injuries of the spleen: a report of 102 patients and a review of the literature, *Surgery*, 40, 615, 1956.
52. **Schwartz, S. S., Boley, S. J., and McKinnon, W. M. P.**, The roentgen findings in traumatic rupture of the spleen in children, *Am. J. Roentgenol.*, 82, 505, 1959.
53. **Abrams, H. L.**., Splenic arteriography, in *Angiography*, Vol.II, 2nd ed., Abrams, H. L., Ed., Little, Brown & Co., Boston, 1971, 1003.
54. **Sadler, R. B. and Chinn, J.**, Negative aortogram not reliable for diagnosis of splenic hemorrhage, *JAMA*, 221, 712, 1972.
55. **Solheim, K. and Aakhus, T.**, Traumatic rupture of the spleen with special reference to angiography, *Injury*, 3, 239, 1972.
56. **Gold, R. E. and Redman, H. C.**, Splenic trauma: assessment of problems in diagnosis, *Am. J. Roentgenol.*, 116, 413, 1972.
57. **Lepasoon, J. and Olin, T.**, Angiographic diagnosis of splenic lesions following blunt abdominal trauma, *Acta Radiol. Diagn.*, 11, 257, 1971.
58. **Jackson, G. L. and Albright, D.**, Splenic rupture, *JAMA*, 204, 930, 1968.
59. **Wener, L.**, Scintiscan diagnosis of splenic hematoma, *Surg. Gynecol. Obstet.*, 134, 430, 1972.
60. **Drapanas, T., Yates, A. J., Brickman, R., and Wholey, M.**, The syndrome of occult rupture of the spleen, *Arch. Surg.*, 99, 298, 1969.
61. **Foster, R. P.**, Delayed haemorrhage from the ruptured spleen, *Br. J. Surg.*, 57, 189, 1970.
62. **Miller, D. W., Jr. and Kelley, D. L.**, Splenic trauma; surgical management in children, *Arch. Surg.*, 105, 561, 1972.
63. **McIndoe, A. H.**, Delayed haemorrhage following traumatic rupture of the spleen, *Br. J. Surg.*, 20, 249, 1932.
64. **Prager, D., Morel, D., and Dex, W.**, The syndrome of chronic, occult rupture of the spleen, *JAMA*, 218, 1824, 1971.
65. **Fontaine, J. L.**, Contribution a l'etude des hematomes enkystes post-traumatiques de la rate, *Presse Med.*, 78, 2069, 1970.

66. **Kloth, H. H. and Spagnuolo, M.**, Aortic ball degeneration with splenic rupture, *N. Y. State J. Med.*, 72, 2664, 1972.
67. **Suitor, E. H., Kim, H. J., and Flynn, J. T.**, Subphrenic hematoma; late complication of traumatic rupture of the spleen, *N. Y. State J. Med.*, 72, 2325, 1972.
68. **Abdel-Moneim, R. I.**, Rupture of the spleen in rural parts of Egypt, *Am. J. Surg.*, 123, 674, 1972.
69. **Kumar, R.**, A case of traumatic rupture of an accessory spleen, *Arch. Dis. Child.*, 37, 227, 1962.
70. **Fink, D. W.**, Scintiphotographic demonstration of rupture of an accessory spleen, *J. Nucl. Med.*, 13, 333, 1972.
71. **Ansigh, H. R. and Stapleton, J. E.**, Epidermoid cyst of the spleen. Diagnosis by photoscanning, *Northwest Med.*, 66, 461, 1967.
72. **Blank, E. and Campbell, J. R.**, Epidermoid cysts of spleen, *Pediatrics*, 51, 75, 1973.
73. **O'Mara, R. E., Hall, R. C., and Dombroski, D. L.**, Scintiscanning in the diagnosis of rupture of the spleen, *Surg. Gynecol. Obstet.*, 131, 1077, 1970.
74. **Witek, J. T. and Spencer, R. P.**, Diagnostic spleen scans in occult splenic injury, *J. Trauma*, 14, 197, 1974.
75. **Slavin, J. D., Jr., Minehan, T. F., and Spencer, R. P.**, Scan demonstration of delayed splenic rupture, *J. Nucl. Med.*, 15, 632, 1974.
76. **Wright, F. W. and Williams, E. W.**, Large post-traumatic splenic cyst diagnosed by radiology, isotope scintigraphy and ultrasound, *Br. J. Radiol.*, 47, 454, 1974.

Chapter 13

ERRORS OF PRODUCTION AND DESTRUCTION OF FORMED BLOOD ELEMENTS

The numbers of circulating blood cells are usually maintained within a fairly narrow range. For each formed element in the bloodstream (leukocytes, erythrocytes, platelets), three types of quantitative information are of importance.

1. Rate of production by synthetic depots, usually in the bone marrow.
2. Quantity circulating in the vascular space.
3. Rate of destruction.

The numbers (or total mass) of circulating leukocytes, erythrocytes, and platelets are of key importance. If any or all of these elements is reduced in amount, and yet there is normal production, then increased destruction is likely.

Production – The simplest and most direct approaches to assaying production of the formed blood elements are the performance of a complete blood count and hematologic evaluation (including a bone marrow examination). Normal numbers and maturation patterns of the precursor cells in the bone marrow are prima facie evidence of normal production of erythrocytes.

Radioisotopic techniques for measuring production rates involve the use of cohort labels. Such radiolabels go to the bone marrow and appear in newly forming red blood cells, white blood cells, or platelets. The use of ^{3}H or ^{14}C amino acids, while a powerful tool for studying hematopoiesis in animal, is often not justified in humans because of the long half-life of these radionuclides and the attendant radiation exposure. Two radiopharmaceuticals have been utilized in clinical studies of production rates of red blood cells. These are ^{59}Fe-ferrous citrate and ^{75}Se-selenomethionine. The physical half-life of ^{59}Fe is 45 days. There are beta ray emissions as well as gamma rays of 1.1 and 1.2 meV. Because of the high energy of the gamma rays, it is difficult to perform whole body scanning if anatomic localization of the radionuclide is of interest. The beta ray emissions, long physical half-life of ^{59}Fe, and minimal iron excretion from the body limit the quantity that can be employed because of the radiation exposure. Another iron radioisotope, ^{52}Fe has a T1/2 of about 8 hr (positron emissions and two gamma rays). This is too short lived to be used in studies of erythrocyte production, although it can be of value in showing sites (such as the spleen) which accumulate iron due to extramedullary hematopoiesis. However, ^{52}Fe is cyclotron produced and relatively difficult to make.[1] Of interest is the finding that the radionuclide ^{111}In is handled much like iron.[2] That is, radioindium (^{111}In, T1/2 = 2.8 days, 173 and 247 keV gamma rays) binds to transferrin, as does iron, and is transported to the bone marrow. Studies have not yet been published on the splenic uptake and turnover of ^{111}In. Surface counting over the spleen has been used to quantify the amount of radioiron present in the organ.[3] However, aside from cases of extramedullary hematopoiesis, such counting may not be of clinical importance. After administration of ^{59}Fe-citrate intravenously, spleen, sacral, and precordial counts are recorded[4] and compared with accepted normal curves. Following use of ^{59}Fe, activity in the sacrum is higher than in the normal liver or spleen. In extramedullary hematopoiesis, this is reversed.

Another cohort label for following production of blood elements is ^{75}Se-selenomethionine (and this is mentioned in another chapter). However, the long physical half-life of ^{75}Se (120 days) and the fact that only 4% of the injected dose appears in formed blood elements make for difficulties in using this radiolabel.

Circulating quantity and destruction – While the rate of production of formed blood elements is measured by cohort labeling, estimation of both the circulating quantity and the rate of destruction is achieved by random labeling. The principal radiolabel for doing this is ^{51}Cr-chromate. In actuality, the labeling may be slightly age dependent, but some cells from all age groups accept the chromate. ^{51}Cr tags the beta chain of hemoglobin.[93] An aliquot of the formed element, whose circulating quantity is to be estimated, is tagged with ^{51}Cr and preferably washed to remove unbound label. It is then injected intravenously, and (unless a significant quantity pools in an area) the circulating amount is measured by radioisotope dilution.

Because ^{51}Cr is not transferred to other formed

elements when a tagged cell is destroyed, a means is available for following the survival of the labeled components. In actuality the picture is more complex then this since some ^{51}Cr is passively eluted from the circulating blood elements, in addition to radiolabel being lost by their destruction. However, until a new and more definitive gamma-ray-emitting radionuclide is found for tagging the formed blood elements, ^{51}Cr will likely continue to be widely employed.

PLATELETS

As platelets age, there is evidence that they change their size and density. By centrifugation, platelet populations of markedly different densities can be separated. The heavier platelets have a volume about twice as large as the lighter ones and are more metabolically active. It therefore appears reasonable that heavier platelets change into lighter ones during their circulation. The large young platelets are referred to as "megathrombocytes."[94] Using ^{75}Se-selenomethionine, Amorosi and co-workers[5] studied the ratio of radioactivity in platelets (heavy/light). Greatest activity was in the heavier fraction initially (after a 24-hr lag). There was then a progression of heavy-large platelets to light-small platelets with time. There is no evidence that the spleen is involved in the platelet progression from heavy to light fractions. Moreover, such studies with selenomethionine can not be used to measure platelet life span because of some reutilization of ^{75}Se.

A second area of study is the function of circulating platelets. Gross morphology has provided little help here, but tests of platelet aggregation and adhesiveness have been more revealing. There is a large literature on the subject of platelet function. For example, Prost-Dvojakovic and co-workers[6] noted that in some leukemias and anemias, with normal platelet counts and hemostasis, disorders of platelet aggregation and adhesiveness were present. Cardamone and associates have presented related data.[7] Again, there is no clear evidence for a role of the spleen in these abnormalities, although a role for the spleen in platelet "activation" has been proposed.[8]

The spleen, however, does play a key role in platelet pooling and likely in platelet destruction. Procedures for following these events have been relatively limited. Immunological techniques, direct-transfusion and blood exchange, as well as ^{51}Cr-platelet labeling, have been the principal methods for looking at thrombokinetics. ^{51}Cr-chromate will bind to hemoglobin within red cells and also to white blood cells and to platelets. Enriched platelet preparations can be labeled with ^{51}Cr, reinjected, and their distribution and survival followed.[91-11] At the extremes are individuals with thrombocytopenia and those with thrombocythemia. We will look at the latter group first. Marsh and associates[12] studied eight patients with thrombocythemia (0.9 to 2.7 million/mm^3) of from 1 to 9 years duration. These individuals had increased megakaryocytes in the bone marrow in addition to the increased platelet count (perhaps a variant of a myeloproliferative disorder). In only two of the eight patients was the spleen palpable below the costal margin. Three of the cases revealed evidence of splenic hypofunction on smears of peripheral blood (Howell-Jolly bodies and occasional target cells). In these three cases, there was delayed clearance of ^{51}Cr-heat-denatured erythrocytes from the bloodstream. The same three cases did not demonstrate a spleen on the ^{51}Cr scan. Why three out of eight of the individuals with thrombocythemia should have splenic hypofunction is unclear. A definite role can not yet be assigned to increased coagulability and blockade of splenic vessels. A slight thrombocytosis follows splenectomy. In some cases it can be severe and has been thought to represent the unmarking of a myeloproliferative disorder[97] (thrombocythemia).

A far more common problem is the finding of thrombocytopenia. Gehrmann and Elbers[13] have presented evidence (including adrenalin-induced platelet release by the spleen) that the thrombocytopenia associated with hepatic cirrhosis was caused by platelet pooling in the spleen and not by splenic inhibition of the bone marrow. Harker[14] studied platelet production and distribution in normal, asplenic, and splenomegalic (methylcellulose-induced) rats. The normal spleen pooled 15% of total platelets, and the value went up to 55% in rats with splenomegaly. However, there was little effect on platelet survival. It appeared that platelets were distributed dynamically between splenic and circulating pools and further that platelet production was seemingly regulated so that circulating levels were kept nearly constant.

Aster[15] had pointed out that after intravenous administration, ^{51}Cr-platelets underwent mixing and splenic pooling; after this, an equilibrium was reached between labeled platelets in the splenic exchangeable platelet pool and those in the circulation. There appears to be a definite relationship between the exchangeable splenic platelet pool and the size of the spleen. Kutti and co-workers[16] measured the exchangeable splenic platelet pool by means of ^{51}Cr-platelets and determined splenic size by use of scintigraphy (after administration of ^{99m}Tc-sulfur colloid) and related the spleenic scan measurements to volume. In 6 normal individuals and 22 patients with polycythemia vera, the recovery (R, in percent) of infused, labeled platelets was related to splenic volume (V in cm^3) by:

$$R = 59 - 0.04\ V. \tag{1}$$

In other words, the larger the spleen, the lower the recovery of platelets. A separate study was carried out by Abrahamsen[17] of 12 patients with Hodgkin's disease, before and after splenectomy. Prior to splenectomy, recovery of infused platelets (R) was given as a function of splenic weight in grams (S):

$$R = 62 - 0.054\ S. \tag{2}$$

The similarity of Equations 1 and 2 is apparent. After splenectomy, platelet recovery increased from about 30% to 90%, showing that considerable splenic trapping had been occurring. Interestingly, aside from a transient postoperative shortening, platelet survival was not affected by splenectomy. The thrombocytosis that followed splenectomy was proportional to the weight of the removed spleen.

In another study of polycythemia vera, Kutti and Weinfeld[18] noted that the platelet half-life was shorter in those with splenomegaly than in individuals with the disease but without splenomegaly (the normal half-life is about 3.8 days, with a production of 23×10^{10} platelets/days). Gehrmann[19] has stated that in hypersplenism, up to 90% of the total number of thrombocytes may be in the splenic pool. This thrombocytopenia may also have an associated slightly shortened platelet survival.

Harker and Slichter[21] studied platelet and fibrinogen consumption in man. There was not a one-to-one correspondence between the two. The commonest finding was combined platelet and fibrinogen consumption (an exaggeration of the hemostatic mechanism). A second class of patients had selective platelet destruction, perhaps related to platelet thrombus formation. A third class of cases had fibrinogen destruction without platelet consumption, and this occurred in fibrinolytic syndromes.

We will take a deeper look at idiopathic thrombocytopenic purpura (ITP). After the introduction of ^{51}Cr as a red cell label[65] and its application in platelet tagging,[66] Cohen and co-workers used ^{51}Cr platelets to classify the thrombocytopenias.[67] There are certainly many mechanisms by which a low platelet count can arise.

1. Decreased production. This occurs in bone marrow failure but does not appear to be of importance in ITP. In fact, platelet production may be increased considerably in ITP, as evidenced by an increased number of megathrombocytes.[94]
2. Production of defective platelets, which are rapidly cleared. Abnormal platelets have not been clearly associated with all cases of ITP, but case reports have appeared.[83]
3. Presence of antiplatelet antibodies.

Over 50 years ago, Bedson[68] produced thrombocytopenia by use of antiplatelet antibodies. Gore and co-workers[69] noted that rabbit antiguinea pig platelet antibodies reduced the platelet count in guinea pigs and also produced ultrastructural changes in capillaries. It was the studies of Harrington and co-workers[70] which established that in over 60% of the cases of ITP, a serum factor was present which resulted in destruction of both autologous and homologous platelets. Later work has confirmed that antiplatelet antibodies occur in ITP,[71,72] and these can be eluted from the spleen removed at surgery.[73] The spleen in ITP shows lymphatic hyperplasia, compatible with antibody formation;[74] the spleen also sequesters platelets in this disorder. Increased immunoglobulin (Ig) synthesis can be shown in the spleens of patients with ITP.[75]

A variant of ITP, referred to as onyalai, is characterized by hemorrhagic bullae of the lips and buccal mucosa. Although thought to be restricted to East Africa,[76] cases have been described in the United States.[77] The disorder occurs in blacks, probably because the purpura of mild ITP is not appreciated in dark skin, and thus only severe cases are seen. Thrombotic thrombocytopenic purpura (TTP) appears to be more severe and perhaps a distinct disease[78,79] whose relationship to ITP is uncertain.

The hemolytic uremic syndrome and some congenital conditions can result in abnormal consumption of platelets. For example, the Klippel-Trenaunay syndrome[80] of flame nevus and bone and limb hypertrophy has been shown to have associated thrombocytopenia and hypofibrinogenemia[81] (likely on the basis of increased consumption: so-called disseminated intravascular coagulation). Heparin administration arrests the defect, and surgical removal of the nevus results in permanent correction[81] (and radiation might also be of help). The abnormal consumption in this disorder was commented upon as likely being related to that in the Kasabach-Merritt syndrome[7] (cavernous hemangioma and purpura).[82] Hamartoma of the spleen has also been associated with thrombocytopenia.[84]

LEUKOCYTES

Radioisotopic studies of leukocyte production, distribution, and destruction have been quite limited. One reason has been that the white blood cells must be separated from the far more numerous erythrocytes. Further, leukocytes themselves are a heterogenous group. ^{32}P-diisopropylfluorophosphate can be injected intravenously (or intramuscularly) to label blood elements, which are then separated from other components.[22] The procedure is not adaptable to external organ counting (^{32}P is a beta ray emitter) and has had relatively little use. Leukocyte labeling by means of ^{14}C and ^{35}S-amino acids has also been reported. Such cohort labeling is limited by the radiation dose of these beta ray emitters and difficulties in counting the labeled cells.

Separated leukocytes can be tagged with ^{51}Cr-chromate and reinjected.[23] The ^{51}Cr has the advantage of allowing external detection. Scott and co-workers[87] studied autologous lymphocytes, tagged with ^{51}Cr, in normal subjects. The recirculating pool of lymphocytes included blood, spleen, and bone marrow. The total pool was about twice the size of the blood pool of lymphocytes and turned over about 12 times a day. The lymphocytes appeared to have a half-life of 18 days. With recognition of the long-lived T lymphocytes, and the shorter-lived B lymphocytes, radiolabel studies should be repeated with each type. Duvall and Perry[24] used ^{51}Cr to study leukocytes in chronic myelocytic leukemia, where the high leukocyte counts make labeling effective. Labeled white cells appeared to be viable, as judged by their morphology, exclusion of trypan blue, and epinephrine-induced leukocyte release from the spleen. External counting revealed trapping of the labeled leukocytes in the lungs of patients with chronic myelocytic leukemia and then pooling in the spleen. Some of the cells could apparently leave the spleen after they entered the organ. It will be recalled that in obstruction to the splenic venous outflow, congestion and splenomegaly can occur. A pancytopenia (Banti's syndrome) or even a depression of the leukocyte count out of proportion to the other blood elements can occur. In Felty's syndrome (rheumatoid arthritis with splenomegaly and depressed granulocyte count), splenectomy may afford some relief from the infections that occur.[85]

At the other extreme, some individuals show an elevated neutrophil count without evidence of systemic disease. In the one case that we studied, there was functional asplenia,[25] suggesting that lack of splenic activity might be related to the elevated white blood count.

ERRORS OF RED CELL PRODUCTION

A red cell volume or hemoglobin concentration lower than that in healthy individuals (anemia) can result from either decreased production or increased destruction of erythrocytes and their contents.

I. Pancytopenia

a. Marrow replacement by tumor or other cells (neuroblastoma, leukemia, myelofibrosis, other diseases).

b. Marrow obliteration by bone (osteopetrosis).

c. Acquired (may be due to an agent capable of destroying marrow such as radiation, chloramphenicol); many cases are idiopathic.

d. Constitutional. These pancytopenias are probably recessively inherited. One of these, associated with congenital anomalies, is Fanconi's syndrome (familial aplastic anemia). Other variants may be pancreatic insufficiency and pancytopenia (Schwachman's syndrome) and dyskeratosis congenita.

II. Deficient erythrocyte production (pure red cell anemia).

a. Congenital: Diamond-Blackfan syndrome.

b. Acquired selected depression of red cell production (etiology often unknown, questionable erythropoietin inhibition, possible thymic tumors).

III. Complex anemias associated with uremia, infection, or inflammation. [There may be a slight increase in hemolysis.]

Radiocolloid scans have an important role to play in evaluating pancytopenia due to bone marrow replacement. When given in sufficient amounts (about 10 millicuries in adults), ^{99m}Tc-sulfur colloid can be visualized in the bone marrow.[26] The limitation, of course, is that the bones near the liver and spleen can not be well defined since these two organs take up the bulk of the radiocolloid and their intense activity obscures the fainter image of the marrow. In neuroblastoma, the bone marrow can be nearly completely replaced by tumor cells (Figure 1). Iron radionuclides can be used (by point counting over the bone, in a search for functional marrow). For example, ^{52}Fe can be employed for marrow localization by means of a rectilinear scanner or a gamma camera. More recently, ^{111}In has been used in marrow visualization since it is an iron analogue (see above).

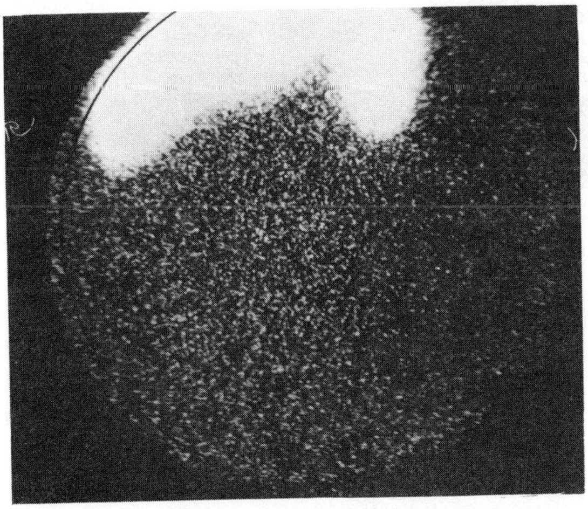

FIGURE 1. Anterior scintiphoto (^{99m}Tc-sulphur colloid) of the abdomen in a 2½-year-old boy with disseminated neuroblastoma. The scan was deliberately overexposed, in terms of the liver and spleen, in an effort to detect radiocolloid uptake in the bone marrow. Despite this, no distinct marrow localization could be seen on the above picture or on multiple other views. The child had replacement of the bone marrow by tumor cells and succumbed some months later. Case 72-678.

Leukemia may present with a pancytopenia. This is probably the result of bone marrow replacement, but inhibition by products of the abnormal cells has not been ruled out. The incidence of leukemia is high in patients with Fanconi's syndrome[27] (constitutional pancytopenia). There is also a common association of splenic atrophy in patients with Fanconi's syndrome. The small spleens and marrow dysfunction might be related to a dystrophy of tissues having a mesenchymal origin.[27] The association of Fanconi's syndrome with other congenital anomalies has been discussed,[28] as well as cytogenetic findings[29] and a possible relationship to diabetes mellitus.[30] We have studied a 4-year-old girl with Fanconi's syndrome by means of both ^{99m}Tc-sulfur colloid and ^{51}Cr-heat-denatured erythrocytes. Both techniques showed a small but functional spleen (case 71-1842). The child had been treated with a synthetic androgen; the typical response to androgens in Fanconi's syndrome is a dramatic rise in the hemoglobin concentration, with a lesser response in leukocytes and platelets.

Another congenital form of pancytopenia (particularly neturopenia) is associated with pancreatic insufficiency and bears the name of Shwachman's syndrome.[31] In the single case we have followed (Figure 2), the spleen has shown

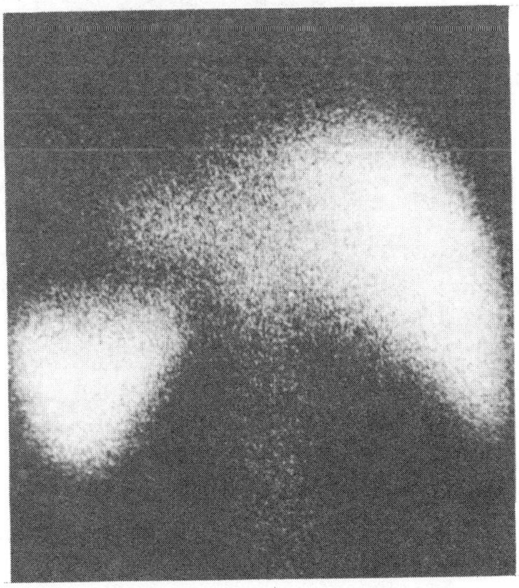

FIGURE 2. Posterior scintiphoto (^{99m}Tc-sulfur colloid) in a 7-year-old boy with Shwachman's syndrome (pancreatic insufficiency and pancytopenia). Case 72-1480.

counts over the liver and spleen are calculated from the fall in the counts over the precordium. Excess counts are the difference between the actual counts and those expected.

4. Another index, the spleen localization index or SLI, was proposed by McCurdy and Rath.[43]

$$\frac{\left(\dfrac{\text{Maximum change in the spleen to precordium counts}}{\text{The initial ratio of spleen to precordium counts}}\right) \times 10}{\text{(The day on which the maximum ratio occurs)}} \qquad (5)$$

Sequestration was said to occur if the SLI was 1.0 or greater or if the maximum spleen-to-precordium ratio exceeded a value of 1.5. Most authors recognize difficulties in absolute separation of groups on the basis of such criteria. Splenic trapping of red cells in myeloid metaplasia, for example, is difficult to quantify because of the often huge size of the organ and the mild degree of sequestration. Splenic uptake of radiomercury-labeled erythrocytes (tagged with 1-mercuri-2-hydroxypropane) has been proposed[64] but appears to offer little advantages over the use of ^{51}Cr.

None of the techniques is foolproof and entirely accurate. Szur[89] has discussed some of the problems involved. Abnormal destruction of erythrocytes occurs if the cells are congenitally abnormal, if they are damaged during their transit through the circulation, or rarely in the course of diseases involving the reticuloendothelial system (erythrophagocytosis). The events occurring in the spleen in such cases are numerous. We will list some of the obvious possible processes, recognizing that the quantification of their time course and extent has still to be achieved.

1. The spleen is a site of erythrocyte trapping and destruction.
2. Iron and other breakdown products of the erythrocytes may be stored in the spleen.
3. In some instances, the spleen can serve as a site of extramedullary hematopoiesis.
4. As a consequence of vascular obstruction, the spleen may suffer from anoxia and segmental infarction (particularly in sickle cell disease).
5. Fibrosis and calcium deposition can occur as a consequence of the infarction.

THE HEMOLYTIC ANEMIAS

A shortened intravascular survival of erythrocytes occurs in a wide variety of diseases. The erythrocyte within the circulatory system does not have a nucleus and cannot readily adapt to changing situations. Hence, its membrane and the contained electrolytes, enzymes, and energy stores must be sufficient to ward off the hazards of passage through the circulation. If the cells are defective or are attacked by exogenous factors, they may be prematurely lysed or trapped (hemolytic anemia).

SOME CAUSES OF HEMOLYSIS OF ERYTHROCYTES

Defects within the Red Cell (All Congenital Except for No. 5)

1. Abnormal hemoglobins (example: hemoglobin S).
2. Abnormal or unbalanced production of hemoglobin chains (example: β-thalassemia, with decreased manufacture of hemoglobin β-chains and excess accumulation of α-chains).
3. Abnormalities of contained enzymes of glycolysis or hexosemonophosphate shunt.
4. Mechanism uncertain (example: hemolysis in erythropoietic porphyria, perhaps related to excess retained prophyrins). Other defects in the red cell wall or metabolism[44,45] should likely be classified here until the specific errors are elucidated.
5. Acquired, such as that occurring when there is vitamin B_{12} deficiency.

Defects within the Red Cell, but Coupled with an Exoerythrocytic Factor

1. Congenital deficiency of glucose-6-phosphate dehydrogenase (when presented with various exogenous drugs).
2. Hereditary spherocytosis (there is a membrane abnormality). The spleen traps many of the abnormal cells; splenectomy is beneficial.
3. Hereditary elliptocytosis (in some instances there can be splenomegaly and hemolytic anemia; splenectomy is helpful in such cases).
4. Paroxysmal nocturnal hemoglobinuria (acquired, in which the red cells are attacked by a part of complement).

Defects Principally Outside the Red Cells (Usually Acquired)

1. Idiopathic, with or without autoantibodies (and the hemolysin of paroxysmal cold hemoglobinuria should likely be classified here).
2. Associated with diseases such as lymphomas, sarcoidosis, renal cortical necrosis (the hemolytic-uremic syndrome).
3. Accompanying infections, particularly those which damage erythrocytes.
4. Erythrocyte damage, such as accompanying burns and cardiac valvular prostheses.
5. Transfusion of incompatible blood.
6. Toxins of many kinds.

We will discuss several of these entities as they relate to the spleen.

Abnormal Hemoglobins

The abnormal hemoglobins may produce symptoms by a number of mechanisms.

1. Some have an altered affinity for oxygen and may result in cyanosis even in the presence of a normal pO_2.
2. Some are unstable and tend to precipitate (inclusion bodies in erythrocytes).
3. Others (particularly hemoglobin S) tend to interact and aggregate. The disorder produced depends both on the nature of the hemoglobin and whether it is found in heterozygous form (often referred to as the "trait"), in double heterozygous form (two abnormal hemoglobins associated, such as S · C), or in the homozygous form (example: S · S).

Sickle cell trait occurs when the host has hemoglobin A S, in the proportions of 35 to 45% hemoglobin S and 55 to 65% hemoglobin A (that is, heterozygous). The person with sickle cell trait is hematologically normal. The hemoglobin, hematocrit, and reticulocyte counts are normal. Red cell survival is also normal, indicating that there is no significant increased hemolysis under physiological conditions. However, under exceptional circumstances imposed by hypoxia, such as high altitudes, in vivo sickling may occur. We have described the exceptional case of a young man with sickle cell trait who experienced a splenic infarct while mountain climbing at a modest altitude and speculated that the lack of physical conditioning and extreme exertion caused sufficient splenic hypoxia to produce infarction.[98]

In homozygous hemoglobin S disease, actual sickling occurs in the circulation under physiologic conditions. Irreversibly sickled cells can be seen in the blood, amounting to 5 to 10% of the red blood cells; there are more of them in venous than in arterial blood.[95] These irreversibly sickled cells are rapidly removed from the circulation, and this is the primary basis for the hemolytic process. The ^{51}Cr-red cell survival half-time in sickle cell disease may be as short as 2 to 10 days.

The spleen in sickle cell anemia is the site of significant pathology. At birth and in early infancy, the spleen is of normal size; splenic reticuloendothelial activity, as measured by ^{99m}Tc-sulfur colloid scans is normal.

Toward the end of the first year of life, after some splenic enlargement in children with sickle cell disease, the spleen looses its ability to "pit" Howell-Jolly bodies and to clear ^{99m}Tc-sulfur colloid. This phenomenon, which we have designated "functional asplenia," is nearly invariable in sickle cell anemia, but unusual in other hemolytic states. In the first 4 or 5 years of life, "functional asplenia" is temporarily reversible by transfusions of normal red cells sufficient to "dilute" the patients own abnormal red cells to less than about 40% of the total.

Finally, with passing time, "functional asplenia" is replaced by anatomic asplenia as repeated episodes of infarction reduce the spleen to a fibrotic, siderotic nubbin which may occasionally be calcified.

In the other sickle hemoglobinopathies (HgbS C, S-thalassemia) function is retained by enlarged organs into later life, although repeated episodes of localized infarction may occur. One exception may be severe variants in which significant in vivo sickling occurs, as in a patient with Hgb S-O Arab disease[96] and documented functional asplenia.

Abnormalities of Contained Enzymes of Glycolysis or Hexosemonophosphate Shunt

There a number of these nonspherocytic disorders. Those involving errors of the glycolytic pathway are usually inherited as autosomal recessives. The heterozygotes do not show hemolysis, while the homozygotes have a hemolytic anemia (which is not cured by splenectomy, although it may be considerably improved). Examples are pyruvate kinase deficiency and hexokinase deficiency. The microscopic picture of the spleen in pyruvate kinase deficiency has been studied.[46]

An error of the hexosemonophosphate shunt, erythrocyte glucose-6-phosphate dehydrogenase deficiency, is a common disorder both among Blacks and certain Caucasians (particularly Greeks and Italians). There are many variants of the enzyme in different populations. The chronic hemolytic anemia can occur in mild form and usually is found in northern Europeans and is not drug related. The more common form, particularly among Blacks and Italians, is exacerbated by exposure to certain drugs (hence, this is also classified under defects of the red cell which are coupled with an exoerythrocytic factor). The enzyme glucose-6-phosphate dehydrogenase is determined by a gene carried on the X-chromosome.[47] Hence, males can have the disorder "full blown" despite only one abnormal gene. Female heterozygotes, with only one of the two X-chromosomes active in any cell, show two cell populations (normal cells and those with the enzyme deficiency) and are usually not affected by drugs. Small numbers of homozygous females can be found.

A number of drugs (primaquine) including 8-aminoquinoline (an antimarlarial) produce hemolysis in patients with glucose-6-phosphate dehydrogenase deficiency. A nearly universal acute finding in drug-induced hemolysis in such cases is the finding of Heinz bodies within the erythrocytes. The Heinz bodies are formed of denatured hemoglobin and perhaps other erythrocyte proteins. They are demonstrable by vital staining of the cells. There are thus two key questions: (1) How are Heinz bodies formed? (2) Why do they contribute to hemolysis? The mechanism is likely related to hydrogen peroxide formation due to drug-hemoglobin interactions or to drug-induced free radial production. Reduced erythrocyte gluthathione (GSH) may then be oxidized to the GSSG form or may couple with other -SH compounds to form mix disulfides. These mixed compounds can be unstable, and the mixed disulfide of hemoglobin probably represents irreversible damage of the hemoglobin, and it appears as Heinz bodies. Erythrocytes from patients with glucose-6-phosphate dehydrogenase deficiency are less able to reduce disulfide bonds due to a reduced production rate of NADPH from NADP. Presence of Heinz bodies decreases the ability of erythrocytes to pass through the splenic pulp.[48] Lubin and Desforges[49] studied erythrocyte filtration in vitro. Heinz bodies were formed by incubation of erythrocytes with acetylphenylhydrazine. The cells with Heinz bodies were noted to be more readily hemolyzed than normal cells. These workers also reviewed some of the literature on the relationship of the spleen to Heinz bodies (sequestration, fragmentation, and pitting).

Some of the mutant hemoglobins (for example, those termed Koln, Zurich, and Genova) are unstable, being denatured to some extent within circulating erythrocytes to form Heinz bodies.[50] These hemoglobins also precipitate at 50°C; hence, there is a real question as to whether they can be tagged with ^{51}Cr and then heat denatured (they might fragment or also undergo hepatic uptake). Most of the unstable hemoglobins involve β-chain substitutions near the heme moiety. Nearly half of the heme may be functionally lost by precipitation to Heinz bodies.[51] Patients with the unstable hemoglobins show what has been called "congenital Heinz body hemolytic anemia." There is chronic hemolysis, Heinz bodies are present in the erythrocytes, and there occurs a large urinary excretion of pyrroles (and the urine is very dark, particularly after splenectomy). This Heinz body formation, due to unstable hemoglobins, must be carefully distinguished from that due to drug exposure in patients with normal hemoglobins.[52]

Mechanism Uncertain

Erythropoietic Uroporphyria

This is an unusual genetically determined error, likely passed on as an autosomal recessive. The key feature is the deposition of pigment in tissues, with photosensitization. Porphyrins also are present in large amounts in erythrocyte precursors. Perhaps this accounts for the increased erythrocyte hemolysis which occurs in erythropoietic porphyria. Splenomegaly is said to occur, and splenectomy may offer amelioration of the excess erythrocyte destruction.

Erythropoietic Protoporphyria

This disorder is more common and is determined as an autosomal dominant.[53] The photosensitivity of skin can be marked ("hydroaestival"), but many individuals do not show the full syndrome. Erythrocyte precursors and circulating erythrocytes have an elevated photoporphyria content and fluoresce under U.V. light. The

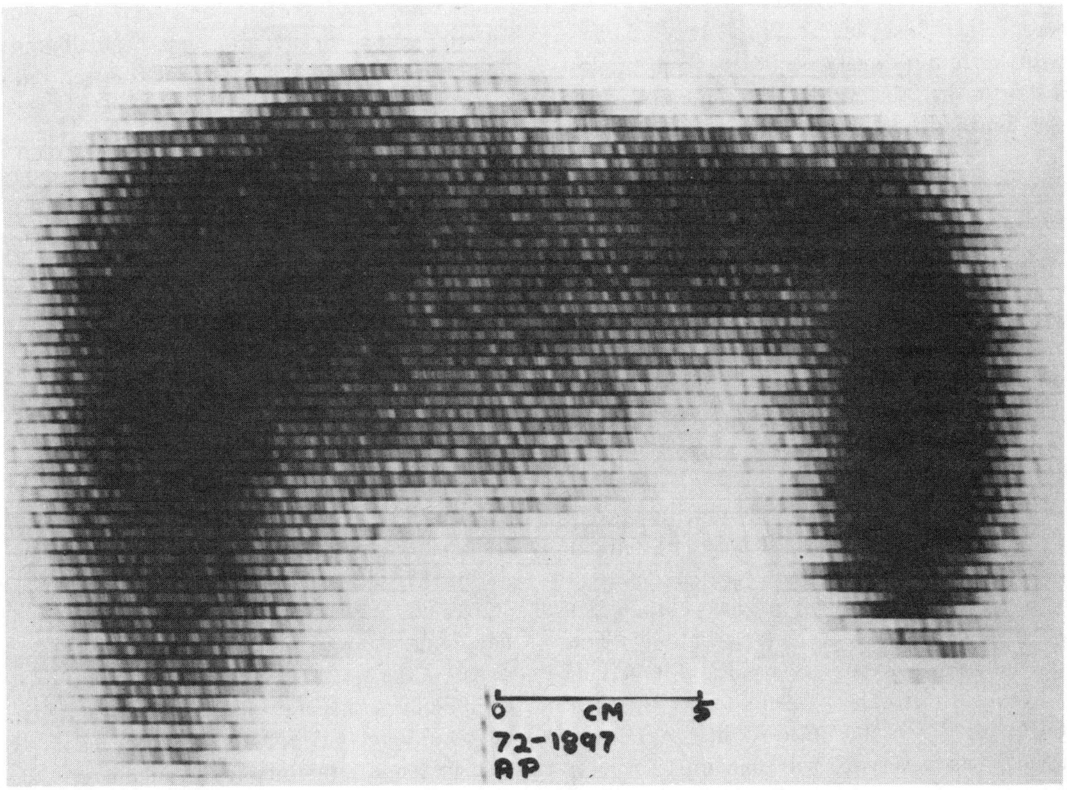

FIGURE 4. Anterior rectilinear scan (^{99m}Tc-sulfur colloid) in a 26-year-old woman with erythropoietic protoporphyria. The spleen is 12 cm in length, and the spleen-to-liver ratio (per unit area) is 90:60. Case 72-1897.

single case we have seen (Figure 4) was characterized by a spleen 12 cm in length, with a shift of radioactive colloid to that organ.

Acquired, Such as in Vitamin B_{12} and Folic Acid Deficiency

The erythrocytes in pernicious anemia are clearly abnormal in size, and likely in biochemical composition as well. ^{51}Cr-red-cell studies show a slightly shortened survival in this disorder, and major hemolysis might occur in bone marrow (ineffective erythropoiesis).

Defects within the Red Cell, but Coupled with an Exoerythrocytic Factor

Congenital Deficiency of Glucose-6-phosphate Dehydrogenase (When Presented with Various Exogenous Drugs)

This was discussed above.

Hereditary Spherocytosis

This is a genetically determined defect (autosomal dominant) of the red cell membrane,[54] which apparently also occurs due to spontaneous mutations in about 20% of the cases. The abnormality is related to increased permeability of the erythrocyte wall to sodium, leading ultimately to loss of plasma membrane lipid, causing the cells to assume a more spherical form than normal. Jaundice, splenomegaly, and increased osmotic fragility are hallmarks of the disease. The spleen is nearly always enlarged, even in the otherwise relatively asymptomatic individual. Indeed, the disorder is often found in multiple members of a family after it is identified in one individual.

Hereditary spherocytosis is of interest since it represents the interaction of an intraerythrocytic factor with the spleen. Splenectomy is almost always followed by a good response in hereditary spherocytosis. Crosby[55] has pointed out that this is a disease in which splenectomy is followed by polycythemia (erythrocyte counts of 6.5 to 7.5 million, without specific symptoms). This is not unique since polycythemia can apparently occur in some cases of thalassemia after splenectomy. Wiley[56] reported on studies utilizing ^{51}Cr-spherocytes. When the ^{51}Cr-spherocytes were transfused into normal recipients, their survival was shorter than that within the circulation of the donor. Further, a mother-to-son transfusion (both of whom had hereditary spherocytosis and intact spleens) of radiolabeled spherocytes showed a shorter survival half-time of the transfused spherocytes than of the recipient's cells. These findings were attributed to a "selective" splenic reticuloendothelial blockade. The selectivity was in the fact that the patient's own spherocytes were less avidly trapped than those of the donor. Wiley[56] concluded that both cell shape and the reticuloendothelial blockade were of importance in determining the degree of hemolysis.

A variation on the usual picture of herediatry spherocytosis has been reported.[57] The patient had anemia, splenomegaly, leg ulcers, and retarded growth as a child. A high median corpuscular fragility was decreased after splenectomy. The autohemolysis observed was atypical for hereditary spherocytosis. The patient's red cells, when tagged with ^{51}Cr and injected into a normal recipient, had a survival half-time of 12.5 min. After splenectomy, the patient's red cells had a survival half-time of 90 min in a recipient (improved, but still quite short). Hence, "splenic conditioning" of erythrocytes (with adverse effects on the cells) may be occurring in hereditary spherocytosis. This patient was also interesting because of the elevated Howell-Jolly body content of erythrocytes.

The fine structure of the spleen in hereditary spherocytosis has been studied.[46,58] Erythrocyte stagnation within splenic cords was stated to be due to lack of deformability since there were no "squeezed" erythrocytes seen passing through the sinus walls. An increased content of macrophages in the cords might also have contributed to impairment of red cell passage. Decreased red cell deformability, in other disorders, can also be expected to result in hemolysis due to decreased ability to traverse the spleen. It has been pointed out that hypophosphatemia can be associated with "rigid red cells" and hemolysis.[59] Spherocytic erythrocytes, with hemolysis, have been noted in a patient with hypothyroidism (and high-sodium, low-potassium erythrocytes)[60] and in magnesium deprivation in the rat.[61] Various congenital nonspherocytic anemias[62] are also known, often based on an enzymatic deficiency.

Hereditary Elliptocytosis

This disorder, also transmitted as an autosomal dominant, appears to be well tolerated by most of its hosts.[63] Perhaps as many as 1 person in 4,000 shows elliptocytes (and the erythrocytes of camels and llamas are said to be elliptocytic). The specific defect in the erythrocytes is unknown, but increased sodium permeability has also been demonstrated, as in hereditary spherocytosis. In perhaps one case in ten, a severe hemolytic anemia can occur. While some cases might represent the exceedingly rare homozygote (carrying two genes for the autosomal dominant), apparently most do not. Splenomegaly can occur in some cases of hereditary elliptocytosis, but massive enlargement does not appear to be necessary for the severe hemolytic form of the disease (Figure 5). Splenectomy results in improvement of the hemolytic form of the disease. Interestingly, splenectomy does not result in an improvement in the elliptical shape of the circulating erythrocytes (and this may even worsen).

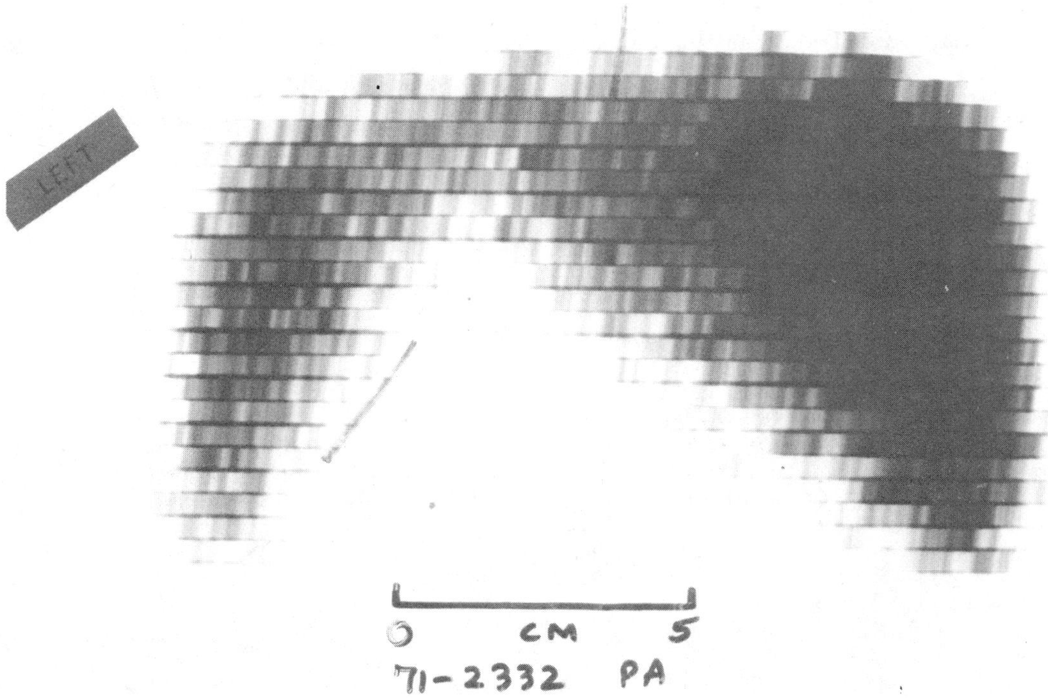

FIGURE 5. Posterior rectilinear scan (^{99m}Tc-sulfur colloid) in a 5-month-old boy with hereditary elliptocytosis. The spleen is slightly enlarged (8 cm). The child had severe hemolytic disease. The hematocrit at birth was 22. This was raised to 33 following transfusion. After discharge he did poorly, and the hematocrit on readmission was 12 (hemoglobin = 4.7). Case 71-2332.

REFERENCES

1. **Greene, M. W., Lebowitz, E., Richards, P., and Hillman, M.,** Production of ^{52}Fe for medical use, *J. Nucl. Med.,* 11, 323, 1970.
2. **Lilien, D. L., Berger, H. G., Anderson, D. P., and Bennett, L. R.,** ^{111}In-chloride: a new agent for bone marrow imaging, *J. Nucl. Med.,* 14, 184, 1973.
3. **Mayer, K., Clarke, L., Ziminski, E., and Laughlan, J. S.,** Application of absolute quantitative scanning of marrow and spleen in a cancer hospital, *J. Nucl. Med.,* 12, 382, 1971.
4. **Wagner, H. N., Jr.,** Technical details of common procedures. Sites of hematopoiesis, in *Principles of Nuclear Medicine,* Wagner, H. N., Jr., Ed., W. B. Saunders, Philadelphia, 1968, 843.
5. **Amorosi, E., Gary, S. K., and Karpatkin, S.,** Heterogeneity of human platelet population with (^{75}Se) selenomethionine, *Br. J. Haematol.,* 21, 227, 1971.
6. **Prost-Dvojakovic, R. J., Doumenc, J., Reva, C., Zittoun, R., and Samama, M.,** Functional platelet study in sub-acute-myelo-monocytic leukemia and resistant anemia, *Sem. Hop. Paris,* 48, 1971, 1972.
7. **Cardamone, J. M., Edson, J. R., McArthur, J. R., and Jacob, H. S.,** Abnormalities of platelet function in the myeloproliferative disorders, *JAMA,* 221, 270, 1972.
8. **Elgjo, R. F. and Hovig, T.,** Ultrastructural studies of platelet activation and aggregation in normal spleen from different species, *Scand. J. Haematol.,* 9, 587, 1972.
9. **Harker, L. A. and Finch, C. A.,** Thrombokinetics in man, *J. Clin. Invest.,* 48, 963, 1969.
10. **Aster, R. H.,** Effect of anticoagulant and ABO incompatibility on recovery of transfused human platelets, *Blood,* 26, 732, 1965.
11. **Paulus, J. M., Ed.,** *Platelet Kinetics: Radioisotopic, Cytological, Mathematical and Clinical Aspects,* American Elsevier, New York, 1971, 447.
12. **Marsh, G. W., Lewis, S. M., and Szur, L.,** The use of ^{51}Cr-labelled heat-denatured red cells to study splenic function. II. Splenic atrophy in thrombocythaemia, *Br. J. Haematol.,* 12, 167, 1966.

13. **Gehrmann, G. and Elbers, C.,** Thrombopenisches Hypersplenies syndrome bei splenomegaler Leberzirrhose, *Dtsch. Med. Wochenschr.*, 95, 1429, 1970.
14. **Harker, L. A.,** The role of the spleen in thrombokinetics, *J. Lab. Clin. Med.*, 77, 247, 1971.
15. **Aster, R. H.,** Pooling of platelets in the spleen: role in the pathogenesis of "hypersplenic" thrombocytopenia, *J. Clin. Invest.*, 45, 645, 1966.
16. **Kutti, J., Weinfeld, A., and Westin, J.,** The relationship between splenic platelet pool and spleen size, *Scand. J. Haematol.*, 9, 351, 1972.
17. **Abrahamsen, A. F.,** Effects of an enlarged splenic platelet pool in Hodgkin's disease, *Scand. J. Haematol.*, 9, 153, 1972.
18. **Kutti, J. and Weinfeld, A.,** Platelet production and platelet survival in polycythaemia vera with special reference to the spleen size, *Scand. J. Haematol.*, 9, 97, 1972.
19. **Gehrmann, G.,** Milz und normaler Thrombocytenhaushalt, in *Die Milz,* Lennert, K. and Harms, D., Eds., Springer-Verlag, Berlin, 1970, 276.
20. **Najean, Y. and Ardaillou, N.,** The sequestration site of platelets in idiopathic thrombocytopenic purpura: its correlation with the results of splenectomy, *Br. J. Haematol.*, 21, 153, 1971.
21. **Harker, L. A. and Slichter, S. J.,** Platelet and fibrinogen consumption in man, *N. Engl. J. Med.*, 287, 999, 1972.
22. **Athens, J. W., Mauer, A. M., Ashenbrucker, H., Cartwright, G. E., and Wintrobe, M. M.,** Leukocyte studies. I. A method for labeling leukocytes with diisopropyl fluorophosphate (DFP 32), *Blood,* 15, 303, 1959.
23. **McCall, M. S., Sutherland, D. A., Eintraut, A. M., and Lanz, H.,** The tagging of leukemic leukocytes with radioactive chromium and measurement of the in vivo cell survival, *J. Lab. Clin. Med.*, 45, 717, 1955.
24. **Duvall, C. P. and Perry, S.,** The use of 51-chromium in the study of leukocyte kinetics in chronic myelocytic leukemia, *J. Lab. Clin. Med.*, 71, 614, 1968.
25. **Spencer, R. P., McPhedran, P., Finch, S. C., and Morgan, W. S.,** Persistent neutrophilic leukocytosis associated with idiopathic functional asplenia, *J. Nucl. Med.*, 15, 224, 1972.
26. **Dibos, P. E., Judisch, J. M., Spaulding, M. B., Wagner, H. N., Jr., and McIntyre, P. A.,** Scanning the reticuloendothelial systems (RES) in hematological diseases, *Johns Hopkins Med. J.*, 130, 68, 1972.
27. **Garriga, S. and Crosby, W. H.,** The incidence of leukemia in families of patients with hypoplasia of the marrow, *Blood,* 14, 1008, 1959.
28. **Beard, M. E. J.,** Fanconi's anaemia: recent advances in diagnosis and treatment, *Proc. R. Soc. Med.*, 65, 747, 1972.
29. **Coutinho, V., Falcao, R. P., and Bottura, C.,** Cytogenetic observations in congenital familial panmyleopathy (Fanconi's syndrome), *Nouv. Rev. Fr. Hematol.*, 11, 781, 1971.
30. **Swift, M., Sholman, K., and Gilmour, D.,** Diabetes mellitus and the gene for Fanconi's anemia, *Science,* 178, 308, 1972.
31. **Shwachman, H., Diamond, L. K., Oski, F. A., and Khaw, K. T.,** The syndrome of pancreatic insufficiency and bone marrow dysfunction, *J. Pediatr.*, 65, 645, 1964.
32. **Taybi, M., Mitchell, A., and Friedman, G. D.,** Metaphyseal dysostosis and the associated syndrome of pancreatic insufficiency and blood disorders, *Radiology,* 93, 563, 1969.
33. **Bottiger, L. E. and Westerholm, B.,** Aplastic anaemia. I. Incidence and aetiology, *Acta Med. Scand.*, 192, 315, 1972.
34. **Bottiger, L. E. and Westerholm, B.,** Aplastic anaemia. II. Drug-induced aplastic anaemia, *Acta Med. Scand.*, 192, 319, 1972.
35. **Bottiger, L. E. and Westerholm, B.,** Aplastic anaemia. III. Aplastic anaemia and infectious hepatitis, *Acta Med. Scand.*, 192, 323, 1972.
36. **Corneo, G., Cortellaro, M., and Maiolo, A. T.,** Aplastic anemia: some clinical and laboratory aspects and an evaluation of the androgen-glucocorticoid treatment, *Acta Haematol.*, 46, 50, 1971.
37. **Diamond, L. K. and Blackfan, K. D.,** Hypoplastic anemia, *Am. J. Dis. Child.*, 56, 464, 1938.
38. **Allen, D. M. and Diamond, L. K.,** Congenital (erythroid) hypoplastic anemia-cortisone treated, *Am. J. Dis. Child.*, 102, 416, 1961.
39. **Hammond, D. and Lieberman, E.,** The hemolytic uremic syndrome: renal cortical thrombotic microangiopathy, *Arch. Intern. Med.*, 126, 816, 1970.
40. **Dameshek, W.,** Hypersplenism, *Bull. N. Y. Acad. Med.*, 31, 113, 1955.
41. **Spencer, R. P., Rockoff, M. L., and Spector, H.,** Studies on quantitation of the ^{51}Cr-erythrocyte spleen-to-liver ratio, *J. Nucl. Med.*, 9, 51, 1968.
42. **Jandl, J. H., Greenberg, M. S., Yonemoto, R. H., and Castle, W. B.,** Clinical determination of the sites of red cell sequestration in hemolytic anemias, *J. Clin. Invest.*, 35, 842, 1956.
43. **McCurdy, P. R. and Rath, G.E.,** Splenectomy in hemolytic anemia: results predicted by body scanning after injection of ^{51}Cr-tagged red cells, *N. Engl. J. Med.*, 259, 459, 1958.
44. **Shohet, S. B.,** Hemolysis and changes in erythrocyte membrane lipids, *N. Engl. J. Med.* 286, 577, 1972.
45. **Cooper, R. A. and Shattil, S. J.,** Mechanisms of hemolysis, the minimal red cell defect, *N. Engl. J. Med.*, 285, 1514, 1971.
46. **Bowman, H. S. and Oski, F. A.,** Splenic macrophage interaction with red cells in pyruvate kinase deficiency and hereditary spherocytosis, *Vox Sang.*, 19, 168, 1970.

47. **Childs, B., Zinkham, W., Browne, E. A., Kimbro, E. L., and Torbert, J. V.,** A genetic study of a defect in glutathione metabolism of the erythrocyte, *Bull. Johns Hopkins Hosp.*, 102, 21, 1958.
48. **Rifkind, R. A.,** Heinz body anemia: an ultrastructural study. II. Red cell sequestration and destruction, *Blood,* 26, 433, 1965.
49. **Lubin, A. and Desforges, J. F.,** Effect of Heinz bodies on red cell deformability, *Blood,* 39, 658, 1972.
50. **Jacob, H. S.,** Mechanisms of Heinz body formation and attachment to red cell membranes, *Semin. Hematol.,* 7, 341, 1970.
51. **Jacob, H. and Winterhalter, K.,** Unstable hemoglobins: the role of heme loss in Heinz body formation, *Proc. Natl. Acad. Sci. U.S.A.,* 65, 697, 1970.
52. **George, J. N., Miller, D. R., and Weed, R. I.,** Heinz body hemolytic anemias, *N. Y. State J. Med.,* 70, 2574, 1970.
53. **Donaldson, E. M., Donaldson, A. D., and Rimington, C.,** Erythropoietic protoporphyria: a family study, *Br. Med. J.,* 1, 659, 1967.
54. **Jacob, H. S.,** Hereditary spherocytosis: a disease of the red cell membrane, *Semin. Hematol.,* 2, 139, 1965.
55. **Crosby, W. H.,** Hyposplenism: an inquiry into normal functions of the spleen, *Annu. Rev. Med.,* 14, 349, 1963.
56. **Wiley, J. S.,** Red cell survival studies in hereditary spherocytosis, *J. Clin. Invest.,* 49, 666, 1970.
57. **Wiley, J. S. and Firkin, B. G.,** An unusual variant of hereditary spherocytosis, *Am. J. Med.,* 48, 63, 1970.
58. **Molnar, Z. and Rappaport, H.,** Fine structure of the red pulp of the spleen in hereditary spherocytosis, *Blood,* 39, 81, 1972.
59. **Jacob, H. S. and Amsden, T.,** Acute hemolytic anemia with rigid red cells in hypophosphatemia, *N. Engl. J. Med.,* 285, 1446, 1971.
60. **Leone, N. T., Narasimhan, P., and Watson-Williams, E. J.,** Hypothyroidism with atypical spherocytic hemolytic anemia with high-sodium, low-potassium red cells, *J. Clin. Endocrinol.,* 33, 548, 1971.
61. **Oken, M. M., Lichtman, M. A., Miller, D. R., and Leblond, P.,** Spherocytic hemolytic disease during magnesium deprivation in the rat, *Blood,* 38, 468, 1971.
62. **Nagaratnam, N.,** Congenital non-spherocytic haemolytic anaemias: study of four cases in Ceylon, *Med. J. Aust.,* 2, 273, 1970.
63. **Jensson, O., Jonasson, T., and Olafsson, O.,** Hereditary elliptocytosis in Iceland, *Br. J. Haematol.,* 13, 844, 1967.
64. **Korst, D. R., Nixon, J. C., Boblitt, D. E., and Quirk, J.,** Studies of selective splenic sequestration of erythrocytes labeled with radioactive mercurihydroxypropane (MHP), *J. Lab. Clin. Med.,* 66, 788, 1965.
65. **Gray, S. J. and Sterling, K.,** The tagging of red cells and plasma proteins with radioactive chromium, *J. Clin. Invest.,* 29, 1604, 1950.
66. **Aas, K. A. and Gardner, F. A.,** Survival of blood platelets with chromium 51, *J. Clin. Invest.,* 37, 1257, 1958.
67. **Cohen, P. F., Gardner, A., and Barnett, G. D.,** Reclassification of thrombocytopenias by the Cr^{51} method for measuring platelet life span, *N. Engl. J. Med.,* 264, 1294, 1350, 1961.
68. **Bedson, S. P.,** Blood-platelet anti-serum: its specificity and role in the experimental production of purpura, *J. Pathol. Bacteriol.,* 25, 94, 1922.
69. **Gore, I., Takada, M., and Austin, J.,** Ultrasound basis of experimental thrombocytopenic purpura, *Arch. Pathol.,* 90, 197, 1970.
70. **Harrington, W. J., Minnich, V., Hollingsworth, J. W., and Moore, C. V.,** Demonstration of patients with thrombocytopenic purpura, *J. Lab. Clin. Med.,* 38, 1, 1951.
71. **Karpatkin, S., Strick, N., and Siskind, G. W.,** Detection of splenic anti-platelet antibody synthesis in idiopathic autoimmune thrombocytopenic purpura (ATP), *Br. J. Haematol.,* 23, 167, 1972.
72. **Karpatkin, S., Garg, S. K., and Siskind, G. W.,** Autoimmune thrombocytopenic purpura and the compensated thrombocytolytic state, *Am. J. Med.,* 51, 1, 1971.
73. **Karpatkin, S., Strick, N., Karpatkin, M. B., and Siskind, G. W.,** Cumulative experience in the detection of antiplatelet antibody in 234 patients with idiopathic thrombocytopenic purpura, systemic lupus erythematosus and other clinical disorders, *Am. J. Med.,* 52, 776, 1972.
74. **Weinreich, J., Milz and Morbus Werlhof,** in *Die Milz,* Lennert, K. and Harms, D., Eds., Springer-Verlag, Berlin, 1970, 285.
75. **McMillan, R., Longmire, R. L., Yelenosky, R., Smith, R. S., and Craddock, C. G.,** Innumoglobulin synthesis in vitro by splenic tissue in idiopathic thrombocytopenic purpura, *N. Engl. J. Med.,* 286, 681, 1972.
76. **Wilkinson, J.,** The nature and classification of Onyalai, *East Afr. Med. J.,* 30, 243, 1953.
77. **Harris, M. B., Murphy, S., and Oski, F. A.,** Onyalai (a form of idiopathic thrombocytopenic purpura) in the United States, *Clin. Pediatr.,* 11, 705, 1972.
78. **Amorisi, E. and Ultmann, J.,** Thrombotic thrombocytopenic purpura, *Medicine,* 45, 139, 1966.
79. **Tartaglia, A. P. and Burkhart, P. T.,** Thrombotic thrombocytopenic purpura: remission following hemodialysis, *JAMA,* 218, 999, 1971.
80. **Klippel, M. and Trenaunay, P.,** Du noevus variquex osteohypertrophique, *Arch. Gen. Med.,* 185, 641, 1900.
81. **Lachmann, D., Lechner, K., Millesi, H., Vinazzer, H., and Zweymuller, E.,** Verbrauchs coagulopathie bei Klippel-Trenanunay-Syndrome in Sauglingsalter, *Monatsschr. Kinderheilkd.,* 118, 592, 1970.
82. **Kasabach, H. G. and Merritt, K. K.,** Capillary haemangioma with extensive purpura, *Am. J. Dis. Child.,* 59, 1063, 1940.

83. **Clancy, R. L., Howard, M., Sawers, R., and Firkin, B. G.,** Qualitative platelet abnormalities in a patient with chronic idiopathic thrombocytopenic purpura (ITP), *Austr. N. Z. J. Med.,* 3, 224, 1971.
84. **Ross, C. F. and Schiller, K. F. R.,** Hamartoma of spleen associated with thrombocytopenia, *J. Pathol.,* 105, 62, 1971.
85. **Crosby, W. H.,** Splenectomy in hematologic disorders, *N. Engl. J. Med.,* 286, 1252, 1972.
86. **Hughes-Jones, N. C. and Szur, L.,** Determination of the sites of red-cell destruction using ^{51}Cr-labeled cells, *Br. J. Haematol.,* 3, 320, 1957.
87. **Scott, J. L., Davidson, J. G., Marino, J. V., and McMillan, R.,** Leukocyte labeling with ^{51}Chromium III. The kinetics of normal lymphocytes, *Blood,* 40, 276, 1972.
88. **Williams, E. D., Ahuja, S., Szur, L., Lewis, S. M., and Glass, H. I.,** Rate of loss of ^{51}Cr from the spleen, *J. Nucl. Med.,* 13, 686, 1972.
89. **Szur, L.,** Surface counting in the assessment of sites of red cell destruction, *Br. J. Haematol.,* 18, 591, 1970.
90. **Schloesser, L. L., Korst, D. R., Clatanoff, D. V., and Schilling, R. F.,** Radioactivity over the spleen and liver following transfusion of chromium-51 labeled erythrocytes in hemolytic anemia, *J. Clin. Invest.,* 36, 1470, 1957.
91. **Goldberg, A., Hutchinson, H. E., MacDonald, E.,** Radiochromium in the selection of patients with haemolytic anaemia for splenectomy, *Lancet,* 1, 109, 1966.
92. **Lewis, S. M., Szur, L., and Dacie, J. V.,** The pattern of erythrocyte destruction in haemolytic anaemia, as studied with radioactive chromium, *Br. J. Haematol.,* 6, 122, 1960.
93. **Pearson, H. A. and Vertrees, K. M.,** Site of binding of chromium-51 to haemoglobin, *Nature,* 189, 1019, 1961.
94. **Gaag, S. K., Amorosi, E. L., and Karpatkin, S.,** Use of the megathrombocyte as an index of megakaryocyte number, *N. Engl. J. Med.,* 284, 11, 1971.
95. **Pearson, H. A., Schiebler, G. L., Krovetz, L. H., Bartley, T. D., and David, J. K.,** Sickle cell anemia associated with tetralogy of Fallot, *N. Engl. J. Med.,* 273, 1079, 1965.
96. **Milner, P. F., Miller, C., Grey, R., Seaking, M., deJong, W. W., and Went, L. N.,** Hemoglobin O Arab in four negro families and its interaction with hemoglobin S and hemoglobin C, *N. Engl. J. Med.,* 283, 1418, 1970.
97. **Jamshidi, K., Ansari, A., Garcia, M. C., and Swaim, W. E.,** Postsplenectomy thrombocythemia: an unmasked myeloproliferative disorder, *J. Am. Geriatr. Soc.,* 21, 419, 1973.
98. **O'Brien, R. T., Pearson, H. A., Godley, J. A., and Spencer, R. P.,** Splenic infarct and sickle-(cell) trait, *N. Engl. J. Med.,* 287, 720, 1972.

Chapter 14

AUTOIMMUNE DISORDERS

It was classically believed that an animal could not produce antibodies against any of its own proteins ("horror autotoxicus"). Evidence for the existence of "autoimmune" disease is convincing. In some cases, "autoimmune" hemolytic anemia occurs, with specific antibodies against red cell antigens. In numerous other instances, antibodies against organs, tissues, or subcomponents can be demonstrated. The evidence in certain of these disorders is well documented, but in some it is less convincing. Utilizing the term "autoimmune" disorders as a focal point, information is included in this section about splenic size and function in several diseases in which autoimmunity against organs, tissues, and tissue components is likely.

GRAFT-VERSUS-HOST REACTION

A host-versus-graft reaction can potentially occur any time a foreign tissue is introduced into a recipient (blood transfusion, organ transplantation). There is some information available as to splenic size and function in these cases (see the section on immunization). A graft-versus-host reaction *can* occur when the introduced or engrafted tissues are immunologically competent (i.e., lymphocytes) and can, themselves, initiate an immune response. There are few cases in which this could occur in man; injection of foreign bone marrow is one instance. Data are almost nonexistent on the response of the human spleen in such cases.

There have been studies on the response of the spleen to various antigenic stimuli such as skin grafting. Gotjamanos[1] noted that mice bearing skin allografts and isografts have splenomegaly; a first peak in size occurred 8 to 12 days after transplantation and a second peak at 22 days. The spleens of isografted mice showed erythropoiesis, with little alteration in lymphatic elements. Allografted mice revealed granulopoiesis and erythropoiesis in the spleen in the course of the first peak of splenomegaly. During the second, there was hematopoiesis and lymphatic activity. Isografted and allografted mice showed increased blood clearance of opsonized ^{32}P-*Salmonella typhimurium* C5.[2] Utilizing carbon as the colloid, there was increased phagocytic activity in mice with small skin grafts, but not in those with large grafts. It was hypothesized that the surgical trauma of large skin grafts depleted serum opsonins, thus limiting splenic phagocytosis. However, Blamey and co-workers[3] noted that reticuloendothelial activity did not parallel lymphoid system activity in transplantation immunity.

E. A. Cornelius and R. P. Spencer studied splenic function by measuring the accumulation of ^{99m}Tc-sulfur colloid in mice undergoing runting (a wasting disease). The mice were BA females, injected intraperitoneally with 200×10^6 spleen cells from strain A mice. On days 7, 8, 11, and 12 post injection two runting animals and two controls were studied. Each was injected with 0.1 ml (90 μCi) of the radiocolloid via a tail vein. Twenty minutes later, the mice were sacrificed and the blood, tail, kidneys, liver, and spleen weighed and counted for radioactivity. There was only slight activity in the blood, tail, and kidneys. Activity in the liver and spleen was expressed as counts/gram, and the mean value of the ratio of spleen (counts/g)/liver (counts/g) was calculated as that of runting mice/control mice. The ratio was less than 1,

Day of runting	7	8	11	12
$\frac{\text{Runt ratio}}{\text{Control Ratio}}$; Ratio = $\frac{\text{Spleen (counts/g)}}{\text{Liver (counts/g)}}$	0.67	0.61	0.37	0.37

indicating that either the liver was becoming more active in trapping radiocolloid (per gram of tissue) or, more likely, that the spleen was becoming less active. These results suggest that some of the newly accumulating cells during runting may not be competent to take up the radiocolloid. Splenic enlargement in the graft-versus-host reaction is followed by contraction of the organ in the preterminal stages of runting. There are data in the literature on the nature of the cells accumulating in the spleen in the graft-versus-host reaction.[4] It has been reported that splenectomy decreases mortality and prolongs survival.[5] The kinetics of splenomegaly in the graft-versus-host reaction have been documented.[30] The time course of splenic enlargement in hydrops fetalis (part of the maternal versus fetal reaction in feto-maternal blood incompatibility) is less well studied, and here most of the splenomegaly is due to extramedullary erythropoiesis.

There is a variant of the runting or wasting syndrome that is of great interest because of its implications in the treatment of human disease. In rodents, shielding the spleen or lower extremities during irradiation of the whole body reduces mortality. It has been shown that the shielded spleen or bone marrow allows regrowth of the hemotopoietic system by proliferation and spread of the remaining cells.

When supralethally irradiated CBA mice are given syngeneic bone marrow and survive the effects of radiation, they eventually develop a wasting syndrome from which they die.[6] Irradiated mice, given midlethal whole body exposures, develop a wasting syndrome some weeks later,[7] which is prevented by injection of syngeneic lymphocytes or bone marrow. It has also been reported that lymphocytes from adults of the same strain also prevent the wasting syndrome.[8] The regrowth of erythroid elements is likely necessary for prevention of early deaths, while lymphoid regrowth is necessary for avoidance of late deaths in the irradiated animals. Although the thymus plays an important role, this will not be discussed. There is some suggestion that splenic transplantation may help prevent radiation-produced wasting disease.[9]

The eventual fate of allografts depends on the genetic relationship of the host and the donor. In particular, one genetic system (termed the HL-A locus) appears to play a principal role in whether tissues are histocompatible in man. A number of tissues, including *spleen and lung,* can be used to obtain antigens of the HL-A system. Of great interest is the finding by Reisfeld and co-workers[10] that these antigens can be extracted from lymphocytes grown from the peripheral blood of donors. The relationship of these antigens to tissue rejection phenomena is slowly becoming clearer, but it is still uncertain whether they are of importance in determining susceptibility to other disease. Zervas and co-workers[11] reported that the frequency of the HL-A5 leukocyte phenotype was higher in patients with Hodgkin's disease than in control individuals. Techniques have been reported for separating spleen cells,[12] and it might eventually be possible to investigate subpopulations of cells for their antigenicity.

Tumors can elicit immunologic responses in their hosts. Mice given syngeneic or allogeneic tumors developed changes in the splenic white pulp.[34] These changes resembled those following introduction of other antigens. The elevated splenic accumulation of radiocolloid, seen in some patients with malignant melanoma, has been related to stimulation of the reticuloendothelial system.[32] The spleen, however, does not play a role in certain other immune phenomena, such as the development of immune thyroiditis in monkeys.[33]

Rheumatoid Arthritis

Rheumatoid arthritis is a generalized disease of unknown etiology in which the joints are especially, but not exclusively, affected. In the rheumatoid variants which will be discussed, a frequent association with splenic abnormalities is noted (Figure 1). Although the precise pathogenesis of the rheumatoid disorders is not understood, a relationship to an antigen which initiates production of an antibody in plasma cells of the synovium is suspected. The antigen-antibody complex may bring about production of rheumatoid factors by plasma cells and by lymph nodes.

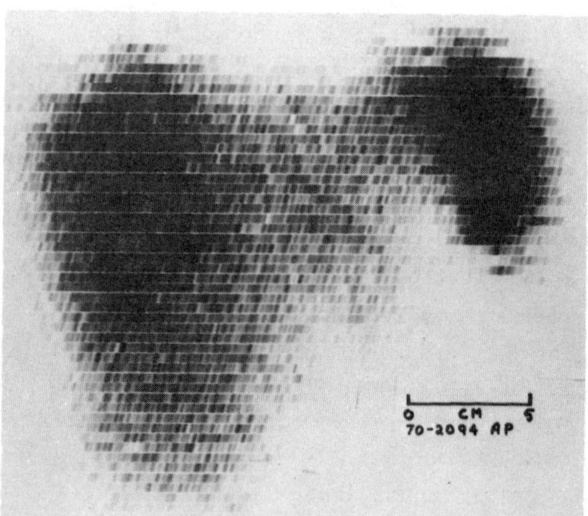

FIGURE 1. Anterior rectilinear scan (^{99m}Tc-sulfur colloid) in a 52-year-old woman. The patient had a long history of rheumatoid arthritis and was on gold therapy. Although the spleen was not enlarged (10 cm), there was a shift of the radiocolloid. Thrombocytopenia was present. There was also a shortened ^{51}Cr-erythrocyte survival (T½ = 14 days). Case 70-2094.

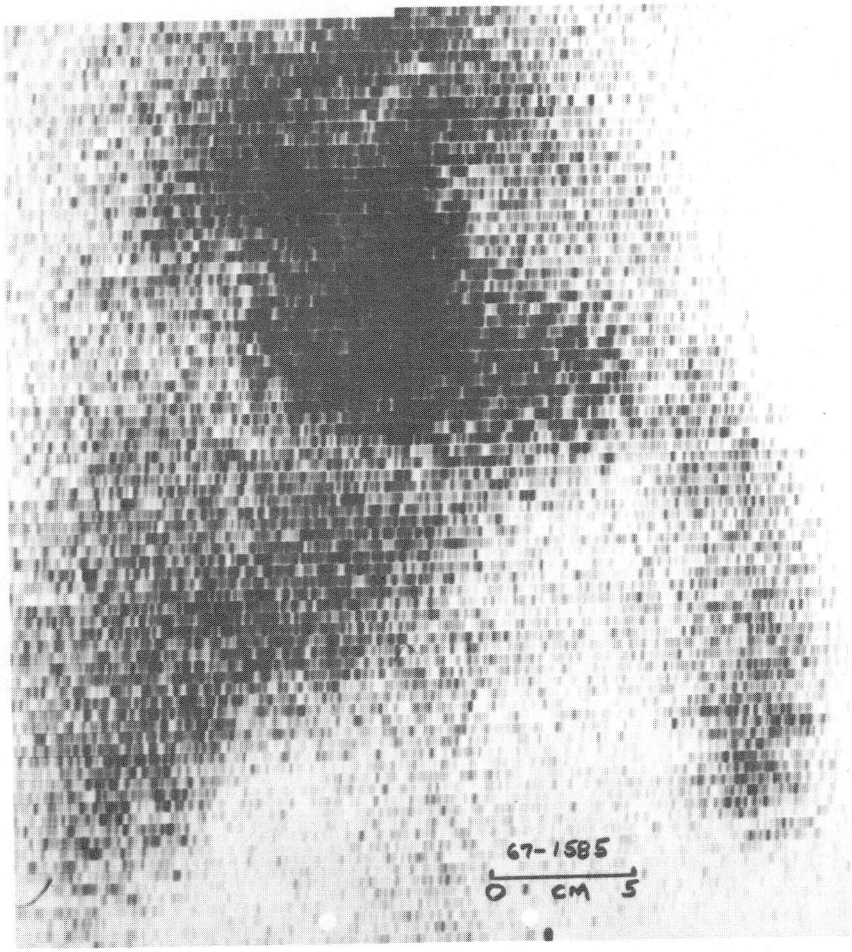

FIGURE 2. Anterior rectilinear scan performed with ^{113m}In-transferrin. The patient is a 63-year-old man with long-standing rheumatoid arthritis. The large splenic blood pool can be seen even from the anterior view. Case 67-1585.

Resultant phagocytosis of these complexes with release of lysosomal enzymes may then produce the characteristic tissue inflammation.

During the active phase of rheumatoid arthritis, anemia is common. This is usually normocytic, although it may be hypochromic. However, iron and splenectomy do not have a beneficial effect. Many patients with long-standing rheumatoid arthritis, particularly rheumatoid spondylitis, have splenomegaly (Figure 2). An interesting variant was described by Felty,[13] consisting of chronic arthritis, splenomegaly, and leukopenia. Although multiple cases have been reported subsequently, and Felty's syndrome is well established as a clinical entity, there is uncertainty as to whether this is truly a distinct disorder (especially since it occurs primarily in far-advanced rheumatoid arthritis). The leukopenia may be associated with pancytopenia. Splenectomy usually ameliorates hematologic abnormalities[14] but has no effect on the arthritis. In a long-term follow-up (1 to 13½ years) of patients with Felty's syndrome who underwent splenectomy, neutropenia was relieved in two thirds of the cases.[15] The histological features of the spleen have been described in this disease[16] as well as spleen weight and values for the red cell survival. Interestingly, after splenectomy in Felty's syndrome, there does not seem to be an increased incidence of infection[15] (perhaps because of improvement of the white cell count). Wimer and Sloan[17] have described the remission of Felty's syndrome with testosterone therapy over a long period.

Arroyo and Aubert[18] in a brief note described

an atrophied spleen in rheumatoid arthritis. Three patients with rheumatoid arthritis showed thrombocythemia and a small spleen. This "obverse" of Felty's syndrome might have been related to the use of corticoids in these cases. Sjogren's syndrome (dry eyes, dry mouth, enlarged lacrimal and salivary glands) is often associated with rheumatoid arthritis, but specific alterations of the spleen have not been reported in such cases. In one series, 11 of 16 patients with Felty's syndrome had Sjogren's syndrome as well.[16]

Rheumatoid arthritis can occur in children, and the disorder beginning prior to puberty is termed Still's disease.[19] Still had stressed the triad of arthritis, splenomegaly, and lymphadenopathy. Schaller and co-workers pointed out the finding of hepatomegaly in juvenile rheumatoid arthritis.[29] In most series of juvenile rheumatoid arthritis, lymphadenopathy is noted in nearly two thirds of the cases, while splenomegaly can be found in about one third of the afflicted children. However, leukopenia is not a feature of juvenile rheumatoid arthritis; indeed, leukocytosis is usual.

Systemic Lupus Erythematosus

Systemic lupus erythematosus (SLE) is a disease which has a predilection for females between 20 to 40 years of age. The disorder is of immense interest because it is characterized by serum proteins which have many features of antibodies. Indeed, serum globulins, which react with erythrocytes, leukocytes, platelets, and systemic tissues, are found. Many patients have a false positive serologic test for syphilis, but the most characteristic antibody is termed the LE factor (likely involved in the phagocytosis of nucleoprotein). In addition, antinuclear factors can frequently be demonstrated. Drugs, especially hydralazine and dilantin, often appear to be associated with the onset of SLE, but this may actually be the unmasking of a latent disease. Enlargement of the lymph glands can be quite prominent in the cervical and axillary regions. Splenomegaly occurs in about one fourth of the cases of systemic lupus erythematosus, but it is rarely massive (Figure 3).

Celiac-sprue Disease

Celiac disease is a disorder of childhood, characterized by malabsorption and diarrhea. There is much evidence that this disease is very similar to nontropical sprue in adults (and the term celiac-sprue is sometimes used). In addition to the malabsorption and diarrhea, there is an abnormal small bowel mucosa as revealed by peroral mucosal biopsy. There can be remission of the disease when gluten and gliadin (wheat proteins) are excluded from the diet. The spleen is often clinically small in sprue.[20] Lymphoreticular dysfunction has been recognized in this disease.[21] It is unclear whether the malabsorption contributes to the lymphoreticular problem or whether it is related to the basic disease process.

The etiology of celiac-sprue is unknown. The disease is aggravated by gluten, a wheat protein

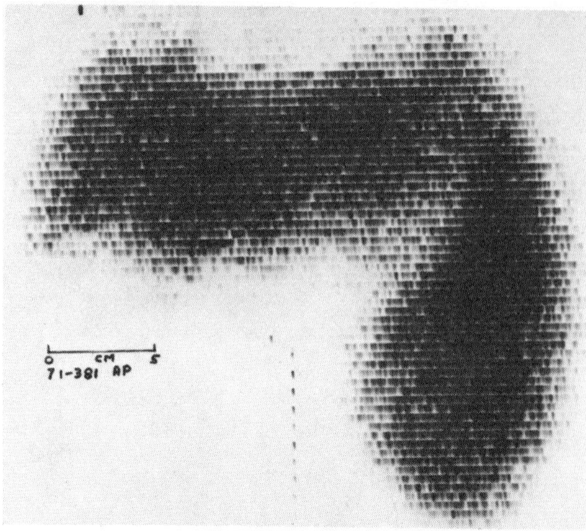

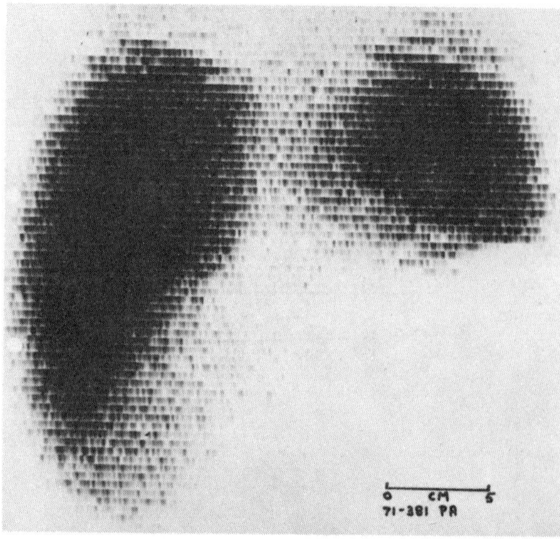

FIGURE 3. Anterior (top) and posterior (bottom) rectilinear scans performed with ^{99m}Tc-sulfur colloid. The patient is a 21-year-old woman with lupus erythematosus and documented lupoid hepatitis. The small liver and large spleen are unusual. Case 71-381.

with a high content of glutamine. The reason for this is unknown. Lack of peptidase in the mucosa has been postulated, allowing the entry of "toxic" products. Hypersensitivity in the intestinal mucosa has also been thought to play a role since antiflammatory drugs often have a beneficial effect, and antibodies to gliadin can be found in the bloodstreams of patients. There is no definitive evidence that immune processes initiate the disease, but it is included in this section because of the associated lymphoreticular dysfunction.

In a retrospective study of blood smears for the presence of Howell-Jolly bodies, Ferguson and co-workers[22] found that all the cases showing a significant number of these intraerythrocytic inclusions had either a prior splenectomy or (in two cases) celiac-sprue disease. It thus appears that not only may the spleen be small in some cases of celiac-sprue disease, but it also may be incapable of removing (the pitting function) Howell-Jolly bodies from erythrocytes. However, the association of a small size with a hypofunctioning spleen in this disease has not been clearly established. In a study of ^{99m}Tc-sulfur colloid uptake by the spleen in various disorders, Spencer and co-workers[23] found that six patients with celiac-sprue disease in remission had normal uptake of the radiocolloid. It has not been determined whether splenic function in celiac-sprue is related to the activity of the disease (that is, whether it is functional during remission and hypofunctional during exacerbation). An interesting observation during the ^{99m}Tc-sulfur colloid studies was that some of the celiac-sprue patients had splenomegaly, rather than a small organ. The incidence of intestinal lymphoma is higher in celiac-sprue disease than in the general population; perhaps some of the cases of splenomegaly in the celiac-sprue disorder represented examples of intestinal lymphoma or other complications.

Marsh and Stewart[24] studied 18 patients with celiac-sprue disease by means of ^{51}Cr-heat-denatured erythrocytes. Fourteen out of the 18 had abnormal clearance of tagged heat-denatured cells from the bloodstream (normal half-time = 10 to 16 min). Four patients had no detectable localization of the altered cells in the spleen, while a fifth case had minimal splenic uptake. These five cases had the most prolonged disappearance half-times for the denatured erythrocytes, and all had the peripheral blood picture of "asplenia." There still has to be a correlative study made of the relationship of these results (utilizing ^{51}Cr-heat-denatured erythrocytes) with ^{99m}Tc-sulfur colloid uptake.

Ulcerative Colitis

This disorder, of as yet unknown etiology, is a chronic inflammatory process involving the colon. All ages, and both sexes, are affected, and the disease may be becoming more prevalent. Because ulcerative colitis has systemic manifestations and tissue responses that include plasma cells and eosinophils, an immune mechanism as the basic defect has been postulated. However, the colon appears to be the primary target organ, and immunologic features may be epiphenomena. In young adults with long-standing disease, autoimmune hemolytic anemia or positive antiglobulin tests are often found.[25] Hepatosplenomegaly is a common physical finding in these patients, and liver disease is a frequent extracolonic complication in ulcerative colitis.[26] Splenomegaly may be secondary to liver disease; products of infection, as well as any underlying immune disease, may all contribute to the splenic problem. In addition, "autoimmune liver disease"[27] has been attracting increased attention; splenic dysfunction might follow the hepatic disease. Recently, Ryan and co-workers have reported on three patients with ulcerative colitis who had evidence of hyposplenism.[31]

Regional Enteritis

This disease, first delineated by Crohn and co-workers,[28] is a granulomatous reaction in the submucosa of the bowel (principally the ileum). There is compromise of the lumen with ulceration of the mucosa, damage to muscle, and formation of fistulae. Some of the patients have a more diffuse involvement than the classical initial limitation to the terminal ileum. Splenomegaly can be prominent in certain instances, perhaps secondary to infection or the hepatic dysfunction that can occur. Lymphatic reaction and the occurrence of granulomas suggest a relationship to sarcoidosis or tuberculosis.

ITP

The probable immunologic basis of ITP is discussed in the prior chapter. There are excellent data that the spleen is both the site of production of an antiplatelet factor in ITP and the locale of platelet phagocytosis.[35] The platelet antibodies are of the IgG class, and the spleen in ITP apparently has a marked capacity for their synthesis.[36]

REFERENCES

1. **Gotjamanos, T.,** The response of the reticuloendothelial system to skin transplantation. The cellular basis of hepatosplenomegaly in mice bearing skin grafts and their significance, *Aust. J. Exp. Biol. Med. Sci.,* 49, 259, 1971.
2. **Gotjamanos, T.,** The response of the reticulonedothelial system to skin transplantation. Phagocytic indices and weights of reticuloendothelial organs of mice bearing primary skin isografts and allografts, *Aust. J. Exp. Biol. Med. Sci.,* 49, 249, 1971.
3. **Blamey, R. W., Baker, J. M., and Crosby, D. L.,** Reticulo-endothelial system activity during homograft rejection and immunosuppression, *Br. J. Surg.,* 59, 62, 1972.
4. **Barchilon, J., Liebhaber, S. A., and Gershon, R. K.,** Significance of cell interactions in production of graft versus host splenomegaly, *Yale J. Biol. Med.,* 48, 519, 1972.
5. **Glucksberg, H. and Fefer, A.,** The effect of splenectomy on graft-versus-host disease (GVHD) in mice, *J. Reticuloendothel. Soc.,* 12, 537, 1972.
6. **Von Bekkum, D. W. and de Vries, M. J.,** 1966. Quoted in Reference 9.
7. **Barnes, D. W. H., Bungay, G. T., and Mole, R. H.,** Delayed mortality after mid-lethal exposures to whole-body irradiation and its modification by treatment with syngeneic lymph-node or bone-marrow cells, *Int. J. Radiat. Biol.,* 11, 409, 1966.
8. **Barnes, D. W. H., Loutit, J. F., and Micklem, H. S.,** "Secondary disease" of radiation chimeras: a syndrome due to lymphoid aplasia, *Ann. N.Y. Acad. Sci.,* 99, 374, 1962.
9. **Sundaram, K., Bains, G. S., and Gopal-Ayengar, A. R.,** Radiation response of newborn mice and the effect of shielding on mortality, in *Radiation Biology of the Fetal and Juvenile Mammal,* Silov, M. R. and Mahlum, D. D., Eds., USAEC CONF-690501, AEC Symposium Series #17, 1969, 475.
10. **Reisfeld, R. A., Dellegrino, A. M., Papermaster, B. W., and Kahan, B. D.,** HL-A antigens from a continuous lymphoid cell line derived from a normal donor. I. Solubilization and serologic characterization, *J. Immunol.,* 104, 560, 1970.
11. **Zervas, J. D., Delamore, I. W., and Israels, M. C. G.,** Leukocyte phenotypes in Hodgkin's disease, *Lancet,* 2, 634, 1970.
12. **Eugster, H.,** Graft-versus-host reactivity of mouse spleen cells separated on discontinuous albumin gradients, *Pathol Microbiol.,* 35, 315, 1970.
13. **Felty, A. R.,** Chronic arthritis in the adult, associated with splenomegaly and leukopenia, *Bull. Johns Hopkins Hosp.,* 35, 16, 1924.
14. **Green, R. A. and Fromke, V. L.,** Splenectomy in Felty's syndrome, *Ann. Intern. Med.,* 64, 1265, 1966.
15. **Moore, R. A., Brunner, C. M., Sandusky, W. R., and Leavell, B. S.,** Felty's syndrome: long-term follow-up after splenectomy, *Ann. Intern. Med.,* 75, 381, 1971.
16. **Barnes, C. G., Turnbull, A. L., and Vernon-Roberts, B.,** Felty's syndrome: a clinical and pathological survey of 21 patients and their response to treatment, *Ann. Rheum. Dis.,* 30, 359, 1971.
17. **Wimer, B. M. and Sloan, M. M.,** Remission of Felty's syndrome with long-term testosterone therapy, *JAMA,* 223, 671, 1973.
18. **Arroyo, H. and Aubert, L.,** Hypotrophie splenique au cours de la polyarthrite rhumatoide, *Nouv. Presse Med.,* 1, 876, 1972.
19. **Brewer, E. J., Jr.,** *Juvenile Rheumatoid Arthritis, Major Problems in Clinical Pediatrics,* Vol. VI, W. B. Saunders, Philadelphia, 1970, 231.
20. **Spiro, H. M.,** *Clinical Gastroenterology,* MacMillan, Toronto, 1970, 444.
21. **McCarty, C. F., Fraser, I. D., Evans, K. T., and Read, A. E.,** Lymphoreticular dysfunction in idiopathic steatorrhea., *Gut,* 7, 140, 1966.
22. **Ferguson, A., Hutton, M. M., and Maxwell, J. D.,** Adult coeliac disease in hyposplenic patients, *Lancet,* 1, 163, 1970.
23. **Spencer, R. P., Pearson, H. A., and Binder, H. J.,** Identification of cases of "acquired" functional asplenia, *J. Nucl. Med.,* 11, 763, 1970.
24. **Marsh, G. W. and Stewart, J. S.,** Splenic function in adult coeliac disease, *Br. J. Hematol.,* 19, 445, 1970.
25. **Bardana, E. J., Jr. and Pirofsky, B.,** Autoimmune hemolytic anemia and ulcerative colitis: a multisystem immunodeficiency disease? *Int. Arch. Allergy,* 37, 325, 1970.
26. Editorial, Liver disease in ulcerative colitis, *Lancet,* 2, 402, 1970.
27. Editorial, Immunological aspects of liver disease, *Br. Med. J.,* 3, 278, 1970.
28. **Crohn, B. B., Ginzburg, L., and Oppenheimer, G. D.,** Regional ileitis: pathologic and clinical entity, *JAMA,* 99, 1323, 1932.
29. **Schaller, J., Beckwith, B., and Wedgwood, R. J.,** Hepatic involvement in juvenile rheumatoid arthritis, *J. Pediatr.,* 77, 203, 1970.
30. **Tigelaar, R. E. and Asofsky, R.,** Kinetics of graft-versus-host splenomegaly in neonatal F_1 recipients of parental strain mouse lymph node cells and/or thymocytes, *Transplantation,* 14, 805, 1972.
31. **Ryan, F. P., Smart, R. C., Preston, F. E., and Holdsworth, C. D.,** Hyposplenism in ulcerative colitis, *Lancet,* 2, 318, 1974.

32. **Goldman, A. B., Braunstein, P., and Song, C.,** Augmented splenic uptake of ^{99m}Tc-sulfur colloid in patients with malignant melanoma, *Radiology,* 112, 631, 1974.

33. **Andrada, J. A., Comini, E., and Premachandra, B. N.,** Studies on thyroid immunity. VII. Splenectomy and monkey immune thyroiditis: thyroidal function and thyroxine transport, *Clin. Exp. Immunol.,* 13, 303, 1973.

34. **Braylan, R. C., Rumi, L., and Pasqualini, C. D.,** Murine splenic changes in response to syngeneic and allogenic neoplasias, *Medicina,* 32, 505, 1972.

35. **McMillan, R., Longmire, R. L., Tarassoli, M., Armstrong, S., and Yelenosky, R.,** *In vitro* platelet phagocytosis by splenic leukocytes in idiopathic thrombocytopenic purpura, *N. Engl. J. Med.,* 290, 249, 1974.

36. **McMillan, R., Longmire, R. L., Yelenosky, R., Donnell, R. L., and Armstrong, S.,** Platelet-binding IgG produced by spleens in idiopathic thrombocytopenic purpura, *N. Engl. J. Med.,* 291, 812, 1974.

Chapter 15

MEDICATION EFFECTS AND RESULTS OF IMMUNIZATION

There are at least three techniques for detecting and following the effects of medications on the spleen.

1. Spleen biopsy, needle or surgical, to observe morphological alterations.
2. Observation of specific indicators of splenic function, such as the presence or absence of Howell-Jolly bodies, and certain immunological responses.
3. Observation of spleen size, configuration, and capacity to concentrate radiocolloids.

Moeschlin[1] has described the use of spleen puncture to document the effects of urethane, nitrogen mustards, and ^{32}P on the spleen. The abnormal granulocytes of chronic myeloid leukemia were found to be particularly susceptible to urethane. Since splenic biopsy is not widely practiced in the U.S.A. and is fraught with danger in the presence of a bleeding diathesis other procedures must be used for following the response of the human spleen to medications. Table 1 summarizes some of the available data on the effects of medications on the human spleen. The section on animal models of splenic diesases should also be consulted; additional medications are discussed there (particularly interesting are

TABLE 1

Effects of Medications on Spleen (Man)

Adrenal steroids, ACTH	The giant splenomegaly of sarcoidosis is benefited by steroids (decrease in splenic size).[5] Administration of ACTH to rats produces a regression of Malphigian bodies of the spleen. A partial escape of the lymphoid tissue can occur.[18] In patients on adrenal steroids or ACTH, we have not noted gross impairment of splenic uptake of radiocolloid (Figure 2). Arroyo and Aubert[26] have reported three cases of small spleen in rheumatoid arthritis. This they attributed to steroid administration.
Alloantiserum	Alloantiserum was given to patients with lymphoproliferative diseases.[24] In two on whom comment was made, the spleen did not appear to change in size.
Antimalarials	Their use results in reduction in the size of the spleen in tropical splenomegaly syndrome.[4]
Other antineoplastic agents	Fifty women having 88 pregnancies while on methotrexate, actinomycin D, or other antineoplastic agents had children without a higher incidence of gross deformities than normal.[11] However, when taken in adequate amounts at the crucial times in gestation, fetal damage can be produced.[12] Specific splenic defects however have not been described. See text for additional discussion.
Carcinostatic agents	A higher incidence of splenic metastases is found in patients with carcinoma, on carcinostatic agents, than in those not on such chemicals.[30]
Diphenylhydantoin	Incidence of lymphoma is 0.5% in the general population. However, 5% of patients with lymphoma had been on diphenylhydantoin in one series.[9] One reaction to the hydantoin drugs consists of fever, lymphadenopathy, and hepatosplenomegaly. Animal studies have also been reported.[10]
Drug addiction	The spleen in drug addicts is larger than that in age, race, and sex controls.[43] Whether this is related to the drugs, or to contaminants, is unknown. Patients on large amounts of analgesics may have splenomegaly.[44]
Epinephrine	Causes apparent transient decrease of splenic size in some children with splenomegaly and sickle cell disease.[6]

TABLE 1 (continued)

Effects of Medications on Spleen (Man)

Estrogens	Numerous studies have shown that estrogens inhibit growth in animals, and the mechanism has been investigated.[14] Estrogens induce a wasting syndrome in neonatal mice,[15] and we have compared the loss of splenic weight to that of body weight at various points in time.[16] As measured by clearance of ^{125}I-microaggregated albumin in man, the rate of blood disappearance of radioactivity was increased after administration of stilbestrol to patients with cancer,[17,25] Radiation therapy depressed the rate of uptake of the radiolabel, and this could be prevented by simultaneous use of stilbestrol.[17] In mice, diethylstilbestrol increases phagocytic clearance of a lipid emulsion by a factor of 8.[19]
Hypertransfusion	In a 2½-year-old girl with thalassemia major, hypertransfusion resulted in a decrease in splenic size.[23] This may be related to suppression of endogenous erythropoietin production.
Hypolipidemic drugs	There was a shift of ^{99m}Tc-sulfur colloid from liver to spleen in three of five patients while on hypolipidemic drug treatment (Clofibrate® and Nafenopin®).[2]
Isonicotinic acid hydrazide (INH)	When given to pregnant rodents, INH can reduce splenic hypoplasia in the offsprings.[13] In man, INH appears to have little gross effect on the spleen. (Figure 1).
L-Asparaginase	Used in a number of hematologic malignancies, L-asparaginase can result in increased hepatic lipid accumulation in man.[20] If hepatic damage is severe, we might expect resultant portal hypertension and splenomegaly. This has not yet been demonstrated. L-asparaginase has an immunosuppressive effect.[21] We have studied only one child on L-asparaginase and did not note any gross change in splenic uptake of ^{99m}Tc-sulfur colloid (Figure 5).
Myleran®	Decreases spleen size when administered for myeloid metaplasia.[3]
Needle puncture	Although not a medication, spleen puncture per se has been reported to cause splenic contraction in dogs;[27] possible significance in human studies has been commented upon.
Testosterone	Three males with Felty's syndrome had a correction of neutropenia after long-term testosterone therapy.[22] Effects on the spleen scan have not been reported.
Thorotrast (thorium dioxide)	The reticuloendothelial blockage and chronic radiation result in splenic hypofunction (functional asplenia has been noted[7] as well as massive pneumococcal septicemia).[8] The high deposition of thorotrast in the spleen and self-radiation may account for the low incidence of splenic tumors.[8]
Vasopressin	Intravenous infusion of vasopressin can result in decreased splenic blood flow.[28] Upon infusion into the splenic artery,[29] the spleen can be effectively excluded from the circulation.
Vincristine	We have had the opportunity to study two patients on this medication. In each case, the spleen was functional, with a shift of radiocolloid to the organ (Figure 3).

ethyl palmitate to produce a "chemical splenectomy," and methylcellulose, which produces splenomegaly when used parenterally).

Two aspects of the effects of medications on the spleen merit particular mention. These are, first, the effects of antineoplastic agents and, second, the use of dynamic radioisotopic techniques. Some antineoplastic agents interfere with reticuloendothelial function as described in the chapter on animal models of splenic diseases. However, such effects have not been fully quantified in man. In a few instances, we have noted loss of splenic uptake of radiocolloid in patients who were receiving antineoplastic agents (Figure 4, see also Reference 7). However, in these cases one could argue that the underlying disease per se perhaps contributes to the lack of splenic function, and the entire process has to be studied in depth.

Once the spleen contains a radiolabel, the organ can be serially visualized as various medications are administered. We have, for example, using a gamma ray camera and computer coupling, noted splenic contraction in two children with splenomegaly, following epinephrine administration.[6] In addition to these rapid changes, slower responses to other medications can occur, and we have shown some of these in graphic form.[6]

IMMUNOLOGICAL FUNCTION OF THE SPLEEN

The spleen has an important role in the immunological response, particularly to injected foreign particulate antigens. Aspects of this have been discussed in several other sections. The present section will focus principally on some of the biochemical events which occur in the spleen upon immunization. That is, the spleen responding to an immune challenge undergoes a series of dramatic changes.

A distinction must be made between the spleen in a previously immunized host and that in a nonimmune individual. In the section on the spleen and its function, it was pointed out that the spleens of immunized and unimmunized animals have different capacities to filter organisms. Using isolated rabbit spleen cells, it has been shown that tissue from immunized rabbits absorbed over 60% of quinacrine-labeled vaccinia virus, whereas spleen cells from nonimmune rabbits absorbed under 25%.[31] In some cases, antigenically active material can be recovered from the spleen after viral infection (equine infectious anemia).[32] Also of great interest are those situations in which an immune response cannot be elicited. For example, prior injection of thorotrast to mice prevents the appearance of plaque-forming cells in the spleen.[33] It was hypothesized that thorotrast inhibits the surface of the immunocompetent cells. Tolerance to injected foreign red blood cells can be produced in mice by massive doses of the red cells.[34] Unresponsiveness was also produced by use of red cells in combination with a cytotoxic chemical (cyclophosphoramide).

Studies using ^{3}H-thymidine in mice that were given sheep red blood cells have shown a metabolic turnover of DNA in the red pulp of the spleen which coincided with the maximal development of cells which produced antibody.[35] Labeled thymidine has also been used to show the increased proliferation of spleen cells following injection of killed *Bordetella pertussis* cells in mice.[36] Changes in splenic ribosomes and cytoplasmic proteins have been documented during the immune response.[37,38]

T cells carrying antigen appear in the spleen within hours of injecting sheep red blood cells into mice.[39] The turnover of splenic lymphocytes has been documented, and the rapid depletion of at least one component following introduction of antigens was noted.[40] The spleen can release antigen-binding cells into the bloodstream, and the event has been especially followed in guinea pigs.[41,42]

An appendix on animal models of splenic disorders, follows the illustrations and figures.

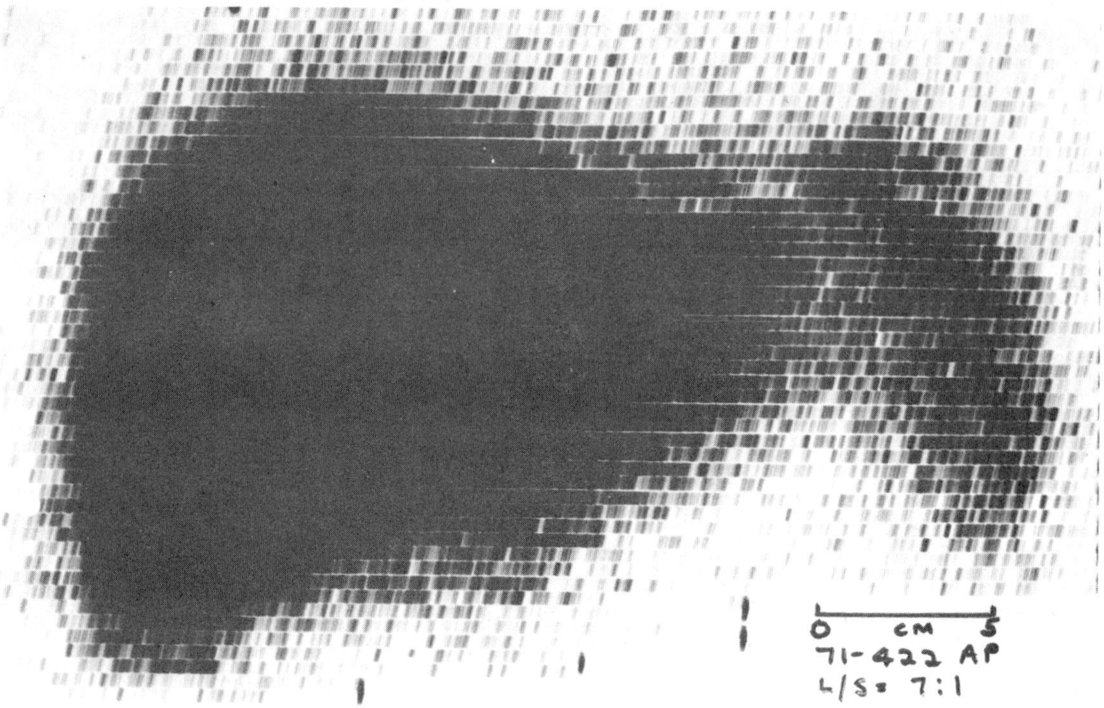

FIGURE 1. Anterior rectilinear scan (^{99m}Tc-sulfur colloid) of a 67-year-old man who had been on INH for many years because of tuberculosis. The liver scan was deliberately saturated in order to show the spleen. The spleen/liver ratio per unit area was 1 to 7; this is slightly low (reduced splenic uptake of radiocolloid). In two other cases we have seen (adults on INH therapy), splenic size and uptake of radiocolloid were both normal. Case 71-422.

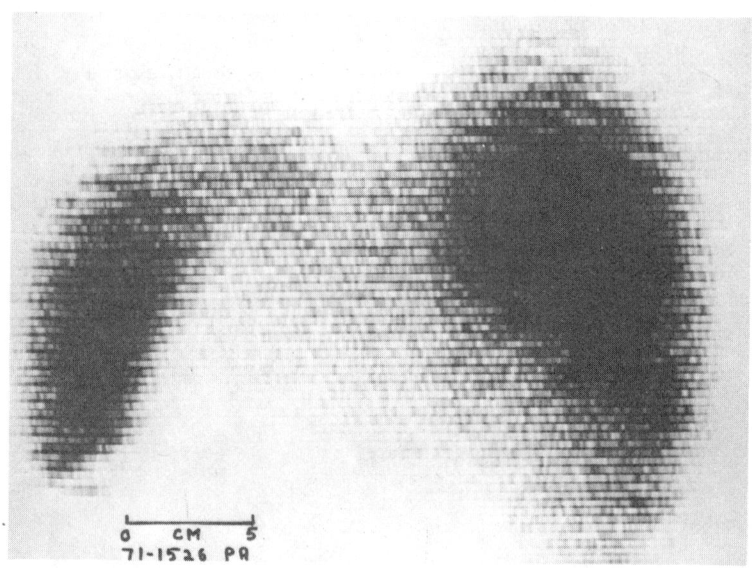

FIGURE 2. Posterior rectilinear scan (^{99m}Tc-sulfur colloid) in a 37-year-old man on intravenous ACTH therapy. The spleen is functional. Case 71-1526.

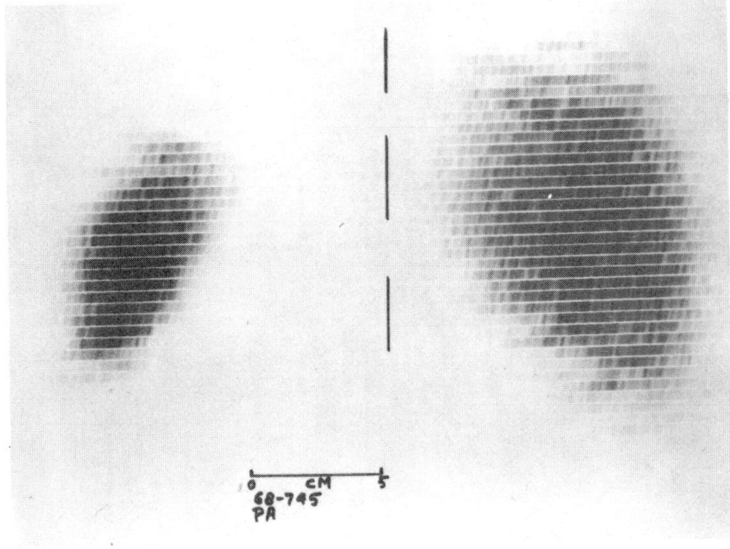

A.

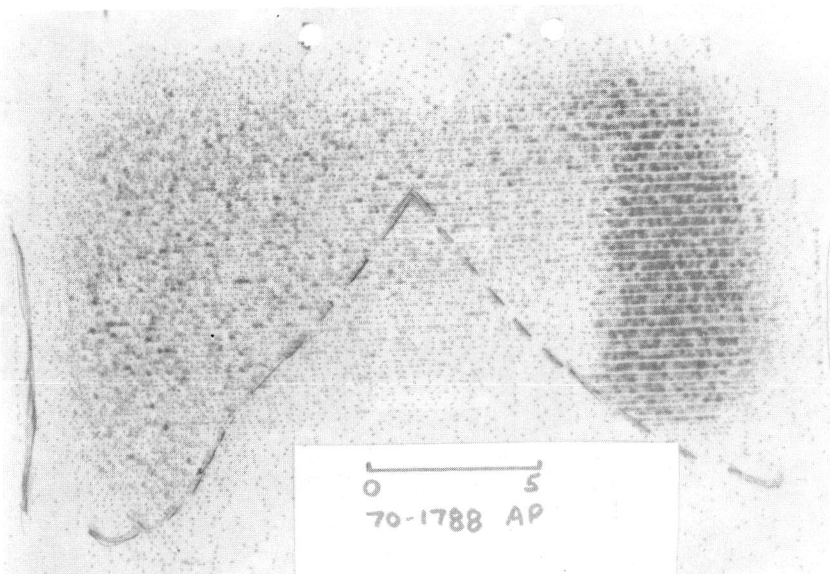

B.

FIGURE 3. (A) Posterior rectilinear scan (^{99m}Tc-sulfur colloid) of a 67-year-old woman. The patient had a right radical mastectomy for carcinoma 25 years ago. Three years ago, abdominal reticulum cell sarcoma was diagnosed. She had radiation therapy to the abdomen. More recently, she had been on a course of vincristine. The spleen is functional. Case 68-745. (B) Anterior rectilinear scan, also with ^{99m}Tc-sulfur colloid, in a 9-year-old girl with acute leukemia and on vincristine therapy. The scan, though clearly suboptimal, reveals that the spleen is functional and that there is a shift of radiocolloid to that organ. Case 70-1788.

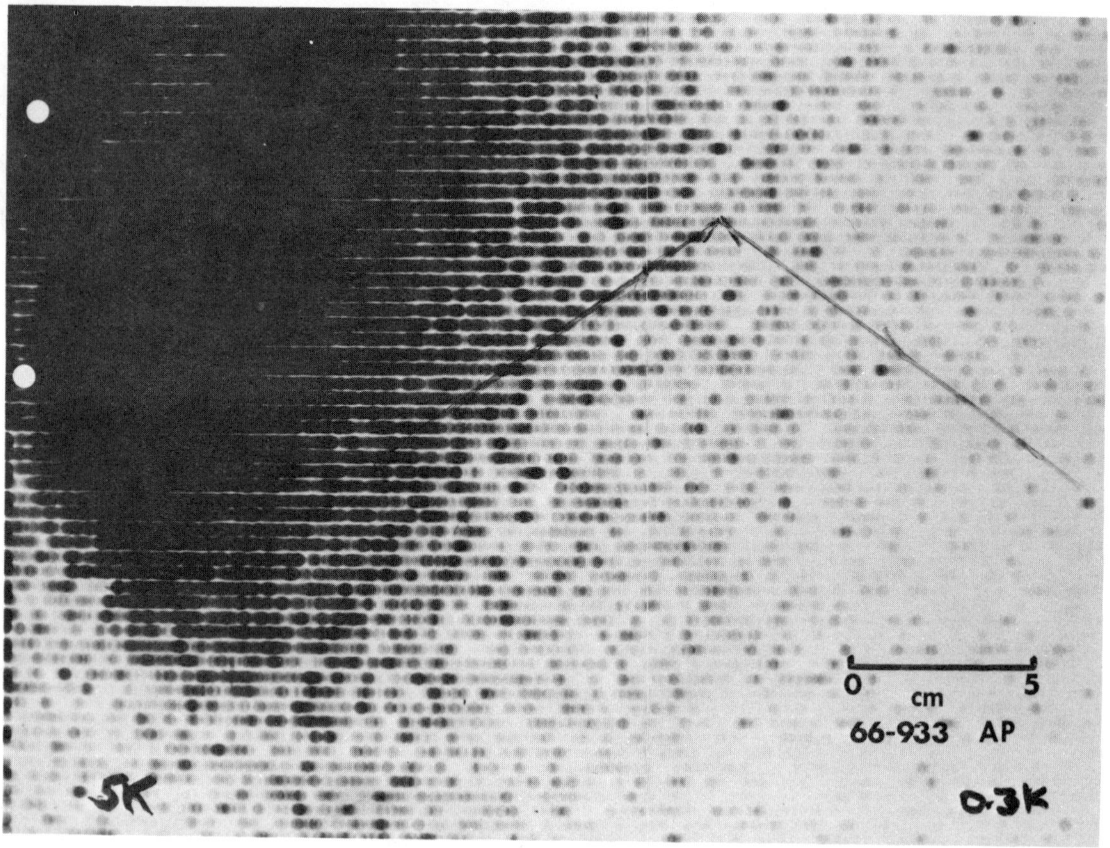

FIGURE 4. Anterior rectilinear scan (^{99m}Tc-sulfur colloid) of an 8-year-old boy who had a posterior fossa tumor (probable ependymoblastoma). This metastasized to a rib on the right; the metastasis was treated by means of external beam radiation. In addition, the patient was placed on chemotherapy. A wide variety of medications had been used prior to the scan (including vincristine, Cytoxan®, prednisone, Dilantin®, and dexamethasone). Perhaps due to one of these, or a combination, no splenic uptake of the radiocolloid could be detected. Case 66-933.

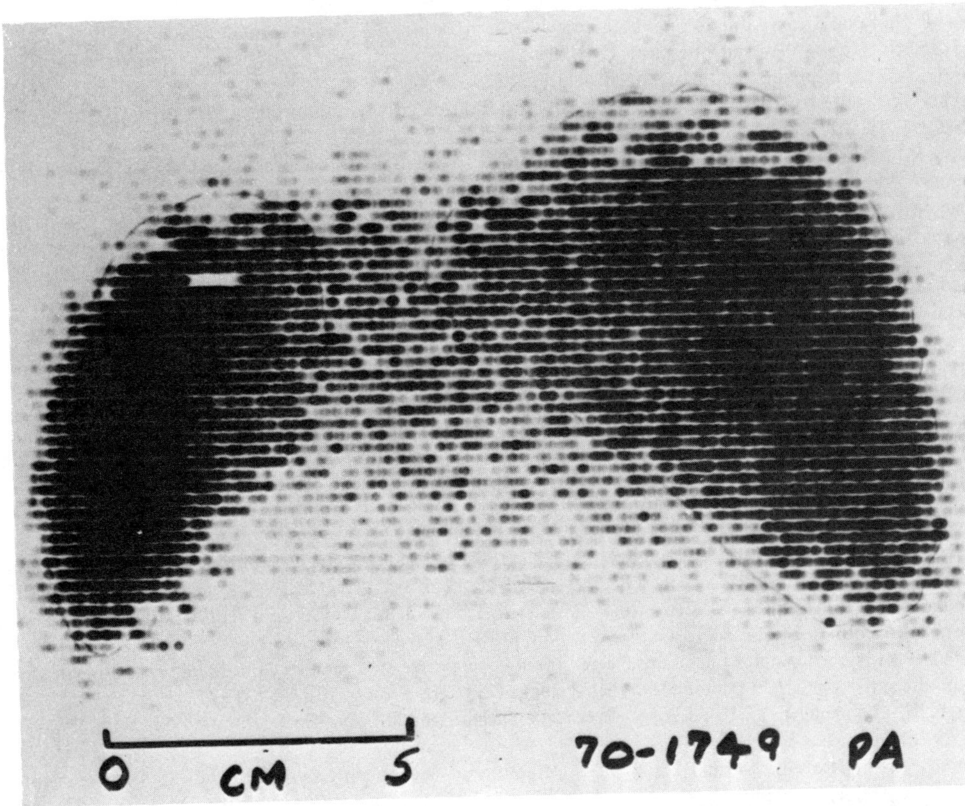

FIGURE 5. Posterior rectilinear scan (^{99m}Tc-sulfur colloid) performed on a 9-month-old girl who was on L-asparaginase therapy. The small (fine) collimator and light pipe were used. The spleen is functional. Case 70-1749.

REFERENCES

1. **Moeschlin, S.,** *Spleen Puncture,* Heinemann, London, 1951, 151, 165, 166.
2. **Dujovne, C. A. and Strauss, H. W.,** Changes in liver and spleen scans of patients during treatment with two hypolipidemic drugs, *Radiology,* 98, 682, 1971.
3. **Dameshek, W., Granville, N. B., and Rubio, F., Jr.,** Therapy of the myeloproliferative disorders with Myleran, *Ann. N.Y. Acad. Sci.,* 68, 1001, 1958.
4. **Stuiver, P. C., Ziegler, J. L., Wood, J. B., Morrow, R. H., and Hutt, M. S. R.,** Clinical trial of malaria prophylaxis in tropical splenomegaly syndrome, *Br. Med. J..* 1, 426, 1971.
5. **Burt, R. W. and Kuhl, D. E.,** Giant splenomegaly in sarcoidosis demonstrated by radionuclide scintigraphy, *JAMA,* 215, 2110, 1971.
6. **Spencer, R. P., Lange, R. C., Schwartz, A. D., and Pearson, H. A.,** Radioisotopic studies of changes in splenic size in response to epinephrine and other stimuli, *J. Nucl. Med.,* 13, 211, 1972.
7. **Spencer, R. P., Pearson, H. A., and Binder, H. A.,** Identification of cases of "acquired" functional asplenia, *J. Nucl. Med.,* 11, 763, 1970.
8. **Bensinger, T. A., Keller, A. R., Merrell, L. F., and O'Leary, D. S.,** Thorotrast induced reticuloendothelial blockade in man: clinical equivalent of the experimental model associated with patent pneumococcal septicemia, *Am. J. Med.,* 51, 663, 1971.
9. **Anthony, J. J.,** Malignant lymphoma associated with hydantoin drugs, *Arch. Neurol.,* 22, 450, 1970.
10. **Kruger, G.,** Effect of dilantin in mice. I. Changes in the lymphoreticular tissue after acute exposure, *Virchows Arch. A,* 349, 297, 1970.
11. **van Phiel, D. H., Ross, G. T., and Lipsett, M. B.,** Pregnancies after chemotherapy of trophoblastic neoplasms, *Science,* 169, 1326, 1970.

12. **Shaw, E. B.**, Fetal damage due to maternal aminopterin ingestion, *Am. J. Dis. Child.*, 124, 93, 1972.
13. **Davis, S. D., Nelson, T., and Shepard, T. H.**, Teratogenicity of vitamin B_6 deficiency: omphalocele, skeletal and neural defects and splenic hypoplasia, *Science*, 169, 1329, 1970.
14. **Herbai, G.**, Studies on the site and mechanism of action of growth inhibiting effects of estrogens, *Acta Physiol. Scand.*, 83, 77, 1971.
15. **Reilly, R., Thompson, J., Bielski, R., and Severson, C.**, Estradiol-induced wasting syndrome in neonatal mice, *J. Immunol.*, 98, 321, 1967.
16. **Spencer, R. P. and Chaudhuri, T. K.**, Quantitative estimates of changes in splenic size during life, *Yale J. Biol. Med.*, 41, 333, 1969.
17. **Magarey, C. J. and Baum, M.**, Oestrogen as a reticuloendothelial stimulant in patients with cancer, *Br. Med. J.*, 2, 367, 1971.
18. **Senelar, R., Catayee, G., Escola, R., Escola, M. J., and Bureau, J. P.**, Light and electron microscopic study of splenic changes in the Wistar rat induced by small doses of ACTH over long periods, *Pathol. Biol.*, 19, 347, 1971.
19. **Trejo, R. A., Loose, L. D., and DiLuzio, N. R.**, Influence of diethylstilbestrol (DES) on reticuloendothelial function, tissue distribution, and detoxication of S·enteritidis endotoxin, *J. Reticuloendothel. Soc.*, 11, 88, 1972.
20. **Pratt, C. B. and Johnson, W. W.**, Duration and severity of fatty metamorphosis of the liver following L-asparaginase therapy, *Cancer*, 28, 361, 1971.
21. **Levin, B. and Merrill, J. P.**, Immunosuppressive activity of L-asparaginase, *Transplantation*, 12, 141, 1971.
22. **Wimer, B. M. and Sloan, M. M.**, Remission of Felty's syndrome with long-term testosterone therapy, *JAMA*, 223, 671, 1973.
23. **O'Brien, R. T., Pearson, H. A., and Spencer, R. P.**, Transfusion-induced decrease in spleen size in thalassemia major: documentation by radioisotopic scan, *J. Pediatr.*, 81, 105, 1972.
24. **Herberman, R. B., Oren, M. E., Rogentine, G. N., and Fahey, J. L.**, Cytolytic effects of alloantiserum in patients with lymphoproliferative disorders, *Cancer*, 28, 365, 1971.
25. **Berstad, T., Liavag, I., and Tamsfoss, S.**, The effect of operative treatment, chemotherapy, and oestrogens on the phagocytic activity of the reticuloendothelial system, *Acta Chir. Scand.*, 138, 557, 1972.
26. **Arroyo, H. and Aubert, L.**, Hypotrophie splenique au cours de la polyarthrite rhumatoide, *Nouv. Presse Med.*, 1, 876, 1972.
27. **Dumont, A. E., Martelli, A., and Biris, L.**, Contraction of the spleen following needle puncture: significance in studies of portal hypertension, *Gastroenterology*, 61, 738, 1971.
28. **Williams, R., Condon, R. E., Williams, H. S., Blendis, L. M., and Kreel, L.**, Splenic blood flow in cirrhosis and portal hypertension, *Clin. Sci.*, 34, 441, 1968.
29. **Sigelman, S. S., Sprayregen, S., Bardfeld, P., and Boley, S. J.**, Vasopressin infusion of the splenic artery: splenic exclusion, *Invest. Radiol.*, 6, 341, 1971.
30. **Watanabe, T. and Tanaka, K.**, Effect of carcinostatic agents on carcinomatous metastasis in the spleen, *Gann*, 60, 611, 1969.
31. **Heiss, J. M. and Stickl, H.**, The antigen-binding capacity of lymphatic spleen cells following immunization, *Med. Microbiol. Immunol.*, 158, 147, 1972.
32. **Nakajima, H., Norcross, N. L., and Coggins, L.**, Demonstration of antigenic identity between purified equine infectious anemia virus and an antigen extracted from infected horse spleen, *Infect. Immun.*, 6, 416, 1972.
33. **Noltenius, H. W. and Chahin, M.**, Inhibition of the primary immune response against sheep red blood cells by short-term reticulo-endothelial system blockage experiments in mice, *Experientia*, 28, 1226, 1972.
34. **Anderson, T. H., Roethle, J., and Auerbach, R.**, Induction of tolerance to sheep red blood cells, *J. Exp. Med.*, 136, 1666, 1972.
35. **Pelc, S. R., Harris, G., and Caldwell, I.**, The relationship between antibody formation and deoxyribonucleic acid (DNA) synthesis in mouse spleen during primary and secondary response to sheep erythrocytes, *Immunology*, 23, 183, 1972.
36. **Stocker, E. and Finger, H.**, Autoradiographic studies on cell proliferation during splenomegaly induced by Bordetella pertussis in mice, *Virchows Arch. Abt. B. Zellpathol.*, 10, 179, 1972.
37. **Storb, U. and Martin, T. E.**, Number and activity of free and membrane-bound spleen ribosomes during the course of the immune response, *Biochim. Biophys. Acta*, 281, 406, 1972.
38. **Bouteille, M.**, Migration of cytoplasmic proteins into nuclei of spleen cells from immunized animals, *Exp. Cell Res.*, 74, 343, 1972.
39. **Hirsch, J. S. and Plescia, O. J.**, Isolation of functional antigen-carrying spleen cells early in the course of the immune response of mice to sheep red blood cells, *Immunol. Commun.*, 1, 199, 1972.
40. **Haas, R. J., Meyer-Hamme, K. D., Trepel, F., and Frolich, D.**, Cytokinetic studies on slowly-renewing bone marrow and spleen lymphocytes in rats during a primary and a secondary immune response, *Acta Haematol.*, 48, 39, 1972.
41. **Sandberg, G.**, Release of lymphocytes from the spleen in neonatally thymectomized guinea pigs, *Scand. J. Haematol.*, 9, 52, 1972.
42. **Sandberg, G.**, Release of antigen-binding cells from the spleen into the blood, *Acta Pathol. Microbiol. Scand. Sect. A*, 80, 477, 1972.
43. **Myers, J. and Segal, R. J.**, Weight of the spleen. II. Range in narcotic addicts, *Arch. Pathol.*, 98, 36, 1974.
44. **Duggan, J. M.**, Splenomegaly in analgesic takers, *Med. J. Aust.*, 2, 580, 1970.

APPENDIX

A number of the results discussed in earlier chapters were obtained through clinical observations. Others, however, had their roots in studies on a variety of animal species. On the following pages we have summarized a number of naturally occurring diseases in animals which involve the spleen, several induced splenic disorders, and a variety of observations on the effects of medication on the spleens of experimental animals. The listing is incomplete but represents an initial introduction to some of the animal models of splenic disorders.

Animal Models of Splenic Disorders

Cat	Hematopoietic neoplasms occur in the cat population; the spleen is frequently involved.[5]
Cat (and other species)	Perfused cat's spleen can be used for studying uptake and liberation of sympathetic transmitters.[39] Storage of noradrenaline and other compounds can be quantified.[40] Splenic strips in many species contract with sympathetic agents.[41]
Cattle, Sheep, Swine	Maternal to fetal transfer (and splenic content) of ^{65}Zn and ^{35}S has been documented.[21]
Chicken (embryo)	Based on decapitation experiments, the pars distalis appears to stimulate splenic white pulp histogenesis but to inhibit spleen growth and red cell differentiation.[4]
Chicken	Bursectomy has little effect on rate of proliferation of lymphoid cells in spleen or differentiation into plasma cells.[6]
Dog	Thioacetamide-induced cirrhosis is of the Laennec type.[13] The spleen was enlarged in all the dogs (personal communication).
Dog	Common bile duct ligation was followed by increased splenic blood flow.[18]
Dog	Dimethylnitrosamine (a toxin for man) produced hepatic cirrhosis in dogs. Elevation of portal pressure occurred. The spleens were large, and one showed evidence of infarction.[14]
Dog	Basophilic stippling of erythrocytes is common in dogs and may have causes other than lead poisoning.[22] Some of the associated diseases are marked by splenic abnormalities.
Guinea pig	After splenectomy, there is early increased release of lymphocytes from the thymus. The spleen may exert abnormal inhibition of lymphocyte production.[8]
Guinea pig	Experimental thrombocytopenia purpura can be produced by rabbit antiguinea pig platelet antibody.[23] Ultrastructural changes have been documented in the spleen.
Hamster	Treating neonatal hamsters with indole and 2-acetylaminofluorene resulted in peliosis of the spleen.[17]
Marmosets and Tamarins	Liver and spleen biopsy procedure for these primate species has been described.[2]
Monkey	The viral agent, *Herpesvirus saimiri,* produces acute lymphocytic leukemia in owl monkeys. Malignant lymphoma can be produced in this primate by intravenous, subcutaneous, or intradermal introduction of the virus.[27]
Mouse	Host-versus-graft reaction is marked by hepatosplenomegaly and an increased phagocytic activity (measured by blood clearance of ^{32}P-labeled *Salmonella typhimurium*).[11] Splenic enlargement is due to white pulp hyperplasia. Host-versus-graft reaction may prevent development of graft-versus-host reaction.
Mouse (also rat, dog, monkey)	A compound that induces interferon, 2,7-bis 2-(diethylamino) ethoxy-fluoren-9-one dihydrochloride, produces vacuolation and granulation of leukocytes as well as changes in fixed macrophages of spleen and lymph nodes.[34]

Animal Models of Splenic Disorders (continued)

Mouse	Vitamin B_6 deficiency in maternal animal is accompanied by multiple defects in the newborn, including splenic hypoplasia.[12]
Mouse	Actinomycin D causes a decrease in the size of the spleen.[15] This effect may be potentiated by acridine orange.
Mouse	Estradiol-induced wasting in neonatal mice is accompanied by decrease in size of spleen.[16]
Mouse	A factor in spleen and serum of mice with amyloidosis has a transferable amyloid-accelerating ability.[42] Spontaneous amyloidosis occurs in animals[44] and the disease can be induced.[45]
Mouse	Serotonin is taken up and stored by the spleen. An assay has been developed to define structure-activity relationship of inhibitors.[36]
Mouse	NZB mouse shows a number of disorders resembling autoimmune disease. "Nude mouse" is congenitally athymic, and the spleen is relatively deficient in T cells.[43]
Pheasants	"Marble spleen disease" might be viral associated. There is splenic amyloid present.[47]
Quail	Splenomegaly occurs in an epizootic reticulum cell sarcoma.[46]
Rabbit	Spleen does not participate in the antibody response to depot antigen of most materials, but does to IgM. The spleen does respond to intravenously administered antigens.[7]
Rabbit	RNA from the human spleen, prepared by phenol extraction, was injected into rabbits. Twenty-five days later, a secondary stimulation was given with human erythrocytes. Antibody titers were measured in the blood. After injection of spleen RNA from blood type B humans and injection of A red cells, anti-A serum of high titer was obtained. Spleen RNA from blood type O humans was apparently able to transfer the factor for anti-A and anti-B.[28]
Rat, Gunn	Erythrocyte and leukocyte counts are lower in Gunn rats than Wistar rats. Females had lower values than males (and leukopenia disappeared after castration). Homozygous female Gunn rats had anemia, shortened erythrocyte survival, and splenomegaly. After either splenectomy or oophorectomy, the erythrocyte survival improved (but oophorectomy alone did not influence splenomegaly or enhanced erythrocyte trapping). Anemia of homozygous female Gunn rats is likely due to increased sequestration of erythrocytes in spleen and a possible estrogen metabolic defect[1] (see also, estradiol-induced wasting in neonatal mice).
Rat (swine, rabbit)	^{59}Fe injected into maternal animal can be found in fetal spleen (and references to other species).[3]
Rat	Methylcellulose induces splenomegaly.[20]
Rat	The spleen may offer some protection against the effects of hyperoxygenation.[26]
Rat	TSH or thyroxin administration produces histological changes in the spleen.[37]
Rat	Selenite and arsenite produce a decrease in splenic weight.[38]
Rat	A Hodgkin's-like tumor is known.[48]
Rodents	Colloidal carbon clearance is a. Enhanced in mice by polyvinylpyridine-*N*-oxide.[29] b. Impaired in mice by antilymphocyte serum.[30,31] c. Enhanced in rabbits by Arvin.[32] d. Enhanced by biotin in rats.[25] e. Enhanced by estradiol, zymosan, and the polysaccharide glucan in mice.[33] f. Impaired by cortisone in mice[35] (but splenic uptake may be more active than hepatic).

Animal Models of Splenic Disorders (continued)

Rodents, principally	A lethal dose of irradiation, followed by injection of hematopoietic cells, is accompanied by the growth of colonies of cells in the spleen. The colony-forming unit assay[9] can be combined with measurement of ^{59}Fe uptake in the spleen colonies.[10]
Rodents	Intravenous ethyl palmitate results in splenic destruction.[19] This is true in mouse, rat, guinea pig, rabbit.
Sheep	Dilution of labeled erythrocytes and albumin was studied in sheep before and after splenectomy.[24] Splenectomy significantly changed all parameters. A good model for following splenic response to epinephrine.[49]

REFERENCES

1. **Lozzio, B. B., McDonald, T. P., Lange, R. D., Cawein, M. J., and Chernoff, A. I.,** Splenomegaly and hematologic disorders of the Gunn rat, *Br. J. Haematol.,* 19, 543, 1970.
2. **Voss, W. R.,** Primate liver and spleen biopsy procedures, *Lab. Anim. Care,* 20, 995, 1970.
3. **Glasser, S. R., McKee, L. C., Jr., and Heyssel, R. M.,** Iron transfer by the fetoplacental unit of the rat in *Radiation Biology of the Fetal and Juvenile Mammal,* Sikov, M. R. and Mahlum, D. S., Eds., USAEC CONF-690501, AEC Symposium Series #17, 1969, 25.
4. **Betz, T. W.,** The developmental endocrinology of the spleen in chick embryos. I. The pars distalis, *J. Embryol. Exp. Morphol.,* 24, 357, 1970.
5. **Nielsen, S. W.,** Spontaneous hematopoietic neoplasms of the domestic cat, *Natl. Cancer Inst. Monogr.,* No. 32, 73, 1969.
6. **Rodak, L.,** Influence of bursectomy on cellular changes in the spleen of immunized chickens. I. An autoradiographic study, *Folia Biol.,* 16, 417, 1970.
7. **Bednarik, T. and Cajthamlova, H.,** Formation of antibodies to immunoglobulins after splenectomy during intravenous and depot immunization, *Physiol. Bohemoslov.,* 19, 135, 1970.
8. **Ernstrom, V. and Sanberg, G.,** Influence of splenectomy on thymic release of lymphocytes into the blood, *Scand. J. Haematol.,* 7, 342, 1970.
9. **Till, J. E. and McCulloch, E. A.,** A direct measurement of the radiation sensitivity of normal mouse bone marrow cells, *Radiat. Res.,* 14, 213, 1961.
10. **Thomas, D. B., Steers, D. J. F., and Riches, A. C.,** A macroautoradiographic method for the demonstration of iron-concentrating spleen colonies, *Transplantation,* 10, 274, 1970.
11. **Gotjamanos, T.,** A comparison of the changes produced in reticuloendothelial organs of mice during host-versus-graft and graft-versus-host reactions, *Aust. J. Exp. Biol. Med. Sci.,* 48, 567, 1970.
12. **Davis, S. D., Nelson, T., and Shepard, T. H.,** Teratogenicity of vitamin B_6 deficiency: omphalocele, skeletal and neural defects and splenic hypoplasia, *Science,* 169, 1329, 1970.
13. **Rodriguez Olleros, A., Taveras, J. E., Irizarry, S., and Landron Becerra, F. M. T.,** Hepatic structure and function, *Am. J. Gastroenterol.,* 52, 127, 1969.
14. **Madden, J. W., Gertman, P. M., and Peacock, E. E., Jr.,** Dimethylnitrosamine-induced hepatic cirrhosis; a new canine model of an ancient human disease, *Surgery,* 68, 260, 1970.
15. **Roth, E. F., Jr. and Kochen, J.,** Acridine orange potentiation of actinomycin D uptake and activity, *Science,* 174, 696, 1971.
16. **Reilly, R., Thompson, J., Brelsk, R., and Severson, C.,** Estradiol-induced wasting syndrome in neonatal mice, *J. Immunol.,* 98, 321, 1967.
17. **Oyasu, R., Sumie, H., and Burg, H. E.,** Neoplasms of urinary bladder of hamsters treated with 2-acetylamino-fluorene and indole, *J. Natl. Cancer Inst.,* 45, 853, 1970.
18. **Ohlsson, E. G., Rutherford, R. B., Haalebos, M. M. P., Wagner, H. N., Jr., and Suidema, G. D.,** The effect of bilary obstruction on hepatosplenchnic blood flow in dogs, *J. Surg. Res.,* 10, 201, 1970.
19. **Prosnitz, L., Kawasaki, S., Cohen, G. S., Dineen, J. L., Perille, P. E., and Finch, S. C.,** Ethyl palmitate-induced splenic destruction, *J. Reticuloendothel. Soc.,* 6, 487, 1969.
20. **Weinberg, E. and Weiss, L.,** Splenomegaly and hemolytic anemia induced in rats by methylcellulose – an electron microscope study, *J. Morphol.,* 122, 35, 1967.
21. **Hansard, S. L.,** Transplacental movement and maternal-fetal organ accretion rates of selected radiominerals in gravid cattle, sheep, and swine, in *Radiation Biology of the Fetal and Juvenile Mammal,* Sikov, M. R. and Mahlum, D. S., Eds., USAEC CONF-690501, AEC Symposium Series #17, 1969, 9.

22. **Zook, B. C., McConnell, G., and Gilmore, C. E.,** Basophilic stippling of erythrocytes in dogs with special reference to lead poisoning, *J. Am. Vet. Med. Assoc.*, 157, 2092, 1970.
23. **Gore, I., Takada, M., and Austin, J.,** Ultrastructural basis of experimental thrombocytopenic purpura, *Arch. Pathol.*, 90, 197, 1970.
24. **Dooley, P. C., Morris, R. J. H., and Harris, L. R. J.,** Distribution volumes of labeled red blood cells and labeled protein and "F-cells" in intact and splenectomized HbA and HbB type sheep, *Aust. J. Exp. Biol. Med. Sci.*, 49, 129, 1971.
25. **Petrelli, F. and Marsili, G.,** Studies on the relationship between the function of biotin and activity of the RES in the rat, *J. Reticuloendothel. Soc.*, 9, 86, 1971.
26. **Cifaldi, S., Marone, G., and DeVivo, P.,** Iperbaria da ossigeno in ratti normali e splenectomizzati, *Bell. D. Soc. Ital. Biol.*, 45, 1631, 1969.
27. **Melendez, L. V., Hunt, R. D., Daniel, M. D., Blake, B. J., and Garcia, F. G.,** Acute lymphocytic leukemia in owl monkeys inoculated with Herpesvirus saimiri, *Science*, 171, 1161, 1971.
28. **Ikemoto, S., Mukoyama, H., Mukoyama, R., and Furuhata, T.,** The primary response of rabbits when immunized with human spleen RNA and the secondary response when further immunized with red cells, *Proc. Jap. Acad.*, 46, 1056, 1970.
29. **Northdurft, W. and Flemming, K.,** Die Wirkung von Polyvinylpyridin-N-oxid auf die Phagocytoseaktivitat des reticulo-endothelialen Systems, *Naunyn-Schmiedebergs Arch. Pharmakol.*, 267, 341, 1970.
30. **Sheagre, J. N., Barth, R. F., Edelin, J. B., and Malmgren, R. A.,** Mechanism of reticuloendothelial system blockade produced by antilymphocyte serum, *J. Immunol.*, 105, 634, 1970.
31. **Gotjamanos, T. and Gill, P. G.,** Changes in phagocytic activity and morphology of reticuloendothelial organs in mice induced by antilymphocyte serum, *Aust. J. Exp. Biol. Med. Sci.*, 48, 461, 1970.
32. **Ashford, A. and Bunn, D. R. G.,** The effect of arvin on reticuloendothelial activity in rabbits, *Br. J. Pharmacol.*, 40, 37, 1970.
33. **Fred, R. K., Dobson, E. L., Kelly, L. S., and Shore, M. L.,** The proliferative and phagocytic capacity of the reticuloendothelial system of sublethally irradiated mice, *J. Reticuloendothel. Soc.*, 7, 453, 1970.
34. **Rohovsky, M. W., Newberne, J. W., and Gibson, J. P.,** Effects of an oral interferon-inducer on the hemotopoietic and reticuloendothelial systems, *Toxicol. Appl. Pharmacol.*, 17, 556, 1970.
35. **Gotjamanos, T.,** Alterations in reticuloendothelial organ structure and function following cortisone administration to mice, *J. Reticuloendothel. Soc.*, 8, 421, 1970.
36. **Lahti, R. A., Platz, P. A., McAllister, B. J.,** Inhibition of (H^3) serotonin uptake by the mouse spleen. A structure-activity study, *J. Med. Chem.*, 13, 681, 1970.
37. **Cirri Borghi, M. B.,** La modificazioni indotte dalla somministrazione dell'ormone tireotropo e della tiroxina sulla struttura della milza, *Sperimentale*, 119, 73, 1969.
38. **Halverson, A. W., Tsay, D. T., Triebwasser, K. C., and Whitehead, E. I.,** Development of hemolytic anemia in rats fed selenite, *Toxicol. Appl. Pharmacol.*, 17, 151, 1970.
39. **Blakeley, A. G. H., Brown, L., Dearnaley, D. P., and Woods, R. I.,** Perfusion of the spleen with blood containing prostaglandin E_1 : transmitter liberation and uptake, *Proc. R. Soc. Lond. B*, 174, 281, 1969.
40. **Schumann, H. J. and Burger, A.,** Effects of calcium on storage of noradrenaline in isolated splenic nerve granules, *Naunyn-Schmiedebergs Arch. Pharmakol.*, 266, 185, 1970.
41. **Takano, S.,** A study of the contraction of spleen strips in kids and dogs, with special reference to the cholinergic and adrenergic receptors, *Jap. J. Pharmacol.*, 19, 563, 1969.
42. **Jakob, W., Hilgenfeld, M., and Karasek, E.,** Beschleunigte Amyloidbildung bei Mausen durch Milzzellkulturen, *Exp. Pathol.*, 6, 141, 1972.
43. **Loor, F. and Roelants, G. E.,** High frequency of T lineage lymphocytes in nude mouse spleen, *Nature*, 251, 229, 1974.
44. **Jakob, W.,** Spontaneous amyloidosis of mammals, *Vet. Pathol.*, 8, 292, 1971.
45. **Cohen, A. S. and Shirahama, T.,** Animal model for human disease: spontaneous and induced anyloidosis, *Am. J. Pathol.*, 68, 441, 1972.
46. **Nishimura, E. T., Ross, E., Leslie, G., Yang, H. Y., and Hokama, Y.,** Epizootic reticulum cell sarcoma in a sequestered colony of Japanese quails, *Cancer Res.*, 30, 2119, 1970.
47. **Wyand, D. S., Jakowski, R. M., and Burke, C. N.,** Marble spleen disease in ring necked pheasants: histology and ultrastructure, *Avian Dis.*, 16, 319, 1972.
48. **Kinns, A. M.,** Growth in the rat's brown fat of a Hodgkin's-like transplantable reticuloendothelial tumour, *Br. J. Exp. Pathol.*, 51, 411, 1970.
49. **Dooley, P. C., Hecker, J. F., and Webster, M. E. D.,** Contraction of the sheep's spleen, *Aust. J. Exp. Biol. Med. Sci.*, 50, 745, 1972.

Chapter 16

RADIATION EFFECTS ON THE SPLEEN

Quantification of the effects of radiation on the spleen is of interest in at least three situations.

1. When the spleen is deliberately irradiated because it is the primary or secondary site of a disease process.
2. When the regions near the spleen are irradiated and the spleen may be subjected to incidental radiation.
3. When the spleen is used as a monitor of the effects of radiation.

Clinical interest perhaps dates from the report of Senn[1] in 1903 that following splenic irradiation, a remission occurs in chronic myelocytic leukemia (which is a systemic disease). The remissions are marked by clinical improvement, a fall in the systemic white blood count, and an increase in the hematocrit. Splenic irradiation in chronic myelocytic leukemia, in addition to destroying many of the leukemic cells in the spleen, may also influence hematopoietic elements far removed from the spleen[2] ("abscopal effects"). The evidence for this is the improved sternal bone marrow picture (determined by operation or biopsy) and the improvement of peripheral blood values. Perhaps part of the explanation lies in the splenic trapping of leukocytes (both normal and abnormal) and erythrocytes and the reversal of this trapping by splenic irradiation. ^{51}Cr-erythrocyte studies indicate an improvement in red cell survival after splenic irradiation (but part of this may be related to the changing blood volume). The possible indirect or distant effects of splenic irradiation ("abscopal effects") have been much debated. Certainly the bone marrow changes (following splenic irradiation in chronic leukemia) are real.[3] In some instances, splenic irradiation may result in a decrease in the number of leukoyctes in the marrow (perhaps related to their massive destruction). This massive destruction can result in the "alarm reaction" (Selye) with depression of lymph nodes, bone marrow, and thymus. For a particular radiation-produced decrease in leukocyte count, direct splenic irradiation is more effective in reducing splenomegaly than total body irradiation.[13]

The exact mechanisms of the abscopal effects of splenic irradiation remain obscure. Maurice and co-workers[4] irradiated the spleen of rabbits (single exposure, 300 rd surface dose) and collected serum. When rabbit serum was collected 2 to 5 hr after irradiation of the hosts, the serum decreased the mitotic activity of suspensions of bone marrow from normal rabbits (and prior studies agreeing with this observation are summarized by Maurice et al.). In patients with chronic myelocytic leukemia, sera obtained 3 hr after 200 to 400 rd to the spleen (surface dose) decreased mitotic activity of erythroblasts.[4]

One of the effects, following splenic irradiation in chronic myelocytic leukemia, is massive destruction of leukocytes. Tischendorf and co-workers[5] showed a massive outpouring of lysozyme in the urine after 4 to 5 courses of 100 rd to the spleen in chronic myelocytic leukemia (the enzyme liberated arises from degradation of the lyosomes of granulocytes and granulocyte precursors).

Comas and associates[6] followed the peripheral leukocyte count in patients with chronic myelocytic leukemia who were given splenic irradiation (doses of 100 to 700 rd). They then quantified the changing white cell count and arrived at a descriptive equation.

$$S_o = \frac{W_o - W}{(1 - e^{-dt})} \qquad (1)$$

The spleen component of circulating white cells could be estimated by taking the white count per unit of blood (W) at some time (t) after irradiation and subtracting it from the original value (W_o) of the white cells. This was then divided by the exponential expression ($1 - e^{-dt}$) for white cell destruction. Indeed, after many days (when t is large), $1 - e^{-dt}$ is approximately equal to 1, and the splenic component is given by:

$$S_o = W_o - W \qquad (2)$$

That is, the difference between the white count at day t and the original white count must have represented the splenic component (since originally the values for white count were given in percent of the original, the results will also be in percent). In the series of Comas and co-workers, the mean value for S_0 was 75%. Despite many simplifying assumptions, this appears a reasonable first approach to elucidating the effects of splenic irradiation on the circulating myelocyte count in chronic myelocytic leukemia.

Irradiation of the spleen, in addition to destroying the radiation-sensitive myelocytes, also has effects on splenic tissue. This topic has not been well quantified. The following observations must be tempered by the fact that the quality of the radiation, host age, and other conditions were not the same from study to study. However, the data may be used as a starting point for further elucidation of the effects.

1. Prenatal irradiation of the male rat fetus produced a spleen smaller in size than normal.[7] However, growth of the irradiated spleens exceeded controls for the first 7 days.

2. Jacobson[40] showed that shielding the spleen during whole body irradiation or introducing spleen homogenates offered a protective effect against irradiation. It is recognized that spleen cells can recolonize other areas. The spleen colony method of Till and McCulloch[8] has provided a powerful tool for determining the number of cells involved in repopulation after irradiation or other treatment. Stem cells usually migrate from bone marrow to lymph nodes, thymus, and spleen. There is some evidence that stem cell division is significantly regulated by that of other cells in division.[9] Following irradiation of animals, if bone marrow depression would be the cause of death, prior shielding of the spleen allows for repopulation of the hematopoietic tissues.[10]

3. The effects of irriadiation on splenic histology have been described in detail.[11] In rats, following irradiation, splenic atrophy is proportional to the fall in blood count.[12] In rats given 600 rd, at 2 weeks the spleen weighed 0.35 g (original weight 1.2 g). In mice after 400 rd, whole body radiation of the spleen decreased in weight up to the 5th day. It then underwent weight gain, peaking at about day 18, then decreasing to preirradiation levels by day 22. Thymectomy had little influence on these events in the spleen.

4. Hotchkiss and Block[2] reported on palpation evidence of the decrease in spleen size following splenic irradiation for chronic myelocytic leukemia. The individuals were given 950 to 2,390 rd over a period of about 17 days. Spleen size was estimated in terms of centimeters below the costal margin at the left midclavicular line. The spleens decreased (in increasing order) 1, 2, 3, 3, 4, 4, 4, 9, 11, and 16 cm in length (mean 5.5 cm) within 24 hr. In two of the patients with rapid destruction of ^{51}Cr-erythrocytes, the red cell survival returned to normal after splenic irradiation.

5. Quantification of the change in spleen size following irradiation by means of spleen scans has not been widely pursued. We can make a few first crude approaches by utilizing the photographs supplied by Sharma and co-workers[14] (spleen scans performed after use of ^{51}Cr-heat-denatured erythrocytes). Using their Figure 1 and assuming the same rotation and magnification in each of the three views, we can attempt to quantify the change in the size of the spleen in a 38-year-old male who had prior irradiation of the spleen because of chronic myelocytic leukemia. After an initial scan, 550 rd were delivered to the portion of the spleen above the costal margin and the spleen rescanned. A third view was taken 7½ months later. Assuming the splenic volume was approximately a function of the length of the organ and the width squared,[21] we can note that the respective volumes were control, 100%; after irradiation, 53%; and 7½ months later, 37%. In another patient studied by these authors, the spleen shrank to two thirds of its original length, following use of 7 mCi of ^{32}P as therapy for polycythemia. We have recently published data on the apparent resistance of the spleen (other than in leukemia) to irradiation.[44]

6. The use of radiation in the treatment of hypersplenism has not been systematically pursued (perhaps in part due to possible damage to the left kidney or other structures). Isolated reports have appeared on the use of radiation in hypersplenism in nonmalignant diseases.[39]

RADIATION EFFECTS ON RETICULOENDOTHELIAL FUNCTION

Since spleen scanning as commonly performed depends on the delivery and accumulation of radioactive colloid, it is of importance to at least briefly inquire as to the effects of irradiation on reticuloendothelial activity. It is soon apparent that the literature abounds with studies, some of which seem to be in conflict with others. There are multiple variables that must be considered. Some of the more obvious of these are as follows:

1. Whether radiation is whole body or regional (and whether the spleen or other organs are shielded).

2. Dose rate and total dose.

3. Time after irradiation that the study is carried out.

4. Whether germ-free animals are used, or whether antibiotics are given.

5. Particle size of colloid used.

6. Whether a tracer dose or a loading dose of colloid is employed (in one study an increase or a decrease of reticuloendothelial activity was found, depending on the dose employed).[18]

7. Whether blood clearance or specific organ uptake is being monitored.

Part of the stimulation of reticuloendothelial activity observed in some experiments,[16] following irradiation, may be related to bacterial invasion and its resultant effects.[17] Reticuloendothelial activity in small animals is usually stimulated by estradiol and zymosan and by the polysaccharide glucan. Whole body irradiation inhibits the glucan-induced response[19] (using colloidal carbon). Irradiation in the range LD_{10} to LD_{50} reduced the ability of the reticuloendothelial system of mice to take up foreign erythrocytes.[20]

Our series of cases is quite limited, but we have not seen functional asplenia in patients given only therapeutic irradiation. However, in several who have had both irradiation and chemotherapy, the spleen has been observed to lose its ability to accumulate radiocolloid. Ariel and Padula[41] have described the delivery of ^{90}Y microspheres to the spleen (by catheterization) in order to give therapeutic radiation. In such a case, complete loss of splenic function might occur (large doses are delivered).

By a mechanism(s) as yet unknown, localized irradiation can stimulate the immune response in mammals. Simic and Petrovic[23] described studies in which female rats were immunized with sheep red blood cells. Five weeks later, their exposed spleens were irradiated. Antisheep cell titers decreased initially following irradiation. By the 5th day post irradiation, the titers began to rise, peaking at about the 10th day. This effect was not obtained if splenectomy was carried out or if there was whole body irradiation. The irradiated spleen[24] or spleen extracts[25] release various materials upon irradiation. Whether this is related to stimulation of the immune response is unknown.

The effect of radiation on the ability to form antibodies depends in part on the time relationship between the antigenic stimulation and radiation. In chicks, at the first week of life, irradiation of the whole body 1 day before antigenic stimulation decreased the plasma cell reaction in the spleen.[26] This type of effect has been attributed to inhibition of DNA turnover.[29] In patients, phagocytic activity of the reticuloendothelial system is depressed by radiation therapy and is stimulated by stilbestrol.[27] The mechanism of estradiol-induced radioprotection has been studied.[28]

The view has been expressed that the reticuloendothelial system of the liver and spleen determines the extent of resistance to shock.[30] Additional data on this topic are discussed in the section on the vascular system. Lethal and wasting effects of radiation in mice are markedly reduced when carbon particles are administered 1 day prior to irradiation.[31] That is, reticuloendothelial blockade has a radioprotective effect. Whether phagocytosis of damaged cells is reduced by the blockade, opsonins are removed, or other actions are involved is unknown. Spleen cells from carbon-injected rats apparently survive less well than those from control animals when injected into irradiated animals.[32]

RADIATION-INDUCED LYMPHOPENIA

Following radiation of part of the body, a lymphopenia occurs. When radiation is carried out for mammary carcinoma, lymphopenia may last for many months. Stjernsward and co-workers[33] noted that in these cases there was a decrease in the T (thymus-dependent) lymphocytes and an increase in B (bone marrow) lymphocytes. The role of the spleen in these changes is uncertain. When germ-free mice were exposed to 700 rd whole body radiation, restoration of the absolute lymphocyte count was delayed in the animals who had been previously splenectomized.[34] Lymphopenia can also be produced by extracorporeal irradiation of blood (and this has been utilized in treating chronic lymphocytic leukemia).[35] How such extracorporeal radiation affects the spleen is not known.

Wilson and Johnson[36] commented on individuals with chronic myelogenous leukemia who were treated by chemotherapy (particularly Busulfan and other agents) and then splenic irradiation. This therapy resulted in a fall in the white count in 19 out of 20 patients. However, hematologic complications occurred in six patients, and five died. The ill effects were likely due to bone marrow depression. Gollerkeri and Shah[38] have expressed the view that oral Busulfan was superior to splenic irradiation during chronic myeloid leukemia in maintaining remission. Salzman and Kaplan[37] noted that splenectomized patients with Hodgkin's disease had fewer episodes of leukopenia during radiation therapy than nonsplenectomized individuals.

CLINICAL DATA

We present a discussion of three cases treated by radiation therapy to the spleen since they raise a number of interesting points.

1. In the first case, the spleen did not decrease in length as judged from the ^{99m}Tc-sulfur colloid scan (despite the fact that clinical notes stated that there was a marked change in size). The case points out the need for *objective* evidence in evaluating spleen size, as well as the relative radioresistance of the spleen in some instances.

2. The second case shows scan-documented evidence of a decrease in spleen size, following external radiation in a case of lymphosarcoma. The decrease, however, did not occur until over 1,075 rd were administered.

3. The third patient, with chronic myelocytic leukemia, was undergoing radiation therapy to the spleen. Left upper quadrant pain suddenly developed. A repeat scan of the spleen revealed a marked decrease in length. The possibility of splenic infarction must be considered as a contributing cause to the diminution of splenic size during irradiation.

Case 1

A 7-year-old boy had acute lymphoblastic leukemia diagnosed 4 years previously (white blood count 39,900, with 79% lymphoblasts). Vincristine, prednisone, and methotrexate administration was followed by a remission. Later, cranial nerve and meningeal involvement was treated by intrathecal methotrexate. Recurrence of the symptoms was treated by 1,050 rd brain radiation and 750 rd to the spinal column. Methotrexate was discontinued when the white cell count fell to 2,000. A minimally palpable spleen in 1969 was stated to be readily palpable in 1971. Hence, the child was started on external radiation to the spleen.[44] Serial scans of the spleen up to a radiation dose of 1,450 rd did not reveal any significant decrease in the length of the organ, despite the clinical impression of some observers that the spleen size had decreased. The scans, however, suggested a slight lateral involution of the organ (perhaps it was bound down and could not decrease in length).

Case 2

A 72-year-old woman with lymphosarcoma was noted to be anemic. The ^{51}Cr-red-cell survival half-life was 8 days (normal = 28 days). Because surgery was contraindicated, anterior splenic irradiation was begun. Serial spleen scans revealed that the organ did not significantly decrease in size until a dose of over 1,075 rd was administered.

Case 3

A 37-year-old woman with chronic myelocytic leukemia had massive splenomegaly and thrombocytopenia (platelet count 5,000). Scan of the spleen (^{99m}Tc-sulfur colloid) revealed the organ to be 30 cm in diagonal length (Case 70-2530). Radiation therapy to the spleen was begun. One evening, the patient described severe, sharp, left upper quadrant pain. A repeat scan of the spleen showed that it had lost nearly 5 cm in length. Obstruction of a major splenic vessel, with infarction, might have contributed to this finding. It has been reported that vascular damage is a prominent component of the effects of radiation on the liver.[15] This might also be true for the spleen.

In multiple cases seen thus far, the spleen has not lost its ability to accumulate radioactive colloid after radiation doses of over 3,000 rd. Szur and co-workers[42] have shown that following irradiation of the spleen possessing erythropoietic activity, ability to accumulate radioactive iron may be lost while radiocolloid accumulation continues. The spleen may also influence the hematologic tolerance to radiation. In a series of patients with Hodgkin's disease, splenectomized individuals had lesser hematologic depression.[43]

REFERENCES

1. **Senn, N.,** Case of splenomedullary leukaemia successfully treated by the use of the roentgen ray, *Med. Rec.,* 64, 281, August 22, 1903.
2. **Hotchkiss, D. J. and Block, M. H.,** Effect of splenic irradiation on systemic hemopoiesis, *Arch. Intern. Med.,* 109, 695, 1962.
3. **Parsons, W. P., Watkins, C. H., Pease, G. L., and Childs, D. S., Jr.,** Changes in sternal marrow following roentgen-ray therapy to the spleen in chronic granulocytic leukemia, *Cancer,* 7, 179, 1954.
4. **Maurice, P. A., Williner, B., Gindrat, J. J., and Brand, A.,** Effect of splenic x-irradiation on bone marrow function: experimental studies of a serum mitotic inhibitor in rabbit and in patients with chronic myelocytic leukaemia, *Br. J. Haematol.,* 17, 543, 1969.
5. **Tischendorf, F. W., Ledderose, G., Muller, D., and Wilmanns, W.,** Heavy lysozymuria after x-irradiation of the spleen in human chronic myelocytic leukaemia, *Nature,* 235, 274, 1972.
6. **Comas, F. V., Edwards, C. L., and Vodopick, H.,** Splenic irradiation in chronic granulocytic leukemia: changes in leukocyte values, *Radiat. Res.,* 42, 413, 1970.
7. **Martin, P. G.,** The postnatal response of four organs to prenatal irradiation as measured by changes in nucleic acids and protein, *Radiat. Res.,* 48, 368, 1971.
8. **Till, J. E. and McCulloch, E. A.,** A direct measurement of the radiation sensitivity of normal mouse bone marrow cells, *Radiat. Res.,* 14, 213, 1961.
9. **Takada, A., Takada, Y., and Ambrus, J. L.,** Proliferation of donor spleen and bone-marrow cells in the spleens and bone marrows of unirradiated and irradiated adult mice, *Proc. Soc. Exp. Biol. Med.,* 136, 222, 1971.
10. **Sundaram, K., Bains, G. S., and Gopal-Ayengar, A. R.,** Radiation response of newborn mice and the effect of shielding on mortality, in *Radiation Biology of the Fetal and Juvenile Mammal,* Sikov, M. R. and Mahlum, D. S., Eds., USAEC CONF-690501, AEC Symposium Series #17, 1969, 475.
11. **Dunlap, C. E.,** Effects of radiation on normal tissues. III Effects of radiation on the blood and the hemopoietic tissues, including the spleen, the thymus and the lymph nodes, *Arch. Pathol.,* 34, 562, 1942.
12. **Clarkson, J. R., Mayneord, W. V., and Parsons, L. D.,** The effect of x-irradiation on the blood and lymphoid tissue of tumour-bearing animals, *J. Pathol. Bacteriol.,* 46, 221, 1938.
13. **Moss, W. T. and Brand, W. N.,** *Therapeutic Radiology,* 3rd ed., C. V. Mosby, St. Louis, 1969, 448.
14. **Sharma, S. M., Patel, M. C., Ramonathan, P., and Ganatra, R. D.,** Role of spleen scanning in planning the treatment and assessement of splenic response in blood dyscrasias, *Am. J. Roentgenol.,* 101, 656, 1967.
15. **Kinzie, J., Studer, R. K., Perez, B., and Potchen, E. J.,** Noncytokinetic radiation injury: anticoagulants as radioprotective agents in experimental radiation hepatitis, *Science,* 175, 1481, 1972.
16. **Sljivic, V. S.,** Radiation and the phagocytic function of the reticuloendothelial system. I. Enhancement of RES function in x-irradiated mice, *Br. J. Exp. Pathol.,* 51, 130, 1970.
17. **Sljivic, V. S.,** Radiation and the phagocytic function of the reticuloendothelila system. II. Mechanism of RES stimulation after irradiation, *Br. J. Exp. Pathol.,* 51, 140, 1970.
18. **Flemming, K., Flemming, C., and Nothdurft, W.,** The phagocytic activity of the reticuloendothelial system of mice following whole-body x-irradiation, *J. Reticuloendothel. Soc.,* 7, 1, 1970.
19. **Fred, R. K., Dobson, E. L., Kelly, L. S., and Shore, M. L.,** The proliferative and phagocytic capacity of the reticuloendothelial system of sublethally irradiated mice, *J. Reticuloendothel. Soc.,* 7, 453, 1970.
20. **Schildt, B. E. and Eriksson, K. H.,** Function of the reticuloendothelial system in whole-body irradiated mice, *Acta Radiol. [Ther.]* (Stockh.), 11, 48, 1972.
21. **Samuels, L. D.,** Estimation of spleen size from posterior spleen scans, *J. Assoc. Can. Radiol.,* 20, 192, 1969.
22. **Takada, A., Takada, Y., Kim, V., and Ambrus, J. L.,** Bone marrow, spleen, and thymus regeneration patterns in mice after whole-body irradiation, *Radiat. Res.,* 45, 522, 1971.
23. **Simic, M. M. and Petrovic, M. Z.,** Enhancement of residual antibody synthesis by irradiation of the spleen in pre-immunized rats, *Nature,* 229, 263, 1971.
24. **Maurice, P. A.,** Release of thymidine from x-irradiated spleen in the rabbit as determined by a new bioassay, *Cancer Res.,* 32, 2799, 1972.
25. **Watkins, D. K. and Deacon, S.,** Comparative effects of electron and neutron irradiation on the release of enzymes from isolated rat-spleen lysosomes, *Int. J. Radiat. Biol.,* 23, 41, 1973.
26. **Rodak, L. and Prochazka, Z.,** Influence of radiation on the pattern of histological changes in the spleen of chickens vaccinated during the early stage of ontogenesis, *Int. J. Radiat. Biol.,* 19, 1, 1971.
27. **Magarey, C. J. and Baum, M.,** Oestrogen as a reticuloendothelial stimulant in patients with cancer, *Br. Med. J.,* 2, 367, 1971.
28. **Thompson, J. S., Simmons, E. L., Crawford, M. K., and Severson, C. D.,** Studies on the mechanisms of estradiol-induced radioprotection, *Radiat. Res.,* 40, 70, 1969.
29. **Harris, G. and Sljivic, V.,** The acute effects of ionizing radiation on antibody producing cells (PFC) in mouse spleen during primary and secondary responses to sheep erythrocytes (SRC), *Immunology,* 23, 147, 1972.
30. **Palmerio, C. and Fine, J.,** The nature of resistance to shock, *Arch. Surg.,* 98, 679, 1969.

31. **Mori, K. J. and Nakamura, S.**, Radioprotective effect of reticuloendothelial system blockade in mice, *Experientia*, 26, 1386, 1970.
32. **Friedman, H. and Sabet, T. Y.**, Effects of RES "blockade" on antibody formation. III. Proliferative capacity of antigen-reactive stem cells in carbon-treated mice after transfer to irradiated recipients, *Immunology*, 18, 883, 1970.
33. **Stjernsward, J., Jondal, M., Vanky, F., Wigzell, H., and Sealy, R.**, Lymphopenia and change in distribution of human B and T lymphocytes in peripheral blood induced by irradiation for mammary carcinoma, *Lancet*, I, 1352, 1972.
34. **Anderson, R. E., Doughty, W. E., and Howarth, J. L.**, Radiation-induced lymphopenia; recovery in thymectomized and splenectomized germ-free mice, *Arch. Pathol.*, 92, 480, 1971.
35. **Field, E. O., Dawson, K. B., Peckham, M. J., Hammersley, P. A., Cooling, C. I., Morgan, R. L., and Smithers, D. W.**, The response of chronic lymphocytic leukemia to treatment by extracorporeal irradiation of the blood, assessed by isotope-labeling procedures, *Blood*, 36, 87, 1970.
36. **Wilson, J. F. and Johnson, R. E.**, Splenic irradiation following chemotherapy in chronic myelogenous leukemia, *Radiology*, 101, 657, 1971.
37. **Salzman, J. R. and Kaplan, H. S.**, Effect of prior splenectomy on hematologic tolerance during total lymphoid radiotherapy of patients with Hodgkin's disease, *Cancer*, 27, 471, 1971.
38. **Gollerkeri, M. P. and Shah, G. B.**, Management of chronic meyloid leukemia: a five year survey with a comparison of oral busulfan and splenic irradiation, *Cancer*, 27, 596, 1971.
39. **Sommer, A. and Kontras, S. B.**, Splenomegaly with hypersplenism in sickle cell anemia treated by radiation-case report, *Pediatrics*, 48, 457, 1971.
40. **Jacobson, L. O.**, Hematopioetic responses to radiation injury, *Annu. Rev. Med.*, 7, 345, 1956.
41. **Ariel, I. and Padula, G.**, Irradiation of the spleen by the intraarterial administration of ^{90}Yttrium microspheres in patients with malignant lymphoma; a preliminary report, *Cancer*, 31, 90, 1973.
42. **Szur, L., Pettit, J. E., Lewis, S. M., Bruce Tagoe, A. A., and Short, M. D.**, The effect of radiation on splenic function in myelosclerosis: studies with ^{52}Fe and ^{99}Tc^{m}, *Br. J. Radiol.*, 46, 295, 1973.
43. **diBella, N. J., Blom, J., and Slawson, R. G.**, Splenectomy and hematologic tolerance to irradiation in Hodgkin's disease, *Radiology*, 107, 195, 1973.
44. **Spencer, R. P. and Knowlton, A. H.**, Radiocolloid scans in evaluating splenic response to external radiation, *J. Nucl. Med.*, 16, 123, 1975.

INDEX

INDEX

A

B

C

D

E

F

G

Q

R

S

T

U

V

W

X

Y

Z